BASIC
VETERINARY
IMMUNOLOGY

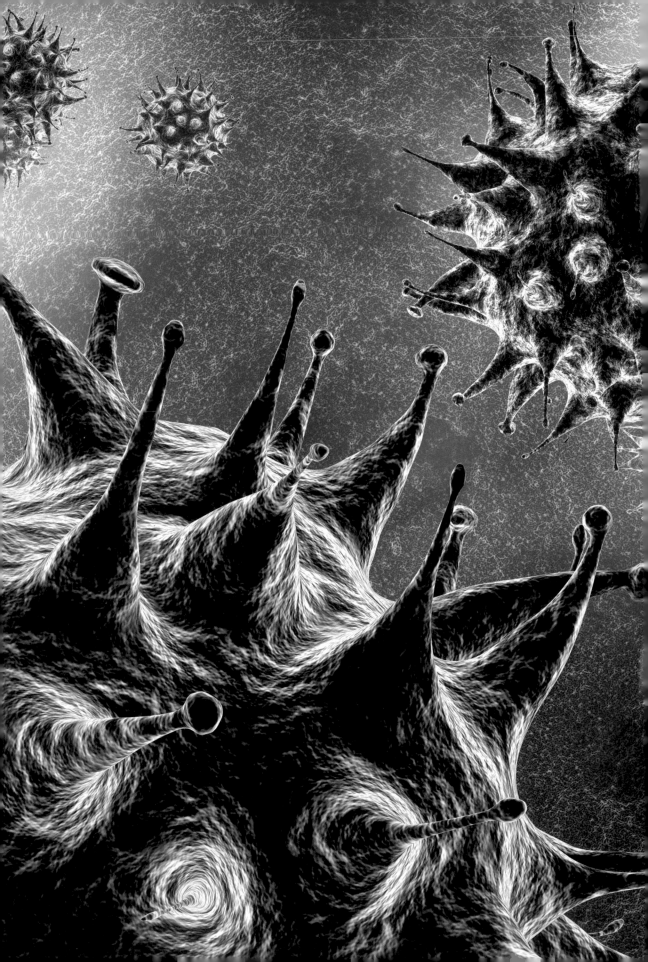

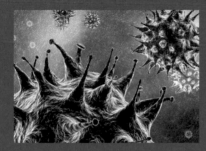

BASIC
VETERINARY
IMMUNOLOGY

Gerald N. Callahan AND Robin M. Yates

VETERINARY CLINICAL LABORATORY IMMUNOLOGY CHAPTER by Amy L. Warren

University Press of Colorado

Boulder

© 2014 by University Press of Colorado

Published by University Press of Colorado
5589 Arapahoe Avenue, Suite 206C
Boulder, Colorado 80303

 The University Press of Colorado is a proud member of
the Association of American University Presses.

The University Press of Colorado is a cooperative publishing enterprise supported, in part, by Adams State University, Colorado State University, Fort Lewis College, Metropolitan State University of Denver, Regis University, University of Colorado, University of Northern Colorado, Utah State University, and Western State Colorado University.

∞ This paper meets the requirements of the ANSI / NISO Z39.48-1992 (Permanence of Paper).

Library of Congress Cataloging-in-Publication Data

Callahan, Gerald N., 1946– author.
  Basic veterinary immunology / Gerald N. Callahan and Robin M. Yates ; Veterinary clinical laboratory immunology chapter by Amy L. Warren.
      p. ; cm.
  Includes bibliographical references and index.
  ISBN 978-1-60732-218-4 (pbk. : alk. paper)
  I. Yates, Robin M. author. II. Title.
  [DNLM: 1. Animal Diseases—immunology. 2. Animal Population Groups—immunology. 3. Immune System Diseases—veterinary. 4. Immune System Phenomena. 5. Veterinary Medicine—methods. SF 757.2]
  SF757.2
  636.089'6079—dc23
                            2013035025

Designed and typeset by Daniel Pratt

23   22   21   20   19   18   17   16   15   14   10   9   8   7   6   5   4   3   2   1

Cover illustrations, top to bottom: Thoroughbred horse © pirita / Shutterstock; Viruses, detailed 3D illustration © nobeastsofierce / Shutterstock; © William Zaun; Chinese shar-pei dog © Waldemar Dabrowski / Shutterstock; © William Zaun.

Contents

BASIC VETERINARY IMMUNOLOGY

Gerald N. Callahan and Robin M. Yates

Overview of Mechanisms of Defense

Chapter 1

10.5876_9781607322184.c001

CLINICAL CORRELATION: SIMIAN ACQUIRED IMMUNE DEFICIENCIES

The story probably began almost 32,000 years ago, but the villain was not discovered until 1985. In that year, M. D. Daniel and his collaborators completed their work on four rhesus macaque monkeys. Table 1.1 lists the symptoms of those monkeys (Figure 1.1).

Four monkeys seriously ill—at least three of them from what appeared to be opportunistic infections—for no apparent reason. Daniel and coworkers began searching for the culprit. What they found in the affected monkeys was a retrovirus—simian T-lymphotropic virus III—a retrovirus very similar to the human T-lymphotropic virus III, the apparent (and later confirmed) cause of human AIDS. The monkey virus was later renamed simian immunodeficiency virus (SIV).

Studies of wild African monkeys revealed that green monkeys had SIV infection rates as high as 30 to 50 percent with no overt clinical syndrome. As with rhesus macaques, however, SIV infection of pig-tailed and crab-eating macaques almost invariably resulted in a chronic wasting disease and severe opportunistic infections, such as oroesophageal candidiasis. What was underlying this clinical syndrome in these monkeys?

LEARNING OBJECTIVES

After reading this chapter, you should be able to

- describe the immune defense system;
- understand how cells of the immune system communicate;
- understand the basic elements of innate immune mechanisms;
- describe the basic elements of adaptive immune mechanisms.

ESSENTIAL INVOLVEMENT OF ANIMAL IMMUNE SYSTEMS IN ALL ASPECTS OF ANIMAL HEALTH

Roughly 4 billion years ago, life on Earth became complex. From the primordial ooze, life coalesced into individual organisms—eubacteria,

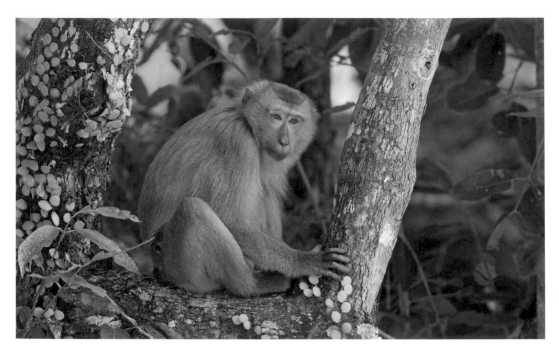

FIGURE 1.1. **Rhesus macaque (© gopause / Shutterstock)**

archaebacteria, and likely others. The brown seas turned azure and the pink skies turned blue. Soon after, the first parasites appeared. Parasitism offered an energy-efficient alternative to survival on one's own. Hosts provided protection and energy with minimal or no investment by the parasite.

By the time metazoan life appeared, almost 3 billion years later, parasitism had become a high art. That constant evolutionary pressure, those threats to the survival of individual organisms, produced immune systems. Both simple and complex mechanisms for defense against parasites had, almost from the outset, become essential components of all life, and still are. Without means for self-defense, no individual plants or animals would exist on Earth.

The proof of that is apparent in both primary and acquired immune deficiencies in animals as disparate as sharks and horses. Immune-deficient animals rapidly disappear, and in their places communities of other living things—bacteria, viruses, fungi, and parasites—abruptly arise. Without immune systems, indi-

TABLE 1.1. Symptoms of macaque monkeys at the New England Regional Primate Research Center (adapted from M. D. Daniel et al., 1985, *Science* 228: 201)

Animal	Symptoms
251–79	Malignant lymphoma
239–82	Macrophage infiltrates in brain, oroesophageal candidiasis, cryptosporidiosis, intestinal trichomoniasis
220–82	Macrophage infiltrates in brain, oroesophageal candidiasis, cryptosporidiosis, intestinal trichomoniasis
142–83	Diarrhea, facial rash, generalized lymphadenopathy, splenomegaly

vidual animals vanish. Because of this critical involvement of immune systems in all animal functions, understanding immunity is essential to understanding animal medicine, including animal behavior.

IMMUNE SYSTEM

Animals have evolved numerous strategies to defend themselves against infections. These mechanisms range from independently acting single proteins to highly trained cellular assassins that can specifically target infected cells. Over evolutionary time, these various mechanisms have coalesced into unified defense systems called immune systems. Collectively, an immune system includes the tissues, cells, and molecules that work together to effect an immune response designed to protect the host animal from a given threat. Immune responses do not only secure the immediate survival of the infected host, but in many cases also better prepare the animal for later exposures to a particular threat.

The immune system is divided into two functional subsystems: the innate immune system and the adaptive (or acquired) immune system. The innate immune system mediates rapid, early-phase responses to threats. These responses include molecular and cellular mechanisms that kill a wide variety of potential pathogens. The adaptive immune system provides a delayed but customized, or specific, response to infectious threats, resulting in the production of antibodies, T-cell responses, and immune memory.

For decades, immunologists considered and studied the innate and adaptive immune systems separately. More recently, it has become clear that these subsystems work together in an overlapping and reciprocating fashion. Generally speaking, without a functional innate immune system, an animal is incapable of generating effective adaptive immune responses. Without a functional adaptive immune system, most innate immune mechanisms are less effective. In truth, animal immunity involves a single collection of cells and their products that act synergistically in defense of their host. How is this synergy orchestrated?

Cells of Defense

The only known vertebrate animals without red blood cells (RBCs) are crocodile icefish, which live in oxygen-rich cold water and absorb gaseous oxygen directly into their blood.

All other vertebrates have both white and red blood cells (RBCs). RBCs, or erythrocytes, transport oxygen to animal tissues and deliver carbon dioxide to animals' lungs. White blood cells, or leukocytes, are, among other things, cells of vertebrate immunity, both innate and adaptive. White blood cells include T and B lymphocytes (often referred to simply as T and B cells and involved primarily in adaptive immune responses), as well as neutrophils, basophils, eosinophils, NK cells (involved primarily in innate immunity), and monocytes, which become, among other things, macrophages and dendritic cells (DCs; involved in both innate and adaptive immune responses). Neutrophils make up about 70 percent of all leukocytes in the blood, followed by lymphocytes at around 20 percent, but the percentages of the various cell types vary among species, as well as with the animal's age and health. T cells can further differentiate into T-helper (Th) and cytotoxic T (Tc) cells. Th cells may differentiate into a variety of Th cell types, including Th1, Th2, Th17, and regulatory T cells, and each of these Th-cell lineages perform specialized functions in adaptive immunity (see chapter 10). B cells ultimately differentiate into plasma cells that secrete antibodies.

Communication between Cells of the Immune System

It takes billions of immune cells to achieve effective defensive responses. Coordination of such massive numbers of cells requires a sophisticated communication system involving multiple cytokines, a variety of other soluble mediators, and direct cell-to-cell communication via intercellular contact.

COMMUNICATION THROUGH CYTOKINES

Essentially, all cells use cytokines (soluble proteins or glycoproteins) to communicate with one another. As with hormones, cytokines may act directly on the cells that produce them (autocrine stimulation); on other nearby cells (paracrine stimulation); or, via the blood, on distant cells (endocrine stimulation). Immune cytokines fall into distinct categories based on structure, function, and origin.

Interleukins (ILs) are a diverse group of cytokines produced predominantly by leukocytes (white blood cells) and act on other leukocytes (*inter,* "between"; *leukins,* "leukocytes"). Activated T lymphocytes secrete the majority of ILs, but many other leukocytes, particularly macrophages and DCs, also produce cytokines to communicate with other cells. The abbreviation *IL* is followed by a number designating the specific IL; for example, IL-2 is an IL that stimulates T-cell division. ILs have a variety of targets and functions within the immune system.

Interferons (IFNs) are a group of cytokines that are particularly important in the coordination of immune responses to infections, particularly viral infections. Because they were first identified as molecules that interfered with viral infection and replication, scientists combined the word "interfere" with the particle suffix "-on" to form *interferon*. They include IFN-α and IFN-β (released by virus-infected cells) and IFN-γ, a proinflammatory cytokine produced predominantly by Th lymphocytes.

Chemokines are a group of cytokines that direct movements of immune cells (*chemo,* "chemical"; *kines,* "kinos or movement"). The movement of leukocytes among various tissues is essential to all immune responses. Chemokines released by other immune cells direct the movements of these leukocytes. Some chemokines can also change the physiology of immune cells so that these cells can perform particular functions (a process commonly referred to as *activation*).

Colony-stimulating factors (CSFs) are cytokines that promote the proliferation and differentiation of leukocyte precursors. The majority of CSFs act on bone marrow stem cells and leukocyte precursors in the bone marrow, although some CSFs also act in peripheral tissues. CSFs were so named because the prolif-

eration of cells in the bone marrow is apparent as new colonies of cells.

OTHER CYTOKINES

Several other immunologically important cytokines do not fit neatly within the preceding categories. These cytokines include transforming growth factor-β (TGF-β; so called because it stimulates [among other things] growth similar to that seen in tumor cells). TGF-β has roles in the regulation of immune reactions and tissue repair. Other significant cytokines include tumor necrosis factors TNF-α and TNF-β (so called because under some conditions these factors can cause tumor cell necrosis), which have roles in mediating inflammation and its systemic effects. Table 1.2 lists some of the more common cytokines and their functions.

COMMUNICATION THROUGH OTHER SIGNALING MOLECULES

Aside from cytokines, the immune system uses several other molecules as messengers. These molecules include the monoamines histamine and serotonin, synthesized and released from mast cells and basophils in response to inflammatory stimuli or allergens, which mediate vascular changes associated with inflammation.

Other important groups of immune signaling molecules derive from cellular lipids. These signaling molecules include the leukotrienes and prostaglandins. Although derived from a common lipid precursor, members of these two molecular families have diverse functions, including vascular changes, immune activation, chemotaxis, and regulation of inflammation and immunity.

COMMUNICATION THROUGH CELL–CELL CONTACT

Much of the communication between immune cells in the adaptive immune system relies on direct molecular interactions between proteins, complexes, and receptors on cell surfaces.

TABLE 1.2. Some of the cytokines involved in innate immunity

	Mass (kDa)	Assembly	Source(s)	Target(s)
IL-1	17	Monomer	Macrophages, endothelia, epithelia	Endothelia (↑ coagulation, ↑ inflammation), hepatocytes (↑ acute phase proteins), hypothalamus (↑ fever)
IL-18	17	Monomer	Macrophages	NK cells (↑ IFN-γ), T lymphocytes (↑ IFN-γ)
TNF	17	Homotrimer	Macrophages, T lymphocytes	Endothelia (↑ coagulation, ↑ inflammation), hepatocytes (↑ acute phase proteins), neutrophils (↑ activation), hypothalamus (↑ fever)
IL-6	26	Homodimer	Macrophages, endothelia, T lymphocytes	Hepatocytes (↑ acute phase proteins), B lymphocytes (↑ proliferation)
IL-15	13	Monomer	Macrophages	NK cells (↑ proliferation), T lymphocytes (↑ proliferation)
IL-12	35/40	Heterodimer	Macrophages, dendritic cells	Th1 lymphocytes (↑ differentiation), Tc lymphocytes (↑ IFN-γ), NK cells (↑ IFN-γ)
IL-23	19/40	Heterodimer	Macrophages, dendritic cells	T lymphocytes (↑ IL-17)
IL-27	28/13	Heterodimer	Macrophages, dendritic cells	Th1 lymphocytes (inhibition and/or differentiation), NK lymphocytes (↑ IFN-γ)
IL-10	18	Homodimer	Macrophages, T lymphocytes	Macrophages, dendritic cells (↓ IL-12)
IFN-α	21	Homodimer	Macrophages	All cells (↑ viral immunity, ↑ MHC class I), NK cells (↑ activation)
IFN-β	25	Homodimer	Fibroblasts	All cells (↑ viral immunity, ↑ MHC class I), NK cells (↑ activation)
Chemokines	8–12	monomer	Macrophages, endothelia, fibroblasts, epithelia	Phagocyte (↑ migration), B lymphocytes (↑ migration), T lymphocytes (↑ migration), ↑ wound repair

Note: MHC = major histocompatibility complex.

This type of communication requires intimate cell–cell contact. T lymphocytes in particular often require contact with other cells for activation and to perform their effector functions.

Innate and Adaptive Immune Systems

Although the innate and adaptive immune systems work together as a functional unit, there are evolutionary and functional differences between these two systems (see Figure 1.2).

Innate immune system

The innate immune system is an evolutionarily ancient system present in one form or another in every animal, from mollusks to humans. In vertebrate animals, the innate immune system represents the first line of defense against invading pathogens, but in invertebrate animals it represents the only line of defense. Over millions of years of evolution, the innate immune system has become amazingly complex and sophisticated. The key feature of this immune system is its ability to distinguish between foreign (often microbial) molecules and molecules normally encountered in healthy host tissue.

Unlike adaptive immune systems, which have to learn the differences between self and nonself, the innate system has evolved to recognize aspects of non-self immediately and to react instantaneously, even before birth. This ability is the result of evolution of the genes encoding

TABLE 1.3. Some cytokines involved in adaptive immunity

	Mass (kDa)	Assembly	Source(s)	Target(s)
Lympho-toxin	21–24	Homotrimer	T lymphocytes	B lymphocytes (↑ development), T lymphocytes (↑ development), neutrophils (↑ migration, ↑ activation)
IL-2	17	Monomer	T lymphocytes	T lymphocytes (↑ survival, ↑ proliferation, ↑ cytokines), B lymphocytes (↑ proliferation, ↑ antibody production), NK cells (↑ proliferation, ↑ activation)
IL-4	17	Monomer	Th2 lymphocytes	B lymphocytes (↑ isotope switch IgE), Th2 lymphocytes (↑ proliferation, ↑ differentiation), macrophages (↓ IFN response), mast cells (↑ proliferation)
IL-5	26	Homodimer	Th2 lymphocytes	B lymphocytes (↑ proliferation, ↑ isotope switch IgA), eosinophils (↑ proliferation, ↑ activation)
IL-13	13	Monomer	Th2 lymphocytes, NK-T lymphocytes, mast cells	B lymphocytes (↑ isotope switch IgE), macrophages (↑ collage), fibroblasts (↑ collage), epithelia (↑ mucus)
IL-17	35/40	Dimer	T lymphocytes	Endothelia (↑ chemokines), macrophages (↑ cytokines/chemokines), epithelia (↑ G-CSF and GM-CSF)
IFN-γ	40	Homodimer	Th1 lymphocytes, Tc lymphocytes, NK cells	B lymphocytes (↑ isotope switch), Th1 lymphocytes (↑ differentiation), macrophages (↑ activation), various cells (↑ antigen processing and ↑ MHC class I)

Note: MHC = major histocompatibility complex.

numerous, highly conserved receptors that recognize molecular patterns specific to pathogens (pattern-recognition receptors [PRRs]) or other receptors specific to the products of host tissue damage and necrosis. Several types of cells express both types of receptors, but they appear in the highest concentrations on the surfaces of the sentinel cells of the innate immune system, including the macrophages and DCs found in practically every animal tissue. Once these cell-surface receptors bind their ligands, the cells release cytokines and chemokines that engage the rest of the immune system, which leads to the activation of antimicrobial effector mechanisms that find and kill invading microbes and parasites as well as dispose of damaged cells.

The simplest of the innate antimicrobial mechanisms involve individual secreted proteins or groups of them. For example, the complement system includes a series of plasma proteins, most of which come from the liver. Activation of the complement system by invading microbes initiates a biochemical cascade that sometimes results in the direct lysis of the microbe and always activates numerous secondary innate and adaptive immune responses.

Specialized groups of cells carry out other innate effector mechanisms. Phagocytes are a group of cells that can, via a process called phagocytosis, engulf and degrade microbes. This ability, plus specific cell-surface receptors, allows phagocytes to selectively ingest individual microbes and, within a cytoplasmic sack called a phagolysosome, eliminate those invading organisms. In this way, phagocytes remove and kill microbes without harming host cells. The phagocytes of the innate immune system include macrophages, DCs, and neutrophils.

In some cases, invading pathogens may be too large or too numerous for phagocytes to handle effectively. In these cases, neutrophils or eosinophils can also release antimicrobial and antiparasitic products directly into extracellular spaces. Although these products can harm bystander cells, they also effectively kill microbes and large parasites such as worms.

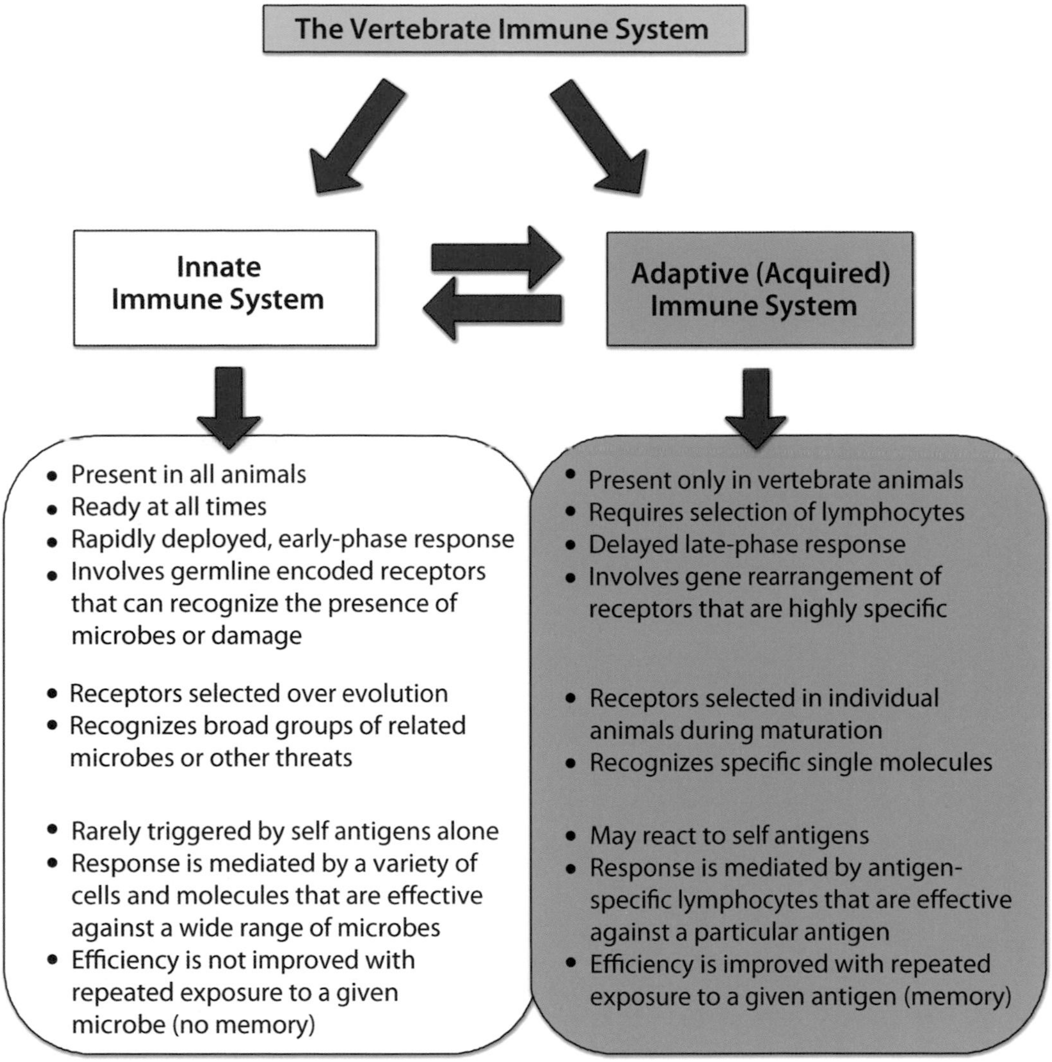

The Vertebrate Immune System

Innate Immune System

- Present in all animals
- Ready at all times
- Rapidly deployed, early-phase response
- Involves germline encoded receptors that can recognize the presence of microbes or damage

- Receptors selected over evolution
- Recognizes broad groups of related microbes or other threats

- Rarely triggered by self antigens alone
- Response is mediated by a variety of cells and molecules that are effective against a wide range of microbes
- Efficiency is not improved with repeated exposure to a given microbe (no memory)

Adaptive (Acquired) Immune System

- Present only in vertebrate animals
- Requires selection of lymphocytes
- Delayed late-phase response
- Involves gene rearrangement of receptors that are highly specific

- Receptors selected in individual animals during maturation
- Recognizes specific single molecules

- May react to self antigens
- Response is mediated by antigen-specific lymphocytes that are effective against a particular antigen
- Efficiency is improved with repeated exposure to a given antigen (memory)

FIGURE 1.2. Major differentiating features of the innate and adaptive immune systems

Other innate immune cells, NK cells, defend against intracellular pathogens such as viruses. NK cells do this by physically touching host cells to determine whether they are healthy or stressed and abnormal (potentially indicating that they may be infected by a virus or are neoplastic). When NK cells detect suspicious cells, they induce apoptosis of those cells and limit viral spread or neoplasia (Figure 1.3).

The entire repertoire of mechanisms that allows the innate immune system to recog-nize and eliminate threats derives from highly conserved genes within the germline chromosomal DNA of animals. Because these systems have been refined over eons of evolution, they regularly and effectively distinguish microbes from normal host tissue. However, the innate system cannot identify subtle differences between strains of microbes and so may be circumvented by evolving pathogens, particularly viruses. Another limitation of the innate immune response is that its efficiency does not

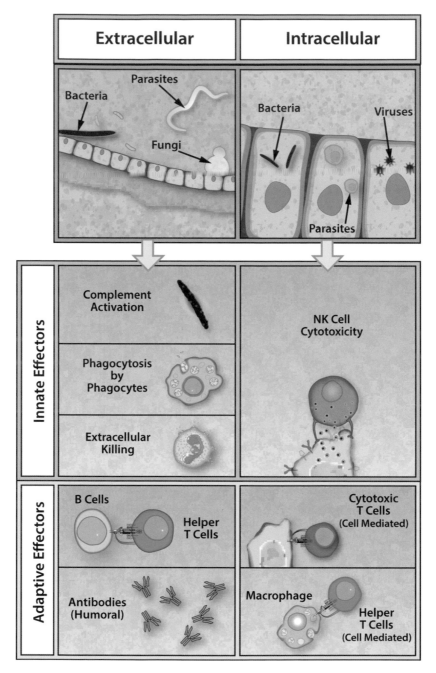

FIGURE 1.3. **Major innate and adaptive defense mechanisms against extracellular and intracellular pathogens**

Different aspects of innate and adaptive immunity have evolved to deal with intracellular and extracellular pathogens. The complement system and phagocytes are especially important aspects of innate immunity that deal with extracellular pathogens. NK cells of the innate response help to eliminate infected cells. During adaptive immune responses (discussed in the Adaptive Immune System section), antibodies and some Th cells act most directly in protecting against extracellular infections, and other Th cells and Tc cells are most effective against intracellular infections.

improve with repeated exposure to a given microbe. Unlike the adaptive immune system, the innate immune system has no memory.

As a result, the innate immune system responds in an identical and predictable manner to microbes, foreign bodies, and trauma. Also, innate responses do not improve with repeated exposures. To escape these limitations, vertebrates have evolved another set of immune mechanisms that are highly specific and evolve over time to deal with ever-changing pathogens: the adaptive immune system.

ADAPTIVE IMMUNE SYSTEM

Beyond innate defenses, vertebrate animals can muster a series of additional protective responses. These responses take longer to develop than innate responses, but add several remarkable defense options. Adaptive responses to infection are adaptive because they are not immediate responses and develop only over time. The adaptive immune response is also referred to as the acquired immune response because the animal does not directly inherit these immune responses but acquires them within its lifetime. Molecules that induce adaptive immune responses are called antigens. In the natural world, antigens are molecular bits of organisms, including pathogens. Some antigens may also induce innate responses, but the term *antigen* is reserved for those molecules that stimulate adaptive immune responses (generally, macromolecules, especially proteins and glycoproteins, but also carbohydrates as well as some lipids and nucleic acids).

Innate immune responses, although rapid and powerful, lack fine specificity. For example, the inflammatory responses (aspects of innate immunity) to type 1 and type 2 parvoviruses are the same. Adaptive immune responses are much more specific and customized to deal with specific pathogens. For example, no matter how many times a dog gets infected with a parvovirus, the innate immune response remains similar, which is not true of the adaptive

immune response. The first time an animal encounters a pathogen, the adaptive immune system generates a primary immune response. During second and subsequent encounters with that same pathogen, adaptive immune responses become more specific, faster, stronger, and longer lasting (see Figure 1.4).

Those differences between primary and subsequent immune responses constitute immunological memory—the adaptive immune system's ability to remember it has seen an antigen before and respond differently on a second encounter with that antigen. Specificity and memory are the hallmarks of adaptive immune responses.

Adaptive immune responses rely on lymphocytes, especially T and B lymphocytes. These cells are the only ones in an animal's body that specifically recognize and respond to antigens. On lymphocytes, antigen recognition occurs through specific molecules called antigen receptors. These molecules are B-cell receptors (BCRs) and T-cell receptors (TCRs; see Figures 1.5 and 1.6).

BCRs and TCRs are exquisitely specific for individual antigens—nearly one BCR or TCR for each potential antigen. Because animals can respond to essentially any antigen inside of an animal, BCRs and TCRs must exist in nearly limitless numbers of specificities. That chemical feat results from a remarkable series of genetic rearrangements.

The genes that encode BCRs and TCRs appear in pieces spread along particular chromosomes. During the development of B cells and T cells, those genetic bits shuffle randomly like a deck of cards to generate a nearly infinite number of possible receptors, including self-reactive receptors. Subsequent processes identify and destroy self-reactive lymphocytes, minimizing the possibility of autoimmunity. Nonetheless, some self-reactive B and T cells can survive selection and may initiate autoimmune disease later in the animal's life.

In spite of their plasticity, specificity, and memory, adaptive responses lack the speed of

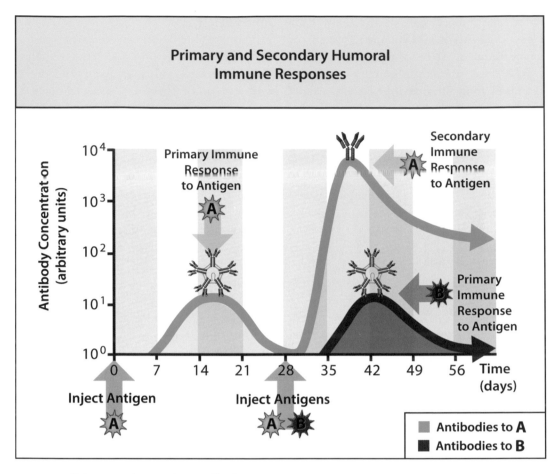

FIGURE 1.4. Primary and secondary antibody responses

After injection of antigen A on day 0, an animal produces a primary antibody response to antigen A. This response lasts for 30–40 days and is dominated by a type of antibody called IgM (pentamers). When again injected with antigen A plus a new antigen B, the animal produces a robust secondary antibody response to antigen A but a primary response to antigen B.

innate responses and can take days to weeks to reach measurable levels. This time lag is the result of a phenomenon called clonal expansion.

After a primary immunization or infection, a special group of cells, called antigen-presenting cells (APCs), ingests and processes pathogens and then presents pathogen-derived antigens to T cells. At the time of immunization or infection, an animal usually has only a few T cells specific for infecting or immunizing antigens. At this stage, these T cells are referred to as "naïve" T cells because they have not yet encountered their specific antigens—they have yet to be ac-

tivated. Once these cells are activated by APCs, they begin to divide rapidly and further differentiate. Ultimately, these waves of cell division lead to a dramatic increase in the number of T cells specific for the immunizing or infecting antigens. This process is clonal expansion—the expansion of a few cells into enormous clones of the originally activated T cell—resulting in thousands to millions of cells that all share the same antigenic specificity. A similar process occurs among B cells. After antigen binding and interaction with T cells, a few antigen-specific B cells rapidly divide to create massive clones

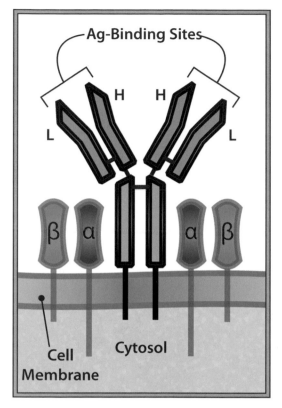

FIGURE 1.5. The B-cell antigen-specific receptor

As B cells mature in the bone marrow, they express a complex of molecules called the BCR. This complex contains two immunoglobulin heavy chains (H) and two immunoglobulin light (L) chains (essentially an antibody molecule) that, together, make up the antigen-specific portions of the BCR. In addition, the BCR contains two other molecules, Igα and Igβ, which participate in signal transduction and B-cell activation. Ag = antigen.

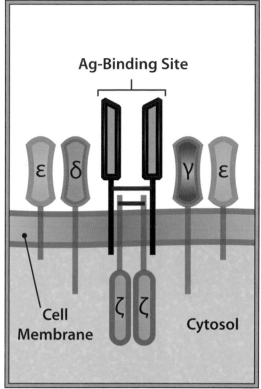

FIGURE 1.6. The T-cell antigen-specific receptor

The antigen-specific portion of the TCR contains two chains, either α/β or γ/δ. Together they make up the single antigen-binding site of the TCR. The TCR also includes γ-, δ-, ε-, and ζ-chain molecules that contribute to signal transduction during T-cell activation. Ag = antigen.

of antigen-specific B cells. Ultimately, these B cells differentiate into plasma cells and secrete antigen-specific antibody. All of this takes time, a week to ten days in a primary adaptive immune response.

Once generated in sufficient numbers, T cells exert their effects directly, especially through destruction of infected host cells and enhancement of other immune responses (see Figure 1.7). B cells, however, provide protection through antibodies. After binding antigen and interacting with certain T cells, B cells differentiate into plasma cells. Plasma cells secrete antibodies (essentially a soluble form of the BCR) into lymph and blood. Antibodies are especially effective in eliminating extracellular pathogens (see Figure 1.8).

As mentioned earlier, unlike the innate immune system, the adaptive immune system remembers its first encounters with antigens. So, in a secondary adaptive immune response, lag times are shorter than primary immune response,

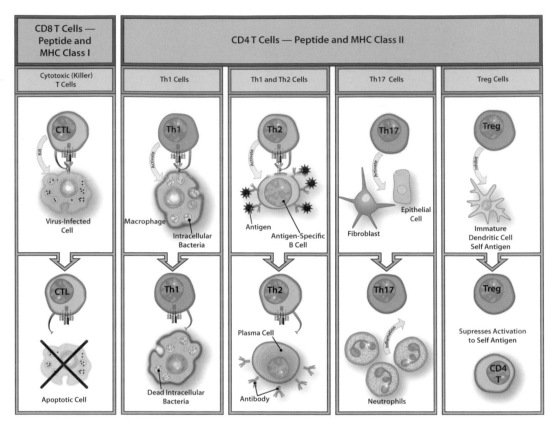

CD8 T Cells — Peptide and MHC Class I	CD4 T Cells — Peptide and MHC Class II			
Cytotoxic (Killer) T Cells	Th1 Cells	Th1 and Th2 Cells	Th17 Cells	Treg Cells

FIGURE 1.7. Some of the actions of effector T cells

After activation by APCs, T cells differentiate into a variety of effector cells that drive the progression of several types of immune responses, including destruction of virus-infected cells (first panel), activation of macrophages to kill ingested bacteria (second panel), activation of B cells to produce antibodies (third panel), stimulation of inflammation (fourth panel), and maintenance of self-tolerance (fifth panel). Treg = regulatory T cell; CTL = Tc cells.

tertiary responses are even faster, and so on. Such immune memory results from the creation of specialized subsets of long-lived B and T cells, called memory cells, which remain after primary adaptive immune responses. This process increases the number of resident antigen-specific cells. The second time an animal encounters the same pathogen or antigen, these memory cells dominate adaptive responses. The result is that secondary and subsequent adaptive immune responses happen much faster, are more specific, are stronger, and last longer (see Figure 1.4).

Also, although innate immune responses may occur nearly anywhere, adaptive immune responses arise at specialized sites in animals' bodies. Those sites include lymph nodes (see Figure 1.9), the spleen, and mucosa-associated lymphoid tissue (MALT).

As mentioned at the beginning of this chapter, separating immune responses and immune systems into innate and adaptive components is primarily a matter of convenience and history. No adaptive response ever occurs in the absence of an accompanying innate response, and most innate responses in vertebrate animals in-

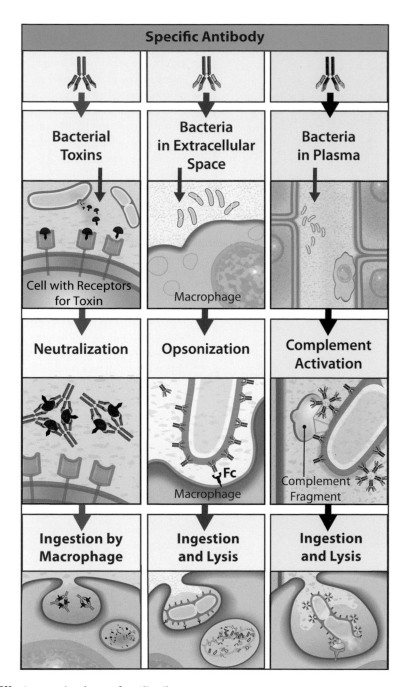

FIGURE 1.8. Effector mechanisms of antibodies

As shown in the left column, when antibodies bind to toxins (or viruses), the toxins can no longer bind to specific receptors on host cells and are neutralized. The center column shows how antibody binding to bacteria (a process called *opsonization*) enhances phagocytosis of pathogens by macrophages. The right column shows a similar process. Once IgM or IgG antibodies have bound to a pathogen, the complex activates complement. Because macrophages and other phagocytic cells also have receptors for complement fragments, this process also leads to more efficient phagocytosis of pathogens.

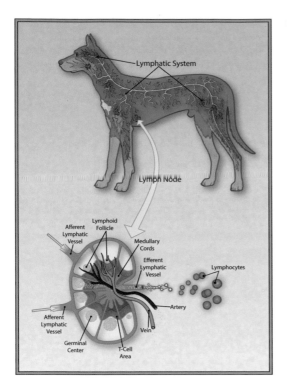

FIGURE 1.10. (FACING PAGE) **Overview of a typical immune response**

Figure 1.10 is a concept map of a typical immune response involving both the innate (yellow) and adaptive (blue) immune systems. These two systems intersect to work together toward a common goal: control or eradication of a threat. Following is a chronological description of the typical immune response depicted. Numbers in parentheses correspond to the circled numbers in the figure.

(1) After recognition of a threat, sentinel innate immune cells initiate immune responses. (2) Recognized threats include microbial products in normally sterile tissues and the products of cellular injury—hallmarks of infection or potential infection. (3) Even without knowing precisely what the threat may be, innate sentinel cells can recruit other innate cells, such as neutrophils, eosinophils, and monocytes, as well as allow serum proteins, such as complement, to permeate the affected tissue through a process called inflammation. (4) Once recruited to the site of infection, innate cells and serum proteins deploy powerful (albeit nonspecific) antimicrobial and antiparasitic mechanisms. (5) During the innate immune response, APCs, such as macrophages and DCs, ingest and process proteins, move to lymph nodes, and present these proteins to lymphocytes, initiating adaptive immune responses. (6) Adaptive immune responses rely on the activation of key antigen-specific lymphocytes (around 1 in each 100,000 lymphocytes). Once activated, these cells undergo rapid replication, expanding a few key lymphocytes to millions of identical cells (clones), a process called clonal expansion. (7) The result is an army of lymphocytes that specifically recognize parts of the invading microbe and effect a targeted attack by producing antibodies or by mobilizing and coordinating other immune processes. Not only do these adaptive immune responses directly kill invading microbes or infected cells, but many of them at the same time enhance the efficiency of innate antimicrobial mechanisms already in play. (8) During clonal expansion, a portion of key antigen-specific lymphocytes differentiate into long-lived memory cells—allowing more efficient adaptive immune responses on repeat exposure to the same threat (immunologic memory).

FIGURE 1.9. Canine lymphatics and lymph nodes

Lymphatics (upper portion) are a system of open-ended vessels that return extravascular fluid from the periphery to the heart and blood. Distributed throughout the lymphatics are a series of small filtering stations called lymph nodes. Each node has both cortical (outer) and medullary (inner) regions in which different aspects of the immune response occur.

duce coincidental adaptive immune responses (see Figure 1.10).

Every day, every animal encounters literally trillions of potential threats in the form of transmissible pathogens—viruses, bacteria, fungi, and parasites. These agents of disease, if unchecked, would quickly destroy us all. Immune systems have evolved to help prevent that. To do this, immune systems recognize specific pieces of pathogens as foreign and, in response, induce a series of protective mechanisms that involve both innate and adaptive reactions. The ability to generate those reactions is why we are all here. The remainder of this book explores

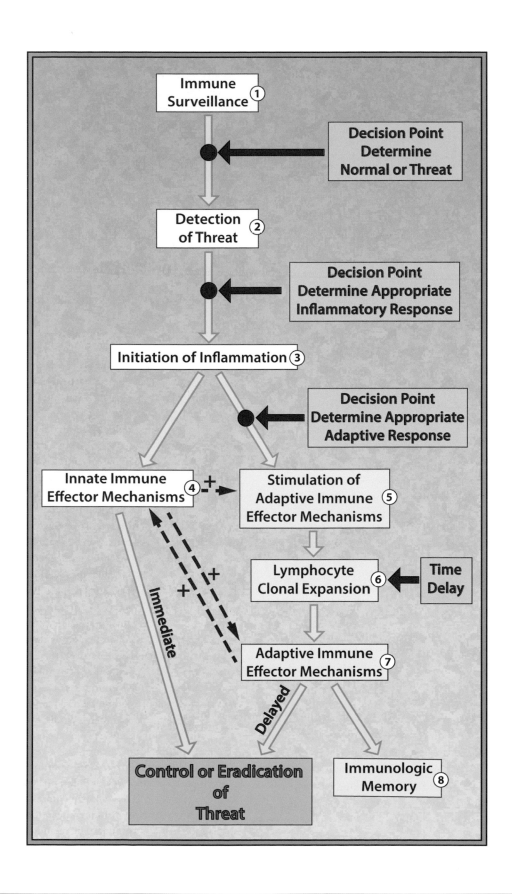

animals' remarkable immune systems and their interactions with the infectious world.

CLINICAL CORRELATION FOLLOW-UP

Student Considerations

Further investigations of the affected monkeys showed that SIV specifically infected T cells, particularly Th cells, a type of T cell necessary for almost all types of adaptive immune responses and for amplification of many innate immune responses.

SIV is a retrovirus, which means that during infection, viral RNA serves as the template for new complementary DNA that, with the help of an integrase, inserts itself into a host's chromosomal DNA. This SIV provirus may remain inactive for years, but once the host T cell activates— for example, during an immune response—viral DNA becomes active, and those host cells begin to produce infectious SIV, which results in host-cell malfunction and often host-cell death.

After reading this chapter, you should be able to propose an explanation for the opportunis-

tic infections apparent in rhesus macaques and other monkeys infected with SIV.

Possible Explanations

As shown in this chapter, T cells are essential components of almost all adaptive immune responses against both intra- and extracellular pathogens. As SIV destroys more and more T cells, these monkeys' immune systems grow weaker and weaker. Eventually, the total number of T cells drops below the levels needed to generate effective immune responses. At that point, the monkeys begin to show signs of an acquired immunodeficiency syndrome. Although the innate immune system is still in play, without help from T cells it is quickly overwhelmed by normally innocuous microbes, such as *Candida albicans,* that become opportunistic pathogens and blossom across mucosal surfaces, causing oroesophageal candidiasis. These and other opportunistic infections quickly overwhelm and kill infected monkeys.

Robin M. Yates

Overview of the Innate Immune System

Chapter 2

10.5876_9781607322184.c002

CLINICAL CORRELATION: CYCLIC NEUTROPENIA IN GRAY COLLIES

An unusual genetic disorder of collies results in gray coat color (Figure 2.1) and increased susceptibility to bacterial infections. Within eight to twelve weeks of age, affected puppies develop a broad range of symptoms, including fever, diarrhea, and joint pain as well as eye, respiratory, and skin infections. As a result, these puppies often die before they reach six months of age. Monitoring the cell composition of the collies' blood over time by means of serial complete blood cell counts reveals an interesting phenomenon. Every twelve to fifteen days, these puppies develop a marked neutropenia (lack of circulating immune cells called neutrophils), after which the number of circulating neutrophils rebounds. During these periods of neutropenia, the animals are extremely susceptible to bacterial infections that often result in illness and dramatically shortened lives. How does a genetic disorder affect neutrophil numbers when other leukocytes seem unaffected? And if the immune system is so complex, why does the periodic loss of one cell type have such devastating effects?

LEARNING OBJECTIVES

After reading this chapter, you should be able to

- describe the anatomical and physical barriers that guard against infection;
- discuss how leukocytes are generated in the bone marrow (hematopoiesis);
- list the major cells in the innate immune system;
- list the basic morphological features of the major innate immune cells;

- outline the origin and anatomical location of the major innate immune cells;
- describe the basic functions of the major innate immune cells;
- list and understand the basic function of the lymphoid innate immune cells.

Only vertebrates have adaptive immunity; in most species in the biome, host defense starts and stops with innate immunity. Starfish, for example, have only innate immune systems, yet they can live in some of the world's most microbe-rich environments and, for the most part, successfully avoid infection. It is interesting that many of the components of the innate immune system in starfish are strikingly similar to those in more complex animals, such as mice, dogs, cats, pigs, horses, and humans.

For most of the twentieth century, immunologists focused on the adaptive immune system; however, the innate immune system is an intricate and sophisticated system in and of itself. In this chapter, we introduce the major cells of the innate immune system of animals and discuss their origins. The following chapters focus on how these components function to immediately protect animals from harm and how the innate and adaptive immune systems work together to form an integrated defense system.

ANATOMICAL AND PHYSIOLOGICAL BARRIERS TO MICROBIAL INVASION

Apart from what one normally thinks of as an immune system, animals have innate anatomical and physiological barriers that are very effective in preventing infection. These barriers are not usually included as bona fide components of the innate immune system, but because their contribution to host defense is so immense, we review them here (Figure 2.2).

Epithelial Barrier

The most obvious barrier to microbial invasion is the skin and the mucous membranes

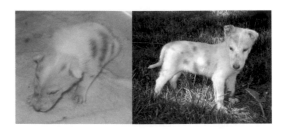

FIGURE 2.1. **Gray-coated collie pup (photograph provided by Michelle Tennis)**
Affected pups are gray (often with a pinkish hue) with pale brown noses.

that coat the exterior surfaces of an animal, including the gastrointestinal, respiratory, and reproductive tracts. Several features of mucous membranes and skin make them ideal barriers (Figure 2.3A–C). First, the flattened epidermal and epithelial cells adhere to one another, forming tight junctions, which create a continuous impermeable shield. Second, in the skin, the outer layer of the epidermis is made up of dead cells that are filled with keratin—a mechanically strong protein that also repels water. Third, the epithelial cells of the skin and mucous membranes continually grow and shed, repeatedly re-creating a fresh, microorganism-free surface. This process is particularly important in the intestine, where epithelial cells in the colon have a turnover rate of approximately six days. During intestinal parasitic infections, the intestinal epithelial cell turnover rate dramatically accelerates to expel the parasites.

Secretions

In addition to the barrier role played by epidermal and epithelial cells, the secretions these cells produce also play a role in innate defense. In the skin, specialized sebaceous glands adjacent to hair follicles produce sebum. Sebum is lipid based and water-repellent. Sebum is also acidic (with a pH of approximately 3 to 5), which inhibits the growth of many microbes.

Numerous other secretions contain antimicrobial proteins that specifically target un-

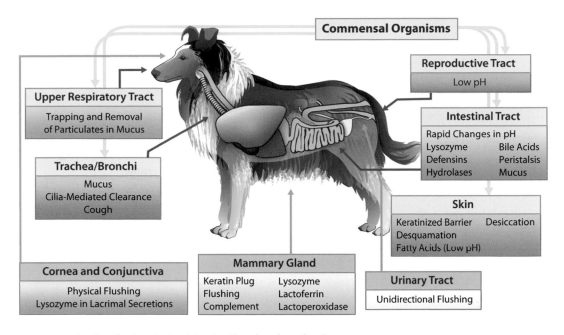

FIGURE 2.2. Anatomical and physiological barriers in animals

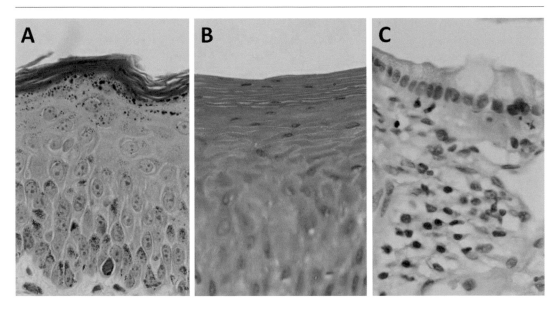

FIGURE 2.3A–C. Epithelial barriers

Skin: keratinized squamous epithelium (panel A); mucous membrane: nonkeratinized squamous epithelium (panel B); epithelium of the large intestine: columnar epithelium (panel C)

wanted microbes at key sites around an animal's body. Lysozyme is one of these secretions. It is found in tears, saliva, milk, and in the mucus in the gut. Lysozyme specifically degrades the peptidoglycan cell walls of bacteria. The cationic peptides defensins and cathelicidins, produced by epithelial cells, also appear in body secretions. These small, positively charged peptides insert themselves into negatively charged microbial membranes and punch holes in them (most

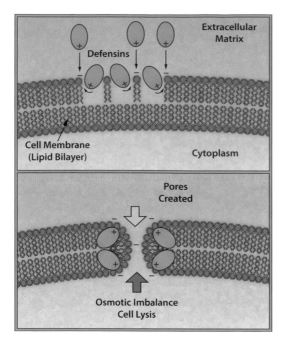

FIGURE 2.4. **Proposed mechanism of action of defensins**

These antimicrobial peptides have clusters of positive charges alongside regions of hydrophobicity that allow them to integrate into negatively charged membranes. Integration of several defensins can destabilize the microbial membrane, creating pores through which water and solutes can pass. In sufficient numbers, these pores can substantially perturb osmoregulation of microbes and cause them to lyse.

membranes in animal cells are positively charged and resistant to these peptides; Figure 2.4). Some leukocytes also synthesize and secrete defensins, as do intestinal crypt Paneth cells. Other antimicrobial proteins can be found in milk, where they help to inhibit microbial growth in the lactating mammary gland. These proteins include lactoferrin, which sequesters iron, making it unavailable for microbial growth, and lactoperoxidase, which generates reactive oxygen compounds that damage microbes.

The gastrointestinal tract produces multiple secretions that not only mediate digestion but also kill many unwanted microbes. The gastric mucosa secretes degradative enzymes as well as hydrochloric acid, which acidifies the gastric contents to a pH of 2 or less. As food moves out of the stomach into the duodenum, the pH is rapidly increased by the addition of bile. Bile also contains numerous detergents that, along with the pancreatic enzymes, act to disrupt microbial membrane integrity.

Aside from the specific antimicrobial actions of many secretions, the physical flushing of milk, tears, saliva, and urine removes many microbes from the mammary glands, eyes, mouth, and urinary tract. The importance of simple unidirectional flushing of surfaces is very evident in animals that cannot fully empty their urinary bladders (as can happen, e.g., in dogs with lower spinal cord injury). In the absence of regular flushing of the lower urinary tract, microbes can more easily colonize and migrate up the tract, predisposing these animals to both lower and upper urinary tract infections.

Mucus and Mucociliary Clearance

Mucosal surfaces (including those lining the respiratory and reproductive tracts as well as the small and large intestines) secrete large amounts of mucus. This sticky, viscous substance coats epithelial cell layers, providing an additional mechanical barrier to microorganisms by preventing them from binding to the epithelial surfaces. It also immobilizes microbes, making them easier to expel.

Although mucus produced by the intestinal mucosa is cleared along with the intestinal contents via peristalsis, mucus in the respiratory tract (along with trapped microbes and debris) is expelled by a process referred to as *mucociliary clearance.* Cilia are minute, fingerlike projections on the apical (lumenal) surface of the respiratory epithelium that move in coordinated waves (Figure 2.5). These waves act to push mucus out of the airway and into the esophagus, inducing swallowing. Inactivation of mucociliary clearance results in the accumulation of microbe-laden mucus in the airways. In a rare heritable disease in dogs called ciliary dyskinesia, affected dogs have an abnormality in the structure of cilia that renders them nonfunctional. Because of this abnormality, these dogs are unable to clear mucus and are prone to upper and lower respiratory tract infections.

Commensal Organisms

The skin and the reproductive, respiratory, and intestinal tracts of healthy animals are colonized by an array of commensal organisms, particularly bacteria. These organisms typically do not cause disease but, among other things, prevent the growth of pathogenic microbes. Prevention is achieved in part by the well-adapted commensal organisms' simply outcompeting foreign microbes for space and nutrients but also by creating a chemical microenvironment that allows some microbes to flourish while others perish. For example, commensal lactobacilli within the vagina create an acidic environment that favors the growth of

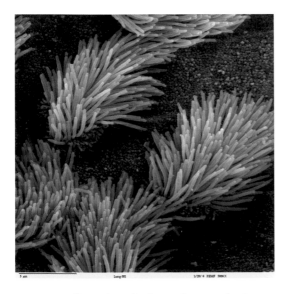

FIGURE 2.5. **Scanning electron micrograph of ciliated epithelium lining the respiratory tract**

These long projections move in coordinated waves that push mucus and ensnared microbes up and out of the respiratory tract. Image by Charles Daghlian.

commensal organisms but inhibits growth of the majority of other microbes.

A growing body of evidence supports the clinical benefits of pro-biotic supplementation of "good" microbes, including protection from gastrointestinal disease, reducing the length of gastrointestinal infections, and reducing the length of antibiotic-induced diarrhea (a side effect of antibiotic-mediated destruction of natural flora). Commensal intestinal bacteria also have a profound influence on the development of the intestine itself and the adaptive immune system.

Overall, the barriers inherent in an animal's anatomy and physiology effectively prevent the invasion of most environmental microbes. These barriers, however, are not impenetrable. Microbial breach is common. The second line of defense faced by invading microbes is the innate immune system.

CELLS OF THE INNATE IMMUNE SYSTEM

The innate immune system is made up of a host of immune cells as well as soluble factors such as complement and acute-phase proteins (APPs, which are discussed in subsequent chapters). Unlike the adaptive immune system, which includes recognizable tissues and organs such as lymph nodes, spleen, and thymus, the innate immune system is spread throughout every tissue of every animal. In spite of this diffuse anatomical distribution, innate immune cells have a common origin in the bone marrow.

Hematopoiesis

The production of immune cells in the bone marrow is termed *hematopoiesis* (literally the ancient Greek words for *blood* and *to make*). As the name suggests, hematopoiesis produces not only immune cells but also red blood cells (RBCs) as well as platelets. Amazingly, all of these arise during a highly coordinated and complex process that produces as many as 10^{11}–10^{12} cells per day from common hematopoietic stem cells.

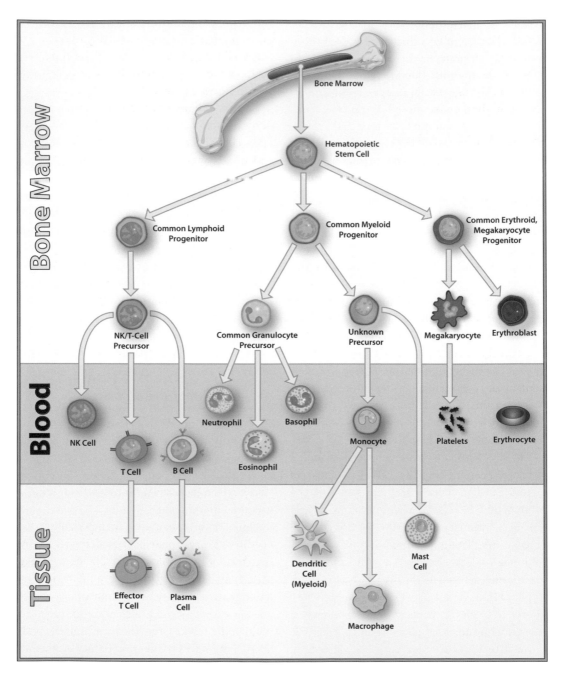

FIGURE 2.6. **An overview of hematopoiesis showing major points of differentiation and anatomical location in healthy animals**

Hematopoiesis has three major lineages: erythroid, myeloid, and lymphoid. The erythroid lineage primarily produces RBCs (erythrocytes) and platelets. The remaining two lineages, myeloid and lymphoid, produce all of the dedicated immune cells in animals (Figure 2.6). Most of the cells of the innate immune system arise from the myeloid lineage. These cells include the granulocytes (neutrophils, eosinophils, and basophils), mast cells, monocytes, macrophages, and myeloid dendritic cells (DCs). The lymphoid lineage predominantly produces lymphocytes (T and B cells) that function in adaptive immune responses. The lymphoid lineage also produces natural killer (NK) cells that, unlike most T and B cells, function in the innate immune system. Other lymphoid cells have innate immune function, but they apparently play only minor roles in innate immune defense, and we consider them only briefly here.

Coordinating Hematopoiesis

With so many different bone marrow lineages, all with quite different roles, it is important that the bone marrow be able to selectively increase or decrease the production of each of the lineages in response to the body's demands. It would be wasteful to increase erythrocyte production during inflammation and, likewise, neutrophil production during anemia. For these reasons, animals have evolved hematopoietic growth factors for specific regulation of bone marrow cell differentiation and division.

The hematopoietic growth factors include a family of proteins known as colony-stimulating factors (CSFs), which include granulocyte–monocyte CSF (GM-CSF), granulocyte CSF (G-CSF), and macrophage CSF (M-CSF). In addition to mediating inflammatory processes (as we discuss in later chapters), several interleukins serve as hematopoietic growth factors (including IL-1, IL-3, IL-4, IL-5, IL-6, and IL-7). These interleukins play important roles in regulating levels of immune cell production to meet the immediate needs of an animal's defense system.

Hematopoiesis in the bone marrow occurs in areas between stromal reticular cells and adipocytes (fat cells). Stromal reticular cells form a very fine meshwork of spindled cells that provide the structural framework of the bone marrow. In addition, stromal reticular cells (along with osteoblasts) produce and bind certain hematopoietic growth factors, increasing their local concentration. This process creates pockets or niches in the bone marrow that favor the differentiation of particular hematopoietic lineages, allowing different areas of the bone marrow to intensively support different hematopoietic activities (Figure 2.7).

Because the majority of innate immune cells derive from the common myeloid precursor stem cell, the activity of each differentiation pathway is what determines the final composition of cells released from the bone marrow. Levels of growth factors (regulated by feedback loops), along with external signals, regulate these pathways. For instance, IL-5, IL-3, and GM-CSF favor eosinophil production; G-CSF, GM-CSF, and IL-3 favor neutrophil production; M-CSF, GM-CSF, and IL-3 favor monocyte production; and IL-4 and IL-9, along with GM-CSF, favor basophil and mast-cell differentiation, respectively. Of course, other cytokines play roles in the differentiation of these cells, but it is easy to see that by varying the levels of cytokines, it is possible to achieve a fine balance of lineage expansion or contraction.

At each step in a cell lineage, precursor cells undergo irreversible commitments to fewer possible cell types. Expression of cell-specific receptors and effector molecules as well as changes in cellular morphology reflect this progressive differentiation.

Once mature, the newly formed leukocytes, erythrocytes, and platelets move from the bone marrow into the blood through highly fenestrated capillary networks. Some of the mature leukocytic cells (particularly neutrophils and, to a lesser extent, eosinophils and monocytes) remain in the blood, circulating through the body and exiting into surrounding tissues as needed. Other cells, such as mast cells, DCs, and macrophages, are mostly directed to other tissues.

Monitoring Hematopoiesis

Normally, the bone marrow of healthy animals releases balanced numbers of mature leukocytes into circulation. But during disease, when demand is high, increased numbers of

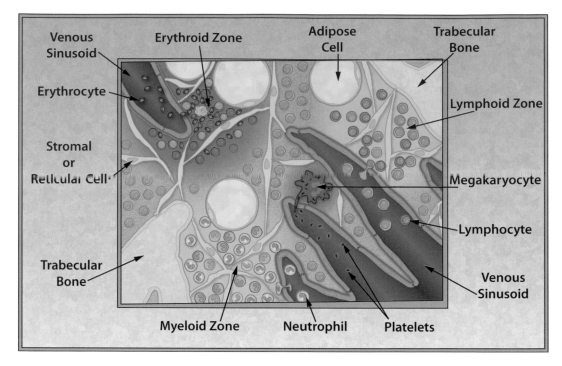

FIGURE 2.7. **Bone marrow**

Representation of localized hematopoiesis in the bone marrow. Hematopoietic precursor cells are enmeshed in a fine stromal network that creates small niches or pockets where growth factors are differentially concentrated. This compartmentalization is thought to support localized growth and differentiation of particular lineages.

certain leukocytes, including their immature forms, appear in the circulation. Blood counts and differentials (the identification and proportion of cell types in blood smears) provide evidence of such changes. Large increases in leukocyte counts, particularly neutrophils (termed *neutrophilia*), often indicate active inflammation. When immature neutrophils (band neutrophils) appear in large numbers in the blood (a phenomenon called a left shift), it is usually indicative of severe, acute inflammation.

In addition, bone marrow aspirates allow practitioners to finely gauge the marrow's response to disease. During inflammation, the number of cells differentiating into leukocytes increases. For example, in allergies, increased numbers of eosinophil precursors appear in the bone marrow. Bone marrow aspiration, however, requires anesthesia and the insertion of

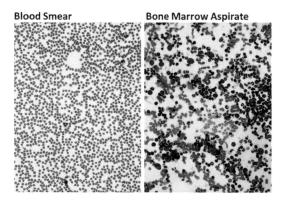

FIGURE 2.8. **Monitoring changes to hematopoiesis can be achieved indirectly through complete blood cell counts or directly by observing changes in bone marrow aspirates.**

a cannula directly into the marrow cavity. Because of that, it is typically used only when the bone marrow is suspected of failing or to diagnose bone marrow neoplasia. More commonly, practitioners exploit changes in circulating blood leukocytes to diagnose certain diseases.

OVERVIEW OF THE CELLS OF THE INNATE IMMUNE SYSTEM

As mentioned earlier, the highly complex hematopoietic process produces different subsets of innate immune cells. Here we provide only a brief introduction to these innate immune cells. More details appear in later chapters.

Myeloid Innate Immune Cells

NEUTROPHILS

These cells make up the majority of circulating leukocytes in many species and are capable of producing a variety of antimicrobial toxins. Under normal conditions, the majority of neutrophils remain in the blood in a resting state for the entirety of their short lives (a few days). However, circulating neutrophils have the ability to swarm in huge numbers into inflamed tissues where they unleash a storm of antimicrobial effectors. In these instances, neutrophils die even more rapidly, often victims of their own effector molecules. The extent of neutrophil recruitment and death is often apparent as pus, which is composed mostly of dead neutrophils.

In their unactivated state in the blood, neutrophils are uniformly spherical. On activation, typically accompanied with extravasation (exit from the bloodstream), the neutrophils assume amoeboid shapes, allowing the cells to crawl (chemotax) in the interstitial spaces. The

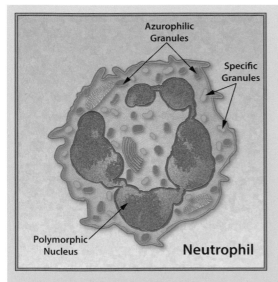
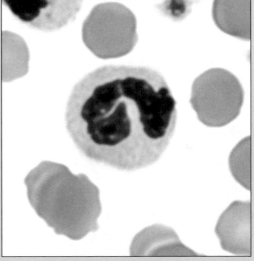

FIGURE 2.9. Canine neutrophil (mature) in a blood smear stained with Wright's Giemsa

Name:	Neutrophils
Other names:	Polymorphonucleocytes; Heterophils (in birds and reptiles)
Classifications:	Granulocyte, phagocyte
Lineage:	Myeloid
Appearance:	Segmented nucleus, granular cytoplasm
Location in health:	Blood
Life span in health:	Forty-eight to seventy-two hours
Primary function:	Antimicrobial effectors, particularly in acute bacterial infection
Mechanism of action:	Phagocytosis; Degranulation; Neutrophil extracellular trap formation

cytoplasm of neutrophils is filled with granules. These granules fail to stain in common hematology and histology stains, resulting in a neutral appearance, hence the name *neutrophil*.

The segmented nuclei of mature neutrophils are unique and hard to miss in a blood smear. The degree of nuclear segmentation is an indicator of neutrophil maturation, with the immature band neutrophils possessing unsegmented nuclei and older neutrophils having highly segmented nuclei.

As stated earlier, the primary function of neutrophils is to kill invading microbes. Neutrophils achieve this through several effector mechanisms. First, neutrophils engulf (eat) microbes via phagocytosis and destroy them in intracellular vesicles called phagolysosomes.

Second, activated neutrophils can kill extracellular microbes by degranulation and secretion of antimicrobial proteins and the release of toxic metabolites. Third, neutrophils release meshlike substances called neutrophil extracellular traps (NETs). These NETs, consisting of DNA and certain proteins, can trap and kill extracellular microbes (literally as a fishing net does). In addition to killing microbes, neutrophils participate in the coordination of inflammation through the release of inflammatory mediators.

EOSINOPHILS

Eosinophils are especially effective in killing multicellular parasites such as parasitic helminths (worms). Eosinophils also have some

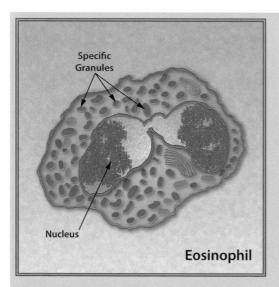
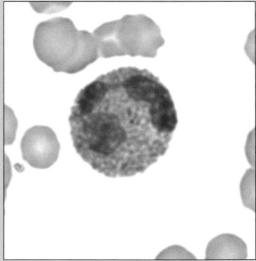

FIGURE 2.10. Canine eosinophil in a blood smear stained with Wright's Giemsa

Name:	Eosinophils
Other names:	Eosinophil granulocytes
Classifications:	Granulocyte
Lineage:	Myeloid
Appearance:	Characteristic eosinophilic granules (staining red with eosin)
Location in health:	Blood and tissues lining gastrointestinal tract and airways
Life span in health:	Days to weeks
Primary function:	Antiparasitic effectors, particularly in helminthic infection; Some antiviral action; Roles in allergy
Mechanism of action:	Degranulation; Limited phagocytosis

antiviral capabilities and are active in certain allergic responses (particularly in cats and horses). Their role in tumor immunity remains unclear.

After release from the bone marrow, mature eosinophils circulate in the blood and make up approximately 0.1 percent to 3.0 percent of leukocytes in most species. In blood smears, their granules stain bright red. The morphology of eosinophil nuclei can range from round to multilobular. Unlike neutrophils, eosinophils normally exit the blood after a brief period of circulation and spend most of their lives in healthy tissues, particularly in the connective tissues underlying mucosal surfaces. It is here that eosinophils are most likely to encounter multicellular parasites. During parasitic infections, eosinophils still circulating in the blood are specifically recruited to the affected tissue.

Once in the tissue and activated by parasite or leukocyte products, resident or newly recruited eosinophils kill invading parasites. Because multicellular parasites are too big to be engulfed by phagocytosis, eosinophils release antiparasitic proteins and toxic metabolites into extracellular spaces to harm or kill these multicellular invaders. They are also active in certain severe allergic responses in cooperation with mast cells and basophils and have roles in antiviral responses. For the most part, however, eosinophils are innate granulocytes and specialists in combating parasitic, particularly helminth, infections.

BASOPHILS

In most domestic species, basophils typically make up less than 0.5 percent of leukocytes

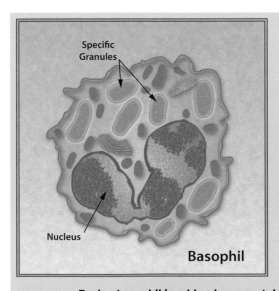
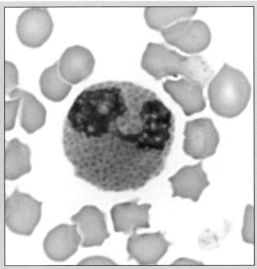

FIGURE 2.11. Bovine basophil in a blood smear stained with Wright's Giemsa

Name:	Basophils
Other names:	Basophil granulocytes
Classifications:	Granulocyte
Lineage:	Myeloid
Appearance:	Characteristic blue-purple basophilic granules with basic dyes
Location in health:	Blood
Life span in health:	Days
Primary function:	Mediator of inflammation
Mechanism of action:	Degranulation

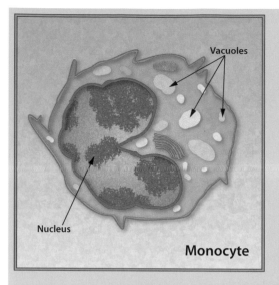

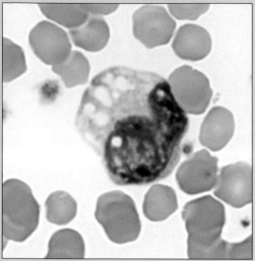

Vacuoles

Nucleus

Monocyte

FIGURE 2.12. **Feline monocyte in a blood smear stained with Wright's Giemsa**

Name:	Monocytes
Classifications:	Mononuclear phagocytes
Lineage:	Myeloid
Appearance:	Large round to kidney-shaped nucleus, diffuse pale blue-gray staining cytoplasm commonly containing vacuoles
Location in health:	Blood
Life span in health:	Days (in circulation)
Primary function:	Precursors of macrophages and DCs
Mechanism of action:	Limited antimicrobial function in blood

circulating in the blood. Although rare, their characteristic dark-staining large cytoplasmic granules (when stained with basic dyes) make it easy to identify them on a blood smear. During multicellular parasitic infections and late-phase allergic reactions, basophils migrate into inflamed tissues. Here, basophils coordinate inflammation (in a manner similar to that of mast cells) and promote the adaptive immune reactions best suited to combating parasites (called a Th-2 response, covered in later chapters). Unfortunately, these functions of basophils also amplify the unwanted effects associated with allergies (type I hypersensitivities). Overall, basophils are mediators of inflammation associated with parasitic infections and allergies.

MONOCYTES

Monocytes are circulating precursors of, among other cell types, macrophages and DCs. In most species, monocytes make up 2 percent to 10 percent of circulating leukocytes. In a blood smear, these cells appear to be 12–20 μm in diameter with diffusely stained cytoplasm and large, round, indented, or kidney-shaped nuclei. Monocytes typically circulate for a few days before exiting the circulation to differentiate into tissue macrophages or DCs. Under normal circumstances, monocytes perpetually replenish tissue macrophages and DCs in all tissues. However, in inflamed tissues, monocytes rapidly exit the blood to quickly populate the area with large numbers of macrophages.

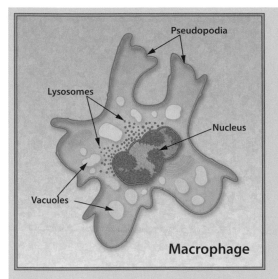
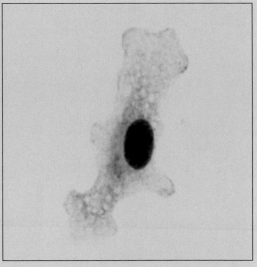

FIGURE 2.13. **Murine tissue macrophage grown in cell culture and stained with Diff-Quik**

Name:	Macrophages
Other names:	Tissue macrophages; Kupffer cells (macrophages in liver); Splenic macrophages (macrophages in spleen); Microglial cells (macrophage equivalents in the central nervous system); Alveolar macrophages (macrophages in airways); Peritoneal macrophages (macrophages in the peritoneal cavity)
Classifications:	Mononuclear phagocyte; Sentinel cell; Antigen-presenting cell
Lineage:	Myeloid
Appearance:	Round nucleus, clear-vacuolated cytoplasm, irregular cell shape
Location in health:	Peripheral tissue
Life span in health:	Months
Primary function:	Immune surveillance, moderate antimicrobial capacity, limited antigen presentation
Mechanism of action:	Detection of threats and release of inflammatory mediators; Phagocytosis

Monocytes themselves are phagocytic and produce some cytokines but are generally not very proficient at these tasks until they fully differentiate into macrophages or DCs after exiting the blood.

MACROPHAGES

Within the immune system, macrophages are sentinel cells, antimicrobial effector cells, and antigen presenting cells (APCs). During health, macrophages also perform numerous housekeeping functions, such as removal of dead and damaged cells and cellular debris, tissue remodeling, and maintenance of iron homeostasis.

As mentioned earlier, macrophages arise from monocytes that exit the circulation. Once monocytes are in a tissue, various tissue factors drive the monocytes' maturation into macrophages. Because this process occurs in practically every tissue and organ, different combinations of tissue factors produce numerous organ- or tissue-specific macrophage types. Although different macrophage types may differ in location, homeostatic function, morphology, and name, most perform similar functions in the immune system. Macrophages are generally larger cells with copious amounts of membrane. They are extremely pleomorphic (i.e., they vary greatly in their size and shape), adopting spherical, spindle, or amoeboid cellular forms.

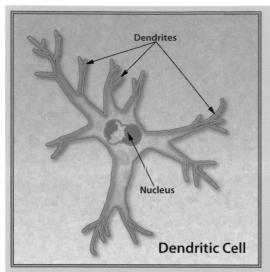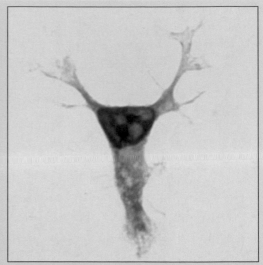

FIGURE 2.14. **Murine DC grown in culture and stained with Diff-Quik**

Name:	Myeloid dendritic cells
Other names:	Inflammatory DCs; Conventional DCs; Langerhaan cells (DCs in skin)
Classifications:	Mononuclear phagocyte; Sentinel cell; Antigen-presenting cell
Lineage:	Myeloid
Appearance:	Round nucleus, clear cytoplasm, irregular shape with long branched projections (dendrites)
Location in health:	Tissue
Life span in health:	Months
Primary function:	Immune surveillance, antigen processing and presentation
Mechanism of action:	Detection of threats and release of inflammatory mediators; Endocytosis and phagocytosis

Macrophages are very active sentinel cells, always on the lookout for signs of danger. They commonly crawl around in the extracellular spaces and have high rates of endocytosis and pinocytosis (two methods of taking up extracellular fluid). These activities allow them to constantly patrol the tissue and sample molecules in the extracellular fluid. Detection of a threat is achieved using a variety of receptors that recognize microbial products as well as products of tissue damage. Once activated, macrophages produce proinflammatory cytokines that engage other aspects of the immune system and promote the recruitment of other leukocytes to the area.

Although macrophages are not as microbicidal as neutrophils, they are reasonably adept at phagocytosis and killing microbes inside of phagolysosomes. Unlike most neutrophils, however, macrophages can also keep pieces of protein from the phagocytosed bacteria and, in a process called antigen presentation, present these pieces to T cells of the adaptive immune system (see chapter 8).

MYELOID DENDRITIC CELLS

The term *dendritic cell* (*DC*) has been applied to a number of different cell types with different origins and functions (see discussion of other innate cells). Thus, the term does not always define a single cell type. However, myeloid DCs (DCs of myeloid origin) are typically just referred to as DCs (as we do here).

DCs are innate sentinel cells that are highly efficient at processing and presenting antigens to T cells. Because antigen presentation is essential for T-cell adaptive immunity, DCs function at the interface between the innate and the adaptive immune systems.

DCs are present in practically every tissue and organ of the body. Like macrophages, DCs derive from circulating monocytes that have exited the blood and migrated into tissues. If given the right stimulus, monocytes mature into DCs that take up residence by extending their long branched cellular projections between cells and connective tissues, which gives the DCs their intricate shape as well as their name (*dendron* is Greek for "tree"). Within tissues, DCs act as sentinel cells. They express numerous receptors that detect tissue damage and infection, and in response they synthesize cytokines that activate other immune cells. Similarly to macrophages, DCs can also endocytose and phagocytose microbes, but unlike macrophages, DCs are not very effective in killing the microbes within the phagolysosome. However, DCs are especially efficient at processing protein antigens, displaying bits of those antigens on their surfaces, and presenting them to T cells. In fact, DCs are the only APCs that can effectively initiate T-cell responses to new antigens. For this reason, DCs are often referred to as professional APCs.

MAST CELLS

Mast cells, like macrophages and DCs, are sentinel cells involved in immune surveillance. On detection of a threat, mast cells rapidly release potent mediators of inflammation, which are usually protective. Mast cells, however, also play a major role in allergies (type I hypersensitivities).

Mast-cell precursor cells arise in the bone marrow and quickly migrate into tissues through-out the body (especially the connective tissues surrounding blood vessels and nerves, as well as in the lamina propria of mucosal surfaces), where they then differentiate into mature mast cells. Because mast cells act as sentinel cells, they express a variety of receptors that can detect innate danger signals. Mast cells also have receptors that recognize IgE, which is important in adaptive immune responses to parasites and allergens.

The cytoplasm of a mature mast cell contains densely packed granules full of proinflammatory mediators. On detection of a threat (either directly or through products released by other leukocytes or by complement activation), mast cells degranulate and release the proinflammatory granule contents into the extracellular space. These granule components, together with the lipid mediators and cytokines synthesized by the mast cells, act on local cells and vasculature, resulting in inflammation (particularly by increasing vascular dilation and permeability). This inflammation not only alerts the immune system to the threat but also assists in the recruitment of effector cells that can combat the threat. Mast cells also play important roles in the coordination of chronic inflammation and tissue repair. Overall, mast cells are specialized sentinel cells strategically positioned in tissues and, when triggered, quickly promote inflammation.

Lymphoid Innate Immune Cells

NATURAL KILLER CELLS

NK cells earn their name because of their ability to innately recognize and kill abnormal host cells without previous sensitization. NK cells do not express either T- or B-cell receptors, which distinguishes them from NK T lymphocytes, which are named for their similarity to both NK cells and T cells but function in both adaptive and innate immune responses.

NK cells arise in the bone marrow from the lymphoid lineage, but go through a second round of maturation (termed *licensing*) in secondary lymphoid tissues (lymph nodes, spleen).

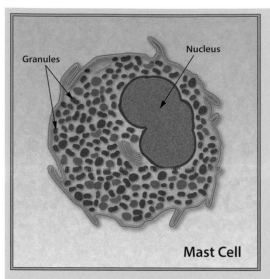
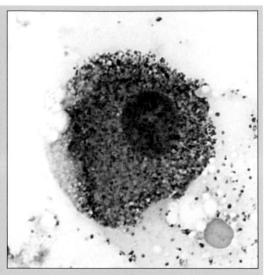

Mast Cell

FIGURE 2.15. **Canine mast cell from a fine-needle aspirate stained with Wright's Giemsa**

Name:	Mast cells
Classifications:	Sentinel cells
Lineage:	Myeloid
Appearance:	Round nucleus, cytoplasm densely packed with granules (purple)
Location in health:	Tissue, particularly connective tissue surrounding vasculature and nerves, and the lamina propria of the mucosa
Life span in health:	Weeks to months
Primary function:	Immune surveillance, mediator and amplifier of inflammation and allergy
Mechanism of action:	Detection of threats and release of inflammatory mediators via degranulation (vasoactive amines) or synthesis of lipid mediators and cytokines

Mature, licensed NK cells then enter the circulation, where they can account for as much as 2 percent to 15 percent of lymphocytes. NK cells are larger than most circulating lymphocytes and have cytoplasms that contain azurophilic granules (hence, they are often described as "large granular lymphocytes"). These granules contain proteins, called granzymes and perforins, that are key to NK cells' cytotoxic abilities. NK cells also appear in normal tissues, particularly underlying mucosal surfaces; however, their function in these locations is less well understood.

NK cells constitute the first line of defense against viral infections and possibly some types of tumor cells. Because viruses replicate inside host cells, the majority of innate immune mechanisms are ineffective against them. Similarly, many tumor cells differ very little from normal host cells. However, both virus-infected and tumor cells often express abnormal molecules on their surfaces or lose markers that normally identify the host cells as self. NK cells use host cell–surface proteins to identify normal and abnormal cells. If a host cell appears abnormal, the NK cell forms a tight adhesion to the target cell and precisely delivers cytotoxic molecules from its granules to the abnormal cell, forcing it into apoptosis (programmed cell death). Antibodies, produced during an adaptive immune response, can also trigger NK cell cytotoxicity in a process called antibody-dependent cell-mediated cytotoxicity.

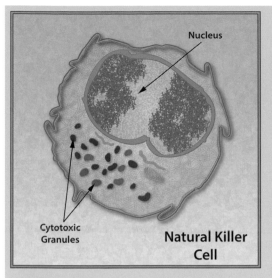
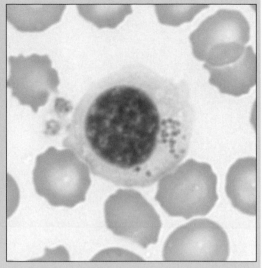

Canine NK cell in blood smear stained with Wright's Giemsa

Name:	Natural killer cells
Other names:	Null lymphocytes
Classifications:	Lymphocyte
Lineage:	Lymphoid
Appearance:	Large lymphoid cell, round nucleus, azurophilic cytoplasmic granules
Location in health:	Blood, spleen
Life span in health:	Weeks to months
Primary function:	Destruction of virally infected or abnormal host cells (including tumor cells)
Mechanism of action:	Recognition of virally infected or abnormal host cells and targeted release of cytotoxic granules

Other Innate Immune Cells

In addition to NK cells, B-1 cells and γδ T cells are innate immune cells of lymphoid origin. Because both of these cell types share much in common with their adaptive immune cousins B-2 cells and αβ T cells, the specifics of these innate lymphocytes are covered in chapters 10 and 12.

As mentioned, DCs also have different subtypes. In addition to myeloid DCs, there are plasmacytoid DCs (pDCs) and follicular dendritic cells (FDCs).

pDCs, named for their resemblance to plasma cells, are of lymphoid origin and circulate in the blood. They are not particularly good at presenting antigen, but during viral infections, they can produce IFN-α, a powerful antiviral agent.

FDCs appear in the B-cell regions of lymph nodes and probably derive from mesenchymal cells. They function to retain unprocessed antigen on their surfaces, which supports B-cell maturation during a humoral immune response (covered in chapter 12).

CLINICAL CORRELATION: FOLLOW-UP

Student Considerations

As described at the beginning of this chapter, collies with cyclic neutropenia go through

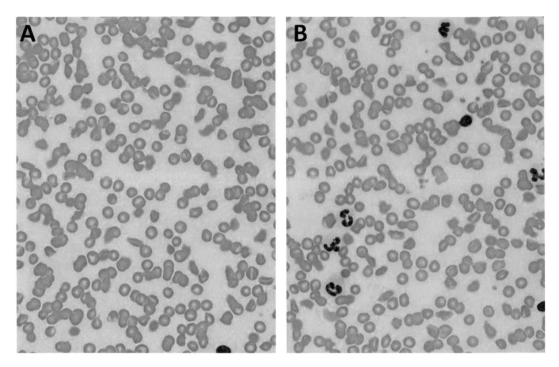

FIGURE 2.17A–B. Cyclic neutropenia

Two blood smears (stained with Wright's Giemsa) taken from a gray collie during (panel A) and after (panel B) a period of neutropenia. Note the difference in mature neutrophils between smears.

cycles of neutrophil depletion that coincide with increased susceptibility to many types of infections, especially bacterial infections. After reading this chapter, you should be able to propose an explanation for the coincidence of neutropenia and susceptibility to opportunistic bacterial infections.

Possible Explanations

Canine cyclic neutropenia is a genetic disorder that affects melanocytes (resulting in the gray coat color) and bone marrow stem cells. Affected puppies exhibit cyclic fluctuations in all their blood cells (RBCs, platelets, and leukocytes), but because neutrophils have the shortest life span of these cells, the most characteristic finding is cyclic neutropenia (Figure 2.17A–B).

A mutation in the gene encoding the protein AP3β1 has been identified as the underlying cause. The mutation disrupts the normal trafficking of granular proteins (such as elastase) to cytoplasmic granules during certain stages in hematopoiesis. This disruption results in a cyclic arrest of maturation of myeloid progenitor cells in the bone marrow followed by their apoptosis—probably the result of buildup of incorrectly trafficked granule proteins in the cell. The end result of this mutation is that these gray collies have compromised production of early myeloid cells.

The understanding behind the cyclic nature of the defect is less clear, with several conflicting theories proposed. However, it is likely that the cyclic nature of the neutropenia is related to feedback loops involving different stages of myeloid precursor cells, which result in oscillating levels of growth factors, apoptosis, or both. Nonetheless, because neutrophils are one of the primary innate defenders against bacterial attack, their depletion in periods of neutropenia most likely underpins the clinical presentation of recurrent bacterial infections.

An interesting finding is that although these puppies usually die at a very young age, there has been some success in the treatment of this lifelong disease. Successful strategies involve bolstering myelopoiesis by increasing the concentration of the hematopoietic growth factor G-CSF through injection of exogenous G-CSF or increasing the expression of G-CSF through gene therapy.

Robin M. Yates

Innate Immune Recognition

Chapter 3

10.5876_9781607322184.c003

CLINICAL CORRELATION: SEPSIS IN NEONATAL FOALS

The medical management of septic foals is a major challenge for equine practitioners. Sepsis is a systemic inflammatory response to infection that in foals is a common sequela of bacteremia (infection of the blood by live bacteria). Neonatal foals are particularly susceptible to bacteremia, especially foals of mares that are sick or experience abnormal or difficult parturition or foals that fail to suckle soon after birth. Bacteria can gain entry to the neonatal foal's blood via wounds, such as the umbilical stump, or after ingestion or inhalation of environmental bacteria. The original infection can also originate in utero.

The most common type of bacteria isolated from septic foals is Gram-negative *Escherichia coli* (*E. coli*), which accounts for 30 percent to 60 percent of reported cases. Bacteremic foals typically present with fever, malaise, and general ill thrift. These symptoms can rapidly progress to life-threatening sepsis, also known as bacteremia-induced systemic inflammatory response syndrome (SIRS). SIRS results from a systemwide uncontrolled activation of multiple proinflammatory reactions. If not aggressively treated, prolonged SIRS and its associated shock (severe hypotension) can lead to multiorgan failure and death (Figure 3.1).

It is easy to rationalize why bacteria in the blood (particularly in an immunocompromised neonate) could result in severe illness. It is interesting, however, that although the bacteria themselves may be the instigators, they are not the pathogenic force behind the symptoms of SIRS.

What is doing all this damage? SIRS resulting from septicemia is primarily propagated by the innate immune system that is overactivated by disseminated bacterial products (not necessarily the bacteria themselves). In the case of sepsis from Gram-negative bacteria such as *E. coli,* one of the most potent activators of the immune system is lipopolysaccharide (LPS). LPS is also commonly referred to as an endotoxin ("inside toxin"). In fact, it is not a toxin in the classic sense

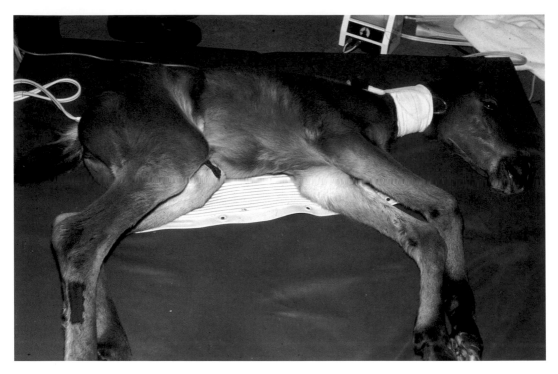

FIGURE 3.1. **A septic neonatal foal undergoing intensive life-supporting therapy (photograph courtesy of Dr. Michel Levy, University of Calgary)**

(such as cholera toxin or botulinum toxin, which have evolved to purposefully cause dysfunction) but a structural component of the outer membranes of Gram-negative bacteria. However, LPS elicits such a strong inflammatory reaction in animals that it is often viewed as toxic, and the reaction is often referred to as endotoxic shock. Experimentally, SIRS can be induced by the injection of purified LPS in the complete absence of live bacteria. How is a chemically inert molecule made up of lipid and sugars able to cause so much damage? Clearly, in the case of septicemia in a neonatal foal, the immune reaction to LPS is detrimental. What is the advantage to the animal, if any, of reacting to LPS at all?

LEARNING OBJECTIVES

After reading this chapter, you should be able to

- describe in general terms how the innate immune system recognizes threats;

- explain the concepts of evolutionarily conserved molecular patterns;
- define the terms *PAMPs*, *DAMPs*, and *PRRs*;
- give examples of PAMPs and DAMPs and the PRRs that recognize them;
- list the general functions and cellular locations of the major PRR families;
- explain the function and formation of the inflammasome;
- list the consequences of sentinel cell exposure to PAMPs and DAMPs.

INTRODUCTION

The immune system of an animal cannot be fully activated in all tissues at all times. Not only would this lead to the depletion of immune components and energy, but it would also cause tissue and organ damage. Instead, the immune system needs to be in a dormant but alert state

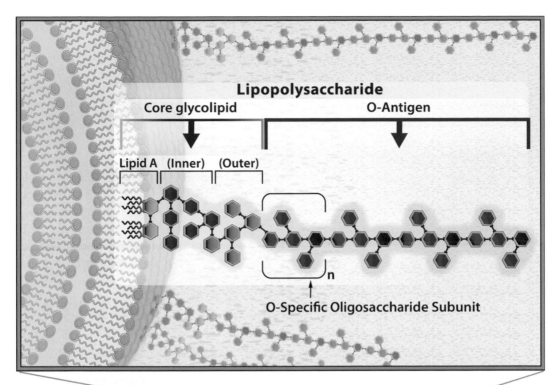

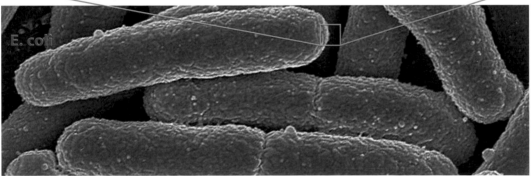

FIGURE 3.2. The structure of LPS

LPS is a macromolecule consisting of a lipid component (lipid A), a core oligosaccharide, and a variable polysaccharide side chain (O antigen). It is an integral component of Gram-negative bacteria, conferring structural stability and chemical resistance to the outer membrane. The scanning electron image of *E. coli* was created in the Rocky Mountain Laboratories, National Institutes of Health.

and be selectively activated when and where it is needed. So, one of the first and most important functions of an animal's immune system is to differentiate between threatening and non-threatening situations. You are probably aware by now that the intricate adaptive immune system can learn over time to differentiate between self and non-self antigens (how it does this has preoccupied the field of immunology for decades). But when an animal is faced with an entity it has never encountered, it needs to be able to instantly and instinctively determine whether it is a threat and be able to act accordingly. The innate immune system has evolved to innately determine whether something is potentially hazardous or not without having to learn how to make that distinction. It can then selectively use offensive strategies to fight this new threat. However, the importance of the innate detection of a threat does not stop with the deployment of innate immune effectors; the innate responses also direct subsequent learned or adaptive immune responses.

Animals encounter countless new foreign antigens every day but only mount an adaptive immune response to some. Moreover, the most effective type of adaptive immune response mounted (e.g., humoral vs. cellular) appears to be directed by the type of infecting agent. For decades, the adaptive immune components were heralded to be the "brains" making these intelligent decisions, but it is now clear that the innate immune system directs most subsequent immune responses. Moreover, the first real advances in this understanding were not achieved by studying the more advanced mammalian system but by looking at the humble fruit fly, which does not have an adaptive immune system at all.

EVOLUTIONARILY CONSERVED MOLECULAR PATTERNS

At the molecular level, viruses, bacteria, fungi, parasites, and animals are all made up of the same elements arranged into similar carbon-based protein, lipid, nucleic acid, and carbohydrate building blocks. At numerous points in speciation, however, divergent evolution generated new arrangements of these molecules and left behind some of the older ones. The result is that certain molecules are peculiar to certain species. These molecules are sometimes so fundamental to the existence of a certain organism that, even if selective pressure against a particular molecule existed, the species could not simply change or eliminate that molecule. Because of that, even over evolutionary time and even in the face of the increasing efficiency of evolving immune systems, all members of

those species continue to express these specific molecules.

Pathogen-Associated Molecular Patterns

The basic structures of microbes (bacteria, fungi, protozoa, and viruses) and mammalian cells have many key differences. For example, most bacteria have a particular cell wall structure that is made up of a substance called peptidoglycan (a network of alternating sugars cross-linked by amino acids). Because mammalian cells do not have cell walls, this arrangement of molecules is absent from normal mammalian tissue, and thus it is a distinguishing molecular feature (or pattern) of many bacteria. Hence, peptidoglycan is an example of a pathogen-associated molecular pattern (PAMP). The term *PAMP* is somewhat misleading because these molecular patterns are present in nonpathogenic microbes as well. The term *microbe-associated molecular patterns* (MAMPs) is more accurate but has not been widely adopted.

In addition to acting as cues to distinguish microbial from host material, different combinations of PAMPs can give an animal's innate immune system an indication as to what type of microbe is present (bacteria vs. virus vs. protozoa, etc.), and thus the subsequent immune reaction can be crafted to best combat the particular type of microbe. Obviously, the ability of the innate immune system to do this relies on its ability to somehow detect these PAMPs.

PATTERN-RECOGNITION RECEPTORS

In subsequent chapters, you will read much about the adaptive immune system's ability to learn to differentiate between self and non-self. This ability involves random and nonrandom recombination of key areas of the chromosome of lymphocytes, together with an accelerated selection process within an individual animal. In contrast, the innate immune system's ability to detect evolutionarily conserved molecular

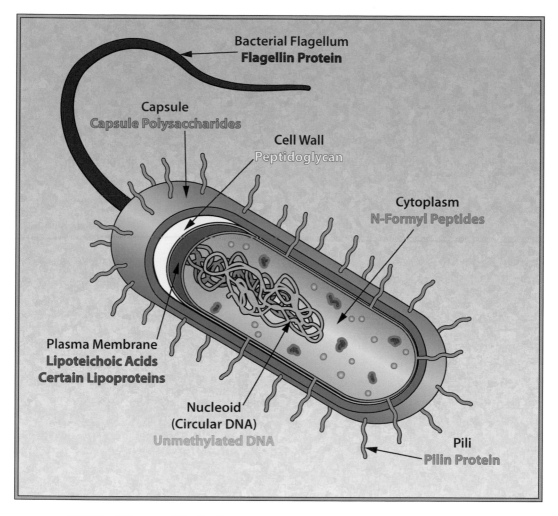

FIGURE 3.3. PAMPs of Gram-positive bacteria

A diagram of a Gram-positive bacterium and associated PAMPs recognized by the innate immune system of mammals.

patterns such as PAMPs relies on numerous receptors that are hardwired into the genome of animals after millions of years of evolution. These receptors are termed pattern recognition receptors (PRRs) and can be found in organisms throughout the biome (they are present in animals, plants, and even some microbes). In essence, PRRs can be considered sensory receptors, but instead of sensing tastes, smells, heat, or pain, they detect PAMPs. Numerous PRRs have been identified in mammals. These PRRs can be divided into families on the basis

of structure and cellular location, but they can also be categorized on the basis of function: signaling PRRs (usually stimulating proinflammatory signaling and cytokine release) and phagocytic PRRs (stimulating uptake of microbes by endocytosis or phagocytosis).

Signaling Pattern-Recognition Receptors

Signaling PRRs (often also referred to as activating or proinflammatory PRRs) appear on a range of cells within the immune system but are particularly concentrated in and on the sentinel cells such as macrophages and DCs. The primary function of these PRRs, after binding to PAMPs, is to initiate intracellular signaling pathways that lead to the activation of the host cell. Activation of sentinel cells by PAMPs usually results in the release of proinflammatory cytokines that alert other immune cells to the presence of microbial products (recall that cytokines are proteins released by cells to communicate to other cells), which in turn can initiate a range of immune defense mechanisms. The three major families of particular note within this functional category are the toll-like receptors (TLRs), the NOD-like receptors (NLRs) and the RIG-like receptors (RLRs).

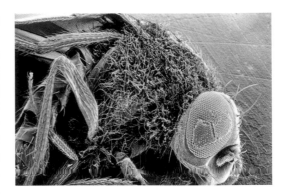

FIGURE 3.4. ***Drosophila* flies that are deficient in the toll receptor are susceptible to fungal infections.**

This image is a scanning electron micrograph of an adult *Drosophila* that has been killed by *Aspergillus* (200× magnification). The hairlike structures over the thorax are actually the germinating hyphae of *Aspergillus*. (Lemaitre et al., 1996, *Cell* 86: 973–83)

TOLL-LIKE RECEPTORS

Mammalian TLRs were actually discovered because of their similarity to the toll receptors of *Drosophila melanogaster* (fruit fly). Flies that were deficient in the toll receptor were extremely susceptible to fungal infections (particularly *Aspergillus* infections) and often died as a result (Figure 3.4). Researchers found that the toll receptor detected fungal PAMPs and stimulated the release of antimicrobial peptides (similar to defensins) that protected fruit flies from fungus. Later, researchers noted that mammals had genes that were similar to the *Drosophila* toll gene, which also mapped to a region of the genome that was known to confer sensitivity to LPS (later found to be the gene for TLR4). This family of related genes was named *TLRs*.

TLRs are a family of numbered, structurally similar transmembrane proteins that detect a broad range of PAMPs derived from bacteria, viruses, fungi, and protozoa. TLRs are expressed predominantly on the sentinel cells of the innate immune system but are also found on many other leukocytes, as well as on key areas of the epithelium exposed to the external environment (such as those lining the intestinal and respiratory tracts). Most TLRs are expressed on the plasma membrane of cells where they can detect extracellular microbes, but some (notably TLR3, TLR7, and TLR9) are expressed on the intracellular endosomal membranes, where they can detect the PAMPs associated with intracellular bacteria and viruses (Figure 3.5). Each individual TLR detects a different set of PAMPs. These PAMPs include LPS, peptidoglycan, unmethylated DNA (nuclear DNA from mammals is methylated, but prokaryotic DNA is unmethylated), single- and double-stranded RNA (some viral genomes are made of these), flagellin (a protein in bacterial flagella), profilin-like protein (a protein found in some protozoan parasites), and various microbial lipoproteins, to name a few. In addition to individual receptor ligands, some TLRs can join forces to detect other PAMPs. For example, TLR2 can dimerize (form a pair) with TLR1 or TLR6 to form a receptor that recognizes microbial diacylated lipopeptides. Some TLRs also cooperate with non-TLR accessory proteins, allowing them to bind to PAMPs that they could not bind to autonomously. As a family, TLRs

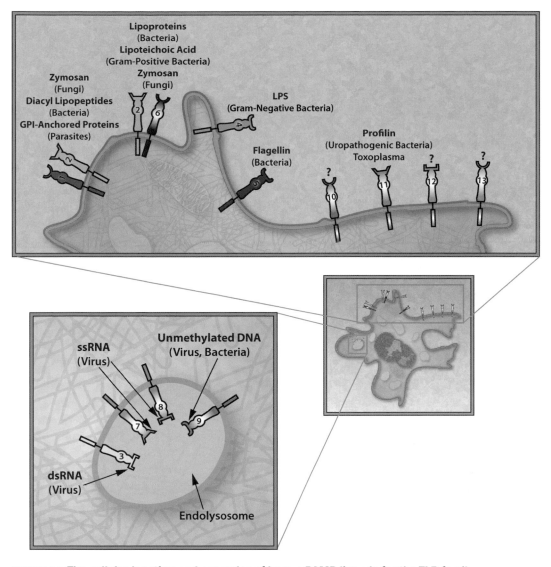

FIGURE 3.5. **The cellular location and examples of known PAMP ligands for the TLR family**

GPI = Glycosylphosphatidylinositol; dsRNA = double-stranded RNA; ssRNA = single-stranded RNA.

collectively detect at least one PAMP from virtually any microbe.

Although the number of TLRs that have been identified varies slightly between different vertebrate species (most mammals have approximately thirteen; chickens have approximately ten), the major individual TLRs (e.g., TLR4) are surprisingly well conserved, displaying little variation between species. The signaling pathways initiated by TLRs are also well conserved. All TLRs have a cytosolic TIR domain that, after detection of a PAMP, recruits signaling adapter molecules (such as MyD88 and TRIF). These adapter molecules initiate signaling cascades involving a slew of kinases, which serve to propagate and amplify the signal. One of the final steps in the signaling pathway is the release of the rapid-acting transcription factor NFκB from its negative regulator (IκB), allowing it to move from the cytoplasm into the nucleus (Figure 3.6). Within the nucleus, NFκB binds specific sequences of DNA (called response elements) and recruits other transcriptional activators as well as RNA polymerase. This process results in the expression of genes that lead to the activation of the cell as well as the expression of numerous proinflammatory cytokines and chemokines. Aside from NFκB, several other signaling pathways can be initiated by TLRs, resulting in the upregulation of a variety of genes associated with immune activation. Without a doubt, the TLR family is one of the most important groups of PRRs in vertebrates. But because TLRs are all transmembrane receptors with their sensing domain always facing outward (detecting extracellular and endosomal PAMPs), infectious invaders of the cytosol can escape their detection.

NOD-LIKE RECEPTORS AND RIG-LIKE RECEPTORS

Two main families of PRRs sense PAMPs within the cytosol of cells: the NLRs, which sense a variety of bacterial PAMPs (as well as damage signals, which we discuss later), and the RLRs, which detect viral RNA. Although TLRs can sense similar PAMPs, these cytosolic PRRs constitute a second line of detection of bacteria and viruses that make their way into the cytosol of the cell.

As with TLRs, the NLRs encompass an evolutionarily conserved family of PRRs with more than 20 to 30 members in mammals (sea urchins are thought to contain upward of 203 different NLR members). NLRs have a common tripartite structure consisting of a leucine-rich pattern-recognition domain, a NOD domain (that facilitates oligomerization after PAMP detection), and a variable protein–protein interaction domain. NLRs are not membrane bound but float in the cytosol of immune cells (although some nonimmune cells can also express certain NLRs).

The PAMPs detected by many of the newly discovered NLR members are currently unknown. The best characterized NLRs are NOD1 (which is expressed in many cell types) and NOD2 (which is expressed predominantly in the sentinel cells). Both NOD1 and NOD2 detect different patterns within peptidoglycan (recall that peptidoglycan is a meshlike component of bacterial cell walls). Because certain pathogenic bacteria actually invade the cytosol of cells (such as *Listeria monocytogenes,* a major problem in dairy and beef cattle), NOD1 and NOD2 have evolved to detect intracellular bacteria that are otherwise hidden from the rest of the immune system. After binding peptidoglycan, NOD1 or NOD2 initiates signaling cascades that result in the activation of NFκB, leading to cellular activation and the expression of proinflammatory cytokines and chemokines, similar to TLR activation.

RLRs are a family of three RNA helicases that sense the presence of viral RNA within the cytosol and hence are important in the detection of certain viruses. The best characterized is RIG-I, which recognizes long double-stranded RNA, as well as single-stranded RNA containing a 5′-triphosphate. Although RNA strands are in normal mammalian cytosol, they are usually single stranded with a 5′ cap (no 5′-triphosphate); hence, RIG-I can differentiate between normal host RNA and RNA that is produced during viral replication. On recognition of viral RNA, RIG-I initiates signaling pathways that not only result in the activation of NFκB but also lead to the expression of type I interferons (cytokines that specifically elicit antiviral responses).

Phagocytic Pattern-Recognition Receptors

All of the phagocytic cells, such as neutrophils, macrophages, and DCs, express a collection of phagocytic PRRs on their surfaces that allows them to autonomously detect microbes and phagocytose them. As you will learn in

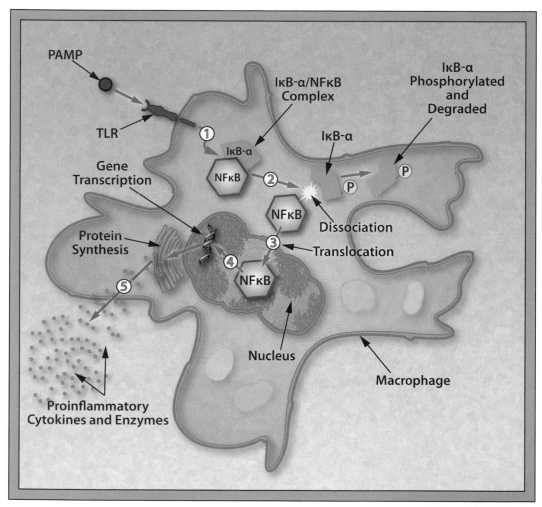

FIGURE 3.6A–C. **Activation of NFκB after binding of PAMPs by PRRs**

Panel A: After PRR activation by PAMPs, intracellular signaling (involving several steps not shown) (1) eventually results in the liberation of NFκB from its inhibitor protein IκB (2), allowing it to move into the nucleus (3) and turn on proinflammatory genes (4). One of the outcomes is the synthesis and release of proinflammatory cytokines (5). Panels B, C: The images show NFκB (green) trapped in the cytosol before exposure to PAMPs (panel B) and its translocation to the nucleus after PAMPs have been detected (panel C). NFκB is green, actin cytoskeleton is red, and nuclear DNA is blue. (Panel B images reproduced courtesy of Cell Signaling Technology, Inc. [www.cellsignal.com].)

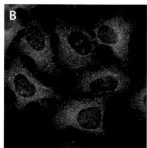

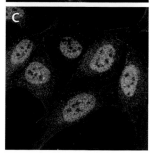

subsequent chapters, phagocytosis of micro-organisms can not only lead to their destruction, but also allow for their protein antigens to be processed and presented to T cells (a critical step in the initiation of the adaptive immune response). Numerous phagocytic PRRs can recognize a wide variety of PAMPs. One of the best-characterized phagocytic PRRs is the mannose receptor (MR; CD206).

The MR is a transmembrane protein expressed on the surface of the macrophages and DCs of mammals. The extracellular domain is a C-type lectin (a lectin is a carbohydrate-binding protein), which allows it to selectively bind terminal mannose, fucose, and N-acetyl-glucosamine residues of modified proteins. These proteins are common on the surface of microbes but absent from normal healthy host cells. As such, the detection of these PAMPs by the MR provides signals to the cell that stimulate phagocytosis (or endocytosis) of the microbes that come into contact with phagocytes, leading to their destruction and the presentation of their antigens to T cells (Figure 3.7).

Other Pattern-Recognition Receptors

Several other PRRs do not fit neatly within the signaling or phagocytic PRR categories. The formyl peptide receptors (FPR) found on the surface of neutrophils and macrophages, although somewhat implicated in cellular activation and phagocytosis, primarily direct chemotaxis. The PAMPs that these receptors detect are *N*-formylmethionine–containing peptides (the amino terminus of bacterial proteins commonly starts with the modified amino acid formylmethionine, which is generally absent from mammalian proteins). On recognition of these bacterial peptides, these G protein–coupled receptors coordinate movement of the neutrophil or macrophage toward the microbes. In this way, these phagocytes can detect, locate, and destroy bacteria.

Another category of PRRs is the secreted PRRs, such as mannose-binding lectin (MBL) and C-reactive protein (CRP). MBL (not to be confused with the membrane-bound MR) is an acute phase protein synthesized primarily by the liver and released into plasma. Here, MBL specifically binds to mannose residues on the surface of microbes and initiates complement activation, resulting in amplification of several innate immune mechanisms. We cover complement activation in greater detail in chapter 4. CRP (the major acute phase protein in primates, rabbits, dogs, and pigs) is another plasma protein that can also be considered a secreted PRR. It selectively binds microbial polysaccharides and glycolipids as well as phosphocholine associated with bacteria or damaged host cells. Once bound, CRP can facilitate complement activation as well as enhance phagocytic clearance of microbes and dead cells.

INNATE RECOGNITION OF DAMAGE-ASSOCIATED MOLECULAR PATTERNS

To this point, we have focused on the innate recognition of microbial products (PAMPs). Recent research, however, has added a second set of molecular patterns recognized by the innate immune system that are not foreign but endogenously derived (made by the host animal). These molecular patterns are associated with cellular and tissue injury, indicating a threat to the animal that may or may not be associated with microbial invasion. The term that has been adopted for these signals is *damage-associated molecular patterns,* or DAMPs, although they have also previously been referred to as *alarmins.*

Irrespective of whether microbes are involved or not, the immune system needs to respond to tissue or cellular trauma. Tissues can be physically damaged (torn, crushed, cut), damaged by heat and cold (burns, frostbite), or chemically damaged (acids, bases, toxins, poisons). Damaged tissues need to be protected from microbial invasion and tissue repair mechanisms deployed; thus, the immune system needs to be alerted. DAMPs are derived from the normal

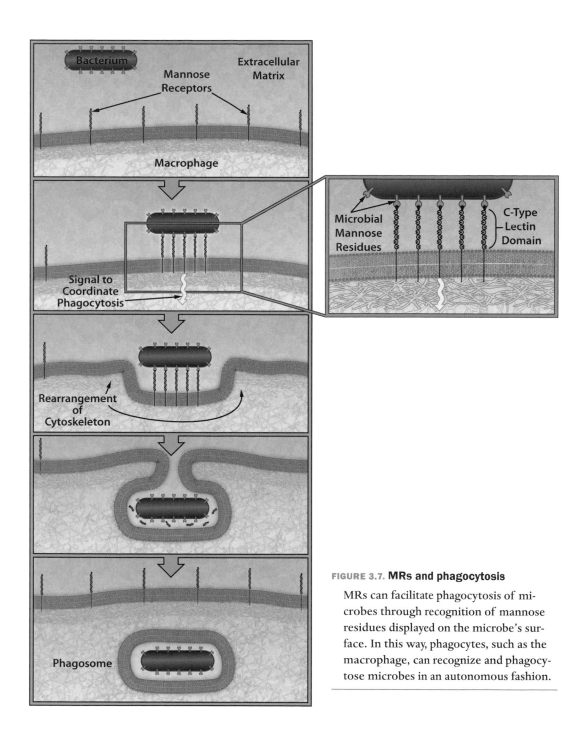

FIGURE 3.7. MRs and phagocytosis

MRs can facilitate phagocytosis of microbes through recognition of mannose residues displayed on the microbe's surface. In this way, phagocytes, such as the macrophage, can recognize and phagocytose microbes in an autonomous fashion.

proteins and metabolites found in the cytoplasm or nucleus of host cells that are released after cellular necrosis (Figure 3.8). The extracellular presence of these molecules indicates cellular injury in the vicinity. Numerous DAMPs have been identified in animals, ranging from nuclear proteins (e.g., high-mobility group box 1 protein [HMGB1]), cytosolic proteins (S100 calcium-binding proteins and heat shock proteins), DNA (particularly mitochondrial DNA),

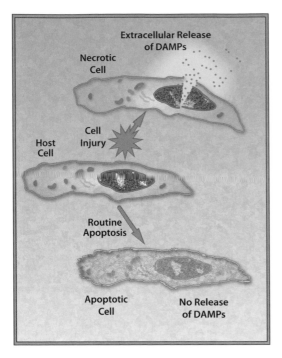

FIGURE 3.8. Endogenous production of DAMPs

As shown, after injury, host cell necrosis can release DAMPs, often leading to inflammation. Programmed cell death via apoptosis does not release proinflammatory DAMPs and will not activate the innate immune system during homeostatic cell turnover.

and purine metabolites (e.g., adenosine triphosphate [ATP], adenosine, and uric acid) (Table 3.1). In addition to DAMP release from necrotic cells, macrophages, neutrophils, and NK cells can actively secrete DAMPs after activation, which can act to amplify danger signals in a tissue after trauma or microbial invasion.

Numerous PRRs specifically recognize DAMPs. For instance, the nuclear protein HMGB1, when released from cells, is recognized by a PRR called the receptor for advanced glycation end products (RAGE), which is expressed on macrophages and certain endothelial cells (cells that line blood vessels and lymphatics). Detection of HMGB1 by RAGE results in signaling pathways that lead to NFκB activation (similar to activation by many PAMPs). Interestingly, some DAMPs are recognized by

PRRs that also recognize PAMPs (e.g., HMGB1 is also recognized by the PAMP receptors TLR2 and TLR4).

Inflammasome

The presence of PAMPs or DAMPs indicates that either a microbial invasion or some sort of tissue damage has occurred, and the immune system is thus stimulated to give a measured response. The presence of both PAMPs and DAMPs indicates both a microbial invasion (most likely pathogenic) and tissue damage have occurred—a serious threat. In addition to the additive effects of PAMPs and DAMPs, they can synergize through the formation of the inflammasome—a signaling cascade that results in the massive production and secretion of IL-1β and IL-18 (both potent proinflammatory cytokines).

Although a variety of inflammasome types exist, most require two separate signals from PAMPs, DAMPs, or both. The best studied is the NALP3 inflammasome (Figure 3.9). This large protein complex is formed in macrophages after stimulation by a PAMP, followed by a second signal provided by ATP (a DAMP). The first signal can originate through the activation of a variety of PRRs (TLRs, NLRs, or RLRs), resulting in the NFκB-mediated expression of inactive (pro-forms) of IL-1β and IL-18. These proteins accumulate in the cytosol in their inactive forms. If damage has occurred to host cells in the vicinity, released ATP, detected through a purinergic receptor (P2X7 receptor), initiates the assembly of a large cytoplasmic complex, activating the protease caspase 1, which efficiently cleaves the inactive IL-1β and IL-18 into their active forms. These potent proinflammatory cytokines are secreted from the macrophage in large quantities, inciting widespread leukocyte activation and inflammation. Aside from ATP, other DAMPs, such as uric acid, as well as alum (a common vaccine adjuvant), can provide the second signal needed for full inflammasome function.

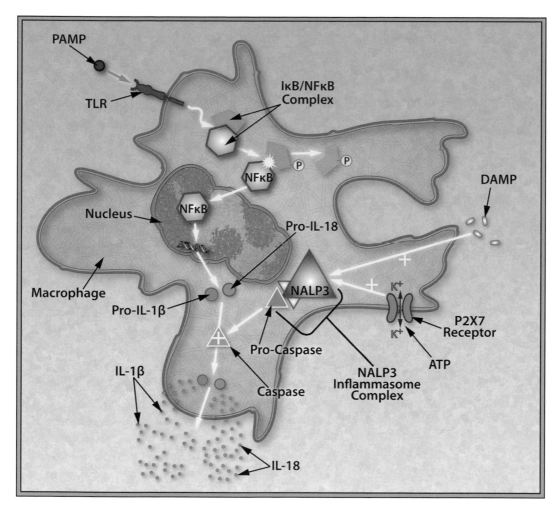

FIGURE 3.9. Intracellular activation of inflammasomes

Full activation of the inflammasome requires activation by a PAMP (e.g., LPS) as well as a DAMP (e.g., uric acid or ATP). This activation indicates that a microbial invasion and cellular damage have occurred. The sentinel cell responds by secreting large quantities of the proinflammatory cytokines IL-1β and IL-18.

TABLE 3.1. Examples of known DAMPs

DAMP	Type	Origin	PRR
HMGB1	DNA-interacting protein	Nucleus and cytoplasm	RAGE, TLR2, TLR4
S100 proteins	Calcium-binding protein	Cytoplasm	RAGE, TLR2, TLR4
Serum amyloid A	Acute-phase protein	Hepatocytes	FPR, RAGE, TLR2, TLR4
DNA	DNA	Nucleus and mitochondria	TLR9
Spliceosome-associated protein 130 (SAP130)	Protein	Nucleus	Mincle
ATP	Adenosine derivative	Cytosol	P2X7 receptor
Uric acid	Adenosine metabolite	Cytosol	NALP3

CONSEQUENCES OF DANGER SIGNAL RECOGNITION BY SENTINEL CELLS

As covered in chapter 2, every tissue within an animal contains innate immune sentinel cells that constitutively express numerous PRRs on their plasma membranes and within their cytoplasm. The majority of these cells are derived from the monocytic lineage, consisting of blood monocytes, tissue macrophages, DCs, and a variety of tissue-specific monocytic cells, including microglial cells (central nervous system), Kupffer cells (liver sinusoids), and Langerhans cells (skin). These relatively long-lived cells patrol the extracellular spaces of the tissue in which they reside, constantly on the lookout for indicators of danger. In healthy tissue, these sentinel cells exist in an unactivated (resting) state. However, binding of PAMPs, DAMPs, or both (via PRRs) activates these sentinel cells, enhancing their abilities to phagocytose and destroy bacteria, to present antigens to the adaptive immune system, and to stimulate the synthesis and release of proinflammatory cytokines and other mediators of inflammation. As you will see in later chapters, this step is the first in initiating both the innate and adaptive immune responses.

Activation of Macrophages

Detection of PAMPs and DAMPs activates macrophages, which allows these cells to better combat microbes. The repertoire of molecules displayed on the surface of macrophages changes, including increased numbers of phagocytic receptors, adhesion molecules, and molecular complexes that are needed to present antigen to T cells. Antimicrobial effectors (covered in chapter 6), such as enzyme complexes that produce oxidative products or proteins that kill microbes directly, are also upregulated during macrophage activation. As a result, activated macrophages more quickly and efficiently find, engulf, and kill microbes in the vicinity. In addition, activated macrophages secrete a variety of proinflammatory cytokines that engage several other aspects of the immune response (Figure 3.10).

Proinflammatory Mediators

Activated macrophages have an extremely high capacity to synthesize and release mediators of inflammation. These mediators are covered in greater detail in chapter 5. However, in brief, they generally include three types of proinflammatory molecules: cytokines, chemokines, and lipid mediators. The major proinflammatory cytokines produced by sentinel cells in response to PAMPs and DAMPs are IL-1β, IL-6, and TNF-α. These cytokines act locally by activating nearby leukocytes and endothelial cells, but when released in large quantities they can also act systemically, producing fever, malaise, and ill thrift. Chemokines are also released by activated macrophages so that additional leukocytes can be recruited to the site of danger (recall that chemokines are proteins that stimulate directed movement of leukocytes). In addition to proinflammatory proteins, the activation of macrophages induces enzymes that can synthesize lipid-based proinflammatory mediators such as prostaglandins, leukotrienes, and platelet-activating factor. These molecules can also assist in the recruitment of leukocytes as well as mediate changes to the local vasculature, which are essential to inflammation.

CLINICAL CORRELATION: FOLLOW-UP

Student Considerations

After reading this chapter, you should understand why LPS, an innocuous bacterial product in and of itself, can cause SIRS in neonatal foals with (Gram-negative) septicemia. You should also be able to reason why animals have evolved to recognize and respond to LPS, even though in cases of septicemia the response itself can be life threatening.

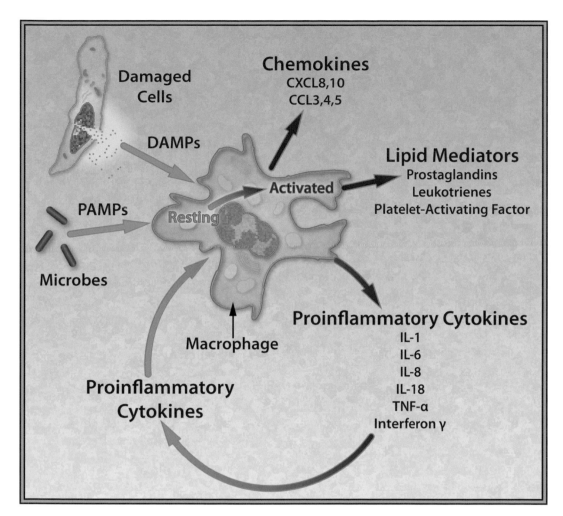

FIGURE 3.10. Inflammatory mediators produced by macrophages after activation by PAMPs, DAMPs, or proinflammatory cytokines

Exposure of a sentinel cell to PAMPs, DAMPs, or proinflammatory cytokines activates the cell, leading to upregulation of cellular antimicrobial defenses as well as release of proinflammatory chemokines, lipid mediators, and cytokines. Many of these proinflammatory products can in turn activate nearby leukocytes.

Possible Explanations

Infection of the blood by live Gram-negative bacteria, such as *E. coli,* would result in massive amounts of LPS being liberated and disseminated throughout the foal's body. Sentinel cells (particularly macrophages) in virtually every tissue will be exposed to LPS in significant quantities. This particular PAMP is detected through the PRR TLR4 (with help from the accessory proteins MD-2 and CD14), which would then initiate intracellular signaling in the sentinel cells, resulting in the expression of multiple proinflammatory cytokines, chemokines, and enzymes that synthesize other proinflammatory mediators. The simultaneous, widespread release of these proinflammatory products, which can in turn stimulate other leukocytes to release the same or similar

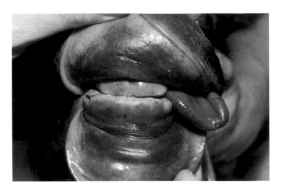

FIGURE 3.11. Oral mucous membranes of a septic foal (photograph courtesy of Dr. Michel Levy, University of Calgary)

Note the marked hyperemia as a result of disseminated PAMPs and proinflammatory mediators.

mediators, can result in a "cytokine storm" (or hypercytokinemia). Ordinarily, the innate immune response to inflammatory mediators in small, localized doses is advantageous to the animal, because it allows the immune system to activate in a focused response to an area of infection (covered in chapter 5). However, systemwide uncontrolled activation of multiple proinflammatory reactions—including vascular changes (see Figure 3.11), clotting and platelet activation, production of oxidative radicals, and leukocyte degranulation—leads to massive disruption to systemic homeostasis and ultimately SIRS.

Although LPS is the most cited initiator of SIRS in sepsis, any PAMP from many varieties of microbes can trigger SIRS in a septic animal. In fact, DAMPs released after severe trauma to an animal, even in the complete absence of infection, can also initiate SIRS. It is important to bear in mind that SIRS is an extreme example of unregulated pattern recognition and response. In a normal, healthy animal and in the majority of those that are diseased, pattern recognition is one of the first and one of the most essential mechanisms by which the immune system, when faced with a threat, can be activated in an appropriate manner.

CLINICAL CORRELATION: C3 DEFICIENCY IN BRITTANY DOGS

During the 1980s, a colony of Brittany dogs, bred for research into hereditary canine spinal muscular atrophy, were noted to have an increased susceptibility to bacterial infections and kidney disease (Figure 4.1). At a young age (younger than two years old, many only a few months old), the dogs developed serious bacterial infections, including sepsis, pyometra, pneumonia, and bacterial myositis at a surgery site. These infections were caused by a variety of different bacteria, including *Pseudomonas, Escherichia coli, Clostridia,* and *Klebsiella.* With veterinary intervention (principally prolonged courses of antibiotics), most of the dogs recovered. Later,

when the dogs reached middle age (four to seven years old), they developed renal disease involving the glomeruli, which was diagnosed as mesangio-proliferative glomerulonephritis. As a result, many of the affected dogs died from renal failure–related illnesses. The dogs in this colony were later discovered to have a genetically determined deficiency in a blood protein called complement C3. How could a deficiency in this one complement component cause the Brittany dogs to develop devastating bacterial infections and renal disease? In this chapter, you will discover that complement forms a very important part of the innate immune system and that C3 in particular is an important player in the effectiveness of the complement system.

LEARNING OBJECTIVES

After reading this chapter, you should be able to

- explain in general terms the arrangement of a biochemical cascade such as the complement system;

- name the major pathways of the complement system in mammals;

- identify the major similarities and differences in the classical, lectin, and alternative pathways of complement activation;

- describe the initiation of the classical, lectin, and alternative pathways of complement activation;

- identify the major convertases in the classical, lectin, and alternative pathways of complement activation;

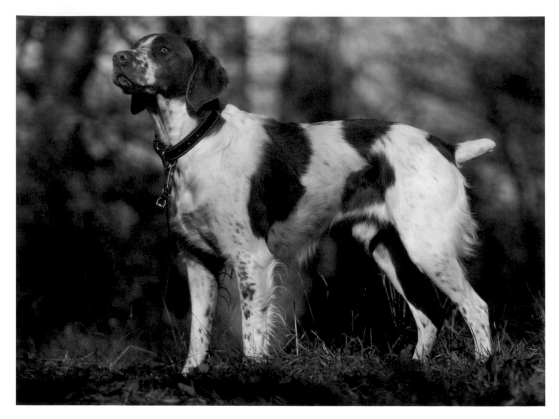

FIGURE 4.1. **A Brittany dog (also referred to as a Brittany spaniel). Photo by Pharaoh Hound.**

- describe in general terms the assembly and function of the membrane attack complex (MAC);
- give an example of how complement activation is regulated;
- list the major outcomes of complement activation and describe the mechanisms leading to them.

COMPLEMENT ACTIVATION

The complement system is made up of a collection of plasma proteins that are individually inert but can interact to create a powerful innate immune response. Complement was originally discovered in the 1890s as a heat-labile serum factor that complemented the bactericidal properties of a heat-stable serum factor (later identified as antibodies). Like most components of the innate immune system, certain triggers and outcomes of the complement system involve parts of the adaptive immune system (such as antibodies). However, the complement system is always present and can act independently as a ready-made, innate immune defense system.

The complement system consists of around sixteen different plasma proteins and glycoproteins that make up around 10 percent of the total serum protein of mammals—a significant investment of energy and resources for an animal. As with most proteins found in plasma, the majority of the complement proteins are synthesized by the liver, but monocytes, macrophages, and certain epithelial cells also contribute. Many of these complement proteins circulate in the blood as (inactive) serine protease proenzymes. Activation of the complement proenzyme to an active serine protease (usually as a result of cleavage by an activated complement protein immediately upstream of it in the pathway) permits it to, in turn, cleave (and activate) downstream complement proteins. This activation forms a biochemical cascade. Activation of the complement cascade results in many outcomes, including release of inflammatory and chemotactic mediators, coating of microbes with complement proteins that "tag" them as foreign (a process called *opsonization*), and also direct lysis of microbes.

But why is this system so overly complex? Why not have a few proteins (such as defensins and C-reactive protein) that can act independently and directly on microbes? The answer lies in the amplification power of a biochemical cascade. Innate proteins (such as defensins) that act on their own cannot amplify. However, an activated complement protein (although it may not be able to effect an immune response by itself) can activate several other complement protein molecules in the next step in the pathway. Each of these activated proteins can in turn activate several complement proteins that follow. Thus, a small inciting stimulus can amplify to a huge response involving billions of complement molecules.

The complement cascade can be activated through three different pathways that are triggered by different stimuli: (1) the classical pathway, (2) the lectin pathway, and (3) the alternative pathway.

The classical pathway is initiated by antibodies (particularly IgM and IgG) complexed to antigens and thus occurs as a consequence of a humoral immune response (the adaptive immune response that produces antibodies to antigens). The lectin and alternative pathways, however, are triggered directly by microbial products or surfaces and thus are purely innate responses. Although each pathway is triggered by different stimuli, they share common features: they all consist of a proteolytic cascade that allows for signal amplification; they all result in the creation of a C3 and a C5 convertase (which can cleave the complement proteins C3 and C5, respectively); and they all end in a com-

mon terminal pathway (also known as a membrane attack pathway).

The nomenclature used to describe each complement component typically uses C (for complement) and a number (e.g., C3). To complicate matters, the numbers are only loosely arranged in the order by which they are activated in the pathway because the specific action of some was discovered after the implementation of the numbering system. Sometimes a letter indicating a subunit or cleavage product of a complement molecule follows the number. For instance, C1 is made up of the proteins C1q, C1s, and C1r. When complement proteins are cleaved into two fragments, the smaller cleavage product is typically (but not always) indicated by the letter *a* and the larger by the letter *b* (e.g., when C3 is cleaved by a C3 convertase, the smaller fragment is named C3a and the larger is named C3b). When several complement proteins or cleavage products form a complex together, the complex is typically named using the complement numbers in the order in which they join the complex (e.g., cleavage products C4b and C2a form a complex C4b2a). Complexes can also be referred to by their function (e.g., C4b2a is also referred to as the classical pathway C3 convertase—the complex formed in the classical pathway that cleaves [converts] C3). Last, other proteins or cofactors integral to the complement pathways are not named according to this system (e.g., factor B). It is easy to get lost in the details of these pathways, so it is important to focus on the salient features common to each of them, particularly the creation of both a C3 and a C5 convertase and the initiation of the terminal membrane attack pathway (Figure 4.2).

Classical Pathway

As mentioned earlier, the classical pathway is triggered by the antibody–antigen complexes produced after an adaptive humoral immune response (covered in chapter 12). So, even though all of the complement components that make up this pathway are always present, the activation of this pathway relies on the production of specific antibodies that may take several days to appear after a new infection. It is also important to note that not all antibody types can activate the classical pathway (sometimes referred to as an antibody's ability to fix complement). In most domestic species, IgM and certain isotypes of IgG are the most potent activators of the classical complement pathway. When one IgM or several IgG molecules are bound to an antigen, the Fc (carboxy-termini of the H chains) portion of the antibodies can be recognized by the large multimolecular complex named C1 (or $C1qr_2s_2$; Figure 4.3). The backbone of C1 is made up of C1q. C1q itself is a massive protein complex that has six globular head domains connected by linear tail domains. Associated with tail domains of C1q are

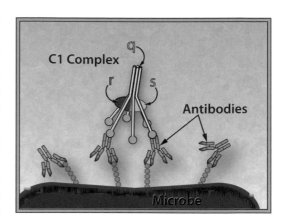

FIGURE 4.3. **Structure of the C1 complex binding to IgG antibodies**

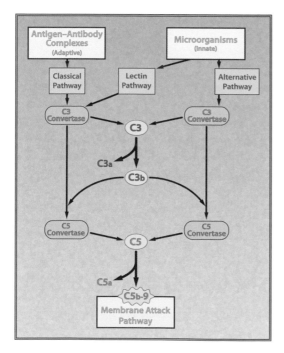

FIGURE 4.2. **A simplified diagram to illustrate the common points of complement activation**

The classical, lectin, and alternative pathways all create a functional C3 convertase and C5 convertase and initiate the terminal membrane attack pathway.

two copies of C1r and two copies of C1s, both serine proteases. For C1 to become activated, at least two globular heads of C1q must recognize and bind to two adjacent Fc regions of antibodies bound to an antigen. This recognition induces conformational change in the C1q protein, which activates the protease activity of C1r through autocatalysis (meaning C1r cleaves itself). The active C1r subunits then cleave the adjacent C1s molecules in the complex, which activates their serine protease activities.

Now activated, C1s of the C1 complex cleaves the nearby complement protein C4 into C4a and C4b (Figure 4.4), revealing a thiolester group on C4b that allows it to covalently attach (through reaction with hydroxyl or amine groups) to a nearby surface. Because thiolesters are extremely unstable, lasting only milliseconds, C4b can only attach to surfaces in the immediate vicinity of the activated C1 complex (with luck, onto the surface of the microbe or antigen complex that is being recognized by the initiating antibodies). The covalently bound C4b can present C2 to C1s, which cleaves it into C2b and the larger fragment C2a (note that for historical reasons the naming of the larger C2 cleavage product C2a goes against the complement nomenclatural convention of labeling the larger fragment *b*). The bound C4b can then bind with the C2a fragment, forming

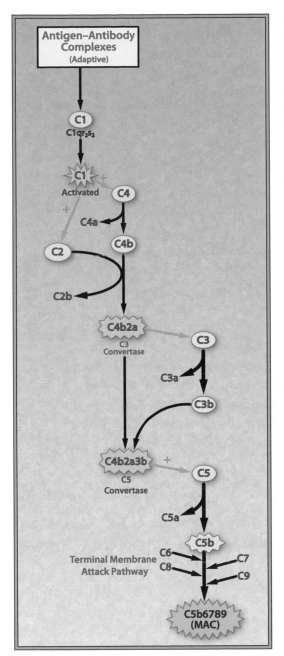

FIGURE 4.4. **The classical pathway of complement activation**

complex C4b2a on the surface of the microbe or antigen.

C4b2a is the classical pathway C3 convertase. Its job is to cleave C3 (the most abundant complement protein) into C3a and C3b. As with C4,

cleavage of C3 reveals a thiolester group in C3b, which allows the fragment to covalently attach to the surfaces in the immediate vicinity. As we discuss later in the chapter, the covalent attachment of C3b to a microbe or other antigen is an important objective of the complement system as it tags (a process called opsonization) the object for phagocytosis and removal. Although the attachment of C3b achieves one goal of the classical complement pathway, the next step is to initiate the terminal membrane attack pathway that can mediate direct lysis of the microbe. For this, a proportion of C3b will complex with the C3 convertase C4b2a to form the classical pathway C5 convertase (C4b2a3b). This complex now cleaves C5 into C5a and C5b. C5b remains associated with the C4b2a3b complex and serves as an anchor that coordinates the assembly of the MAC in the terminal membrane attack pathway (as detailed in the Terminal Membrane Attack Pathway section).

Lectin Pathway

The lectin pathway of complement activation is not reliant on any products of the adaptive immune response; thus, it is an independent innate immune response. Lectins are proteins that bind particular carbohydrate (sugar) residues. The lectin complement pathway is driven by lectins found in plasma, such as the mannose binding lectin (MBL) and ficolins that can recognize microbial-specific carbohydrates displayed on the surface of various microbes. MBL is a tetrameric member of the C-type lectin family and shares structural similarities with C1q. Instead of recognizing bound antibodies (as does C1q), however, MBL binds mannose, fucose, and N-acetylglucosamine PAMPs that are commonly present in the cell walls of bacteria and fungi, as well as on some protozoa and viruses. Essentially, as mentioned in chapter 3, MBL can be considered an extracellular PRR. Binding to a microbial cell wall induces a conformational change in MBL, which promotes activation of MBL-associated serine proteases

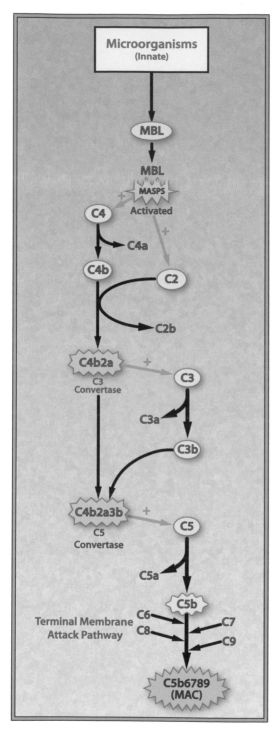

FIGURE 4.5. The lectin pathway of complement activation

(MASPs) via autocatalysis (Figure 4.5). Similarly to C1s, MASPs can in turn cleave C4 and C2 to create the C3 convertase C4b2a, which is assembled on the surface of the microbe. From here on, the lectin pathway resembles the classical pathway, with C4b2a cleaving C3, leading to deposition of covalently bound C3b on the surface of the microbe and the creation of the C4b2a3b C5 convertase, which initiates the terminal membrane attack pathway. Ficolins are a family of lectins that, like MBL, bind microbe associated carbohydrates and activate MASPs. In essence, the lectin pathway is homologous to the classical pathway but uses the innate recognition of microbial products (PAMPs) and surfaces using lectins instead of the recognition of antibodies by C1.

Alternative Pathway

The alternative pathway of complement activation is unlike the classical and lectin pathways because it does not require specific recognition of a microbial surface by antibodies or lectins. It relies on the nonspecific, low-level hydrolysis of C3 (remember, C3 is the most abundant complement protein and a key player in all pathways). In plasma, C3 is inherently slightly unstable, with a small portion of it spontaneously degrading into its C3a and C3b components. As you recall, this cleavage reveals the reactive thiolester group on C3b, which allows it to covalently bind to surfaces in the immediate vicinity. If C3b binds to a healthy host cell membrane, it is rapidly degraded to prevent any further complement activation. This degradation occurs because host membranes are rich in sialic acid residues that promote binding of C3b to factor H (a negative regulator of complement activation; Figure 4.6A). Factor H, along with factor I, inactivates and degrades inappropriately bound C3b. Hence, on those surfaces on which complement activation is not wanted, spontaneously bound C3b is destroyed as fast as it is deposited. However, microbial membranes and cell walls are typically rich in polysaccharides that do not

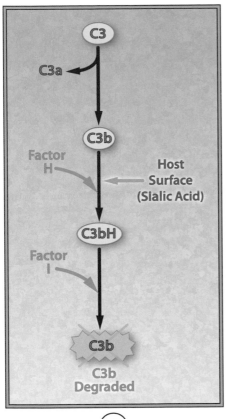

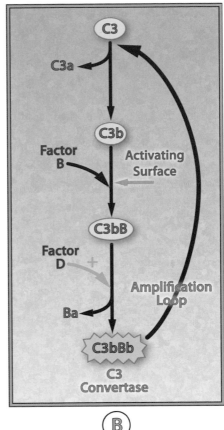

Alternative Pathway

FIGURE 4.6A–B. The alternative pathway of complement activation

Panel A: In the presence of sialic acid residues, which are abundant on the surface of host cells, bound C3b preferentially binds factor H and is degraded by factor I. Panel B: On activating surfaces, bound C3b can bind factor B, which can be cleaved by factor D, resulting in the activation of the alternative C3 convertase C3bBb. C3bBb can now catalyze C3 proteolysis into C3a and C3b, eventually leading to more C3bBb, thus creating an amplification loop.

contain sialic acid. Should C3b happen to covalently bind to one of these so-called activating surfaces, C3b does not bind the regulatory factor H and instead adopts a conformation that allows it to preferentially bind factor B, forming the complex C3bB (Figure 4.6B).

Another serum factor, factor D, cleaves the factor B component of the C3bB complex, releasing Ba and creating the active proteolytic complex C3bBb. C3bBb is the alternative C3 convertase. Now, instead of relying on the low level of spontaneous hydrolysis of C3, this C3 convertase efficiently catalyzes the cleavage of plasma C3, resulting in the rapid deposition of C3b onto the activating surface. A portion of this bound C3b will recruit factor B and, with the help of factor D, will create more of the alternative C3 convertase C3bBb. As you can

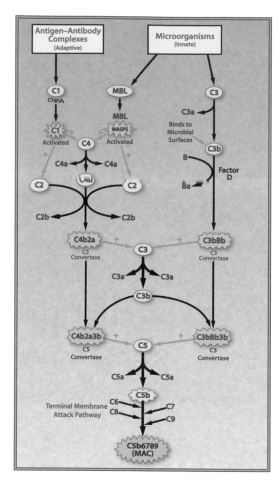

FIGURE 4.7. **The classical, lectin, and alternative pathways of complement activation**

pathways (C4b2a3b), the alternative C5 convertase (C3bBb3b) cleaves C5, which initiates the terminal membrane attack pathway.

Terminal Membrane Attack Pathway

All complement activation pathways can initiate the common terminal membrane attack pathway (Figure 4.7). The goal of this particular pathway is to construct a protein complex that essentially punches a hole in the target membrane and thus can directly lyse and kill the microbe (Figure 4.8). This protein complex is aptly named the membrane attack complex (MAC). The terminal membrane attack pathway is initiated by the activating pathways' C5 convertase (C4b2a3b, generated by the classical and lectin pathways, and C3bBb3b, generated by the alternative pathway). These C5 convertases cleave C5 into C5a and C5b. C5b recruits C6 and C7 to the target membrane, forming the complex C5b67. This complex can bind and partially unfold C8, exposing a hydrophobic region of the protein that allows it to wedge itself deep in the target membrane. With C8 now inserted into the membrane, the complex can recruit and insert ten to sixteen copies of C9 into the membrane to create a cylindrical pore (using C9 much like the wooden staves that make up a barrel). The completed MAC breaches the cell membrane of the microbe, allowing water to rush into the cell. If sufficient numbers of MAC form on the membrane, the microbe is destroyed by osmotic lysis.

REGULATION OF COMPLEMENT ACTIVATION

One downside of an amplifying biochemical cascade is that it can easily get out of hand. Thus, it is not surprising that the system of complement activation is highly regulated by an equally complex system of complement control proteins (see Table 4.1) that not only increases the complement system's selectivity for non-self but also limits activated comple-

see, this process initiates an amplification loop leading to the accelerated deposition of C3b on the activating surface. (As a side note, because C3b deposition is common to all pathways, the alternative C3 convertase C3bBb and the amplification loop that results are also inherent in the classical and lectin pathways.) The C3 convertase C3bBb is itself relatively unstable but can complex with a plasma protein called factor P (also known as properdin), which helps stabilize the complex. The alternative C5 convertase is created when an additional C3b molecule complexes with the C3 convertase C3bBb to form C3bBb3b (Figure 4.7). As with the C5 convertase formed in the classical and lectin

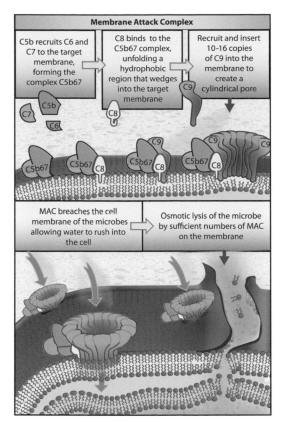

Membrane Attack Complex

C5b recruits C6 and C7 to the target membrane, forming the complex C5b67	C8 binds to the C5b67 complex, unfolding a hydrophobic region that wedges into the target membrane	Recruit and insert 10-16 copies of C9 into the membrane to create a cylindrical pore

MAC breaches the cell membrane of the microbes allowing water to rush into the cell	Osmotic lysis of the microbe by sufficient numbers of MAC on the membrane

FIGURE 4.8. Assembly of the MAC by the terminal membrane attack pathway

The final MAC consists mostly of ten to sixteen molecules of C9 arranged into a barrel-shaped pore within the target membrane. The diameter of the inner pore is around ten nanometers and allows fluid to rush into the target cell.

ment cascades from continuing indefinitely. The classical, lectin, alternative, and terminal membrane attack pathways can all be stopped or downregulated at key points by soluble or membrane-associated complement control proteins. Many of these control proteins function by inhibiting the protease activities or facilitating the degradation of activated complement complexes or convertases.

An example of an inhibiting protein is the acute phase protein C1 inhibitor. As the name suggests, the C1 inhibitor inhibits the protease function of C1 (specifically C1r and C1s), which prevents excessive or inappropriate cleavage of

C4 and C2. C1 inhibitor can also inhibit MASPs that have been activated by MBL; hence, it plays a role in the regulation of the early stages of both the classical and lectin pathways.

Other complement control proteins found in plasma include factor H and C4b-binding protein. As mentioned earlier, factor H enhances the degradation of C3b bound to membranes rich in sialic acid and can thus (along with factor I) directly influence the formation and stability of the alternative C3 convertase (C3bBb). The C4b-binding protein, as its name suggests, preferentially binds C4b. Binding results in the accelerated degradation of the C3 convertase C4b2a; hence, it is a regulator of the classical and lectin activation pathways.

In addition to plasma proteins, many complement control proteins are displayed on the surfaces of host cells. Decay-accelerating factor (CD55) is displayed on the surfaces of erythrocytes, circulating leukocytes, platelets, and endothelia, where, as its name suggests, it acts to accelerate the decay of the alternative C3 convertase (C3bBb), thus providing an extra level of security against inappropriate activation of the alternative pathway on host cells that are continually exposed to plasma. Similarly, complement receptor 1 (CR1 or CD35) and membrane cofactor protein (CD46) are membrane proteins that can inhibit either the alternative or the classical and lectin C3 convertase by interacting with C4b or C3b. Several other complement control proteins found on the cell membranes of host cells also specifically act to prevent formation of the MAC. One of these control proteins, protectin (CD59), acts to prevent MAC formation on host cells by binding the C5b678 complex and preventing the binding and oligomerization of C9. Several other host membrane glycoproteins act in a similar fashion.

Together, the complement control proteins act to prevent the complement innate defense system from acting on inappropriate targets and also from acting in perpetuity. The inability of the control proteins to halt complement

TABLE 4.1. A summary of known complement control proteins and their function

Complement control protein	Location	Pathway regulated	Action
C1 inhibitor	Plasma, serum	Classical and lectin	Inactivates C1r, C1s, and MASPs
C4b-binding protein	Plasma, serum	Classical and lectin	Binds C4b; accelerates decay of the classical and lectin C3 convertase (C4b2a)
Factor H	Plasma, serum	Alternative	Binds C3b and accelerates decay
Decay-accelerating factor (CD55)	Cell membrane of erythrocytes, neutrophils, lymphocytes, monocytes, platelets, and endothelial cells	Alternative	Accelerates decay of C3 convertase (C3bBb)
Complement receptor I (CD35)	Cell membrane of erythrocytes (primates), neutrophils, lymphocytes, monocytes, and macrophages	Classical, lectin, and alternative	Binds C3b and C4a and inhibits alternative and classical/lectin C3 convertases
Membrane cofactor protein (CD46)	Widely expressed on cell membrane of host cells	Classical, lectin, and alternative	Binds C3b and C4a and inhibits alternative and classical/lectin C3 convertases
Protectin (CD59)	Predominantly expressed on cell membrane of erythrocytes, leukocytes, and vascular endothelium	Terminal membrane attack	Binds to C5b678 and prevents C9 recruitment and MAC formation

cascades can have devastating consequences. An interesting fact is that venom from the cobra snake contains a C3b analogue (called cobra venom factor) that can complex with factor Bb and factor P to form a stable C3 convertase (cobra venom factor Bb). This convertase is not recognized by the regulatory proteins factor H and I, and thus it will continually hydrolyse C3 (and C5), leading to complement depletion and severe local tissue damage.

OUTCOMES OF COMPLEMENT ACTIVATION

Aside from the direct complement-mediated lysis of cells by formation of a MAC, numerous products of complement activation act to enhance immune defense within an animal (see Table 4.2). These products include those promoting inflammation, chemotaxis of leukocytes, phagocytic uptake of targets, humoral immune responses, and the clearance of immune complexes.

Inflammation and Chemotaxis

As you recall, two major points of all complement activation pathways are the assembly of C3 and C5 convertases. These convertases mediate the cleavages of C3 and C5, respectively, resulting in the attachment of the large fragments C3b and C5b to microbial surfaces. It is easy to discount the two smaller fragments C3a and C5a as useless by-products, but they actually play important roles in their own right. Because both C3a and C5a are small (around 10 kDa), they readily diffuse away from the site of complement activation. Numerous leukocytes detect local complement activation through the recognition of C3a and C5a by surface complement receptors, which alerts these cells to a potential threat in the vicinity. Mast cells react to both C3a and C5a by degranulating, thus dumping loads of vasoactive amines into the extracellular space, which in turn leads to dilation and increased permeability of the local vasculature (both hallmarks of acute inflammation, covered in chapter 5).

TABLE 4.2. A summary of outcomes of complement activation

Outcome	Complement products	Action
Direct target lysis	MAC	Osmodysregulation and lysis of target cells
Tissue inflammation	C3a and C5a	Activation of mast-cell degranulation leading to release of vasoactive amines (histamine and serotonin)
Endothelial activation	C3a and C5a	Increased expression of adhesion molecules
Chemotaxis	C3a and C5a	Promotes migration of neutrophils, eosinophils, and macrophages toward site of complement activation
Leukocyte activation	C5a (C3a and C4a)	Upregulation of adhesion molecules, phagocytic receptors, and antimicrobial effectors by neutrophils and monocytes
Opsonization	C3b and iC3b	Enhancement of particle phagocytosis by macrophages and neutrophils
Promotion of humoral responses	C3dg	Enhanced B-cell activation, retention of antigen complexes in B-cell follicles
Immune complex clearance	C3b (and iC3b)	Blocking of growth and facilitation of dissociation of immune complexes; immobilization and clearance of immune complexes through interaction with CR1 on erythrocytes

With a small localized response, complement-mediated vascular dilation and permeability act to enhance the delivery of leukocytes and immune proteins to the site of complement activation. C3a and C5a can also help recruit circulating leukocytes by prompting endothelial cells lining the local vasculature to express adhesion molecules. But when generated in large amounts systemically, C3a and C5a can cause systemic anaphylactic shock. For this reason, C3a and C5a are sometimes referred to as anaphylotoxins.

In addition, C3a and C5a in particular stimulate the chemotaxis (movement) of many leukocytes, including neutrophils, eosinophils, and macrophages. Diffusion of C3a and C5a away from the site of complement activation establishes a chemotactic gradient, up which leukocytes can migrate toward the potential threat. These complement products also activate leukocytes such as neutrophils, allowing these cells to upregulate their receptors, adhesion molecules, and the antimicrobial arsenal needed to find and combat microbes and other threats in the tissue.

Enhancement of Phagocytosis (Opsonization)

A major outcome of complement activation is the covalent attachment of C3b to target surfaces, which essentially tags these surfaces as foreign, hazardous, or simply abnormal. Particles with C3b and its breakdown product iC3b on their surfaces are recognized by macrophages and neutrophils through complement receptors (specifically CR1, CR3, and CR4), which mediate phagocytosis of the particles. Although microbes can be recognized by macrophages and neutrophils without complement (e.g., via the MR), the presence of C3b and iC3b on their surfaces dramatically enhances their phagocytosis. This binding of C3b and iC3b to microbial surfaces is termed *opsonization* (covered in greater detail in chapter 6).

Promoting Humoral Immunity

Another breakdown product of bound C3b is C3dg, which can be recognized by the CR2 expressed on both B cells and follicular dendritic cells (FDCs). When a B cell recognizes a specific antigen through its B-cell receptor, it is stimulated to activate and proliferate (covered in chapter 12). Recognition of C3dg by CR2, in association with the specific antigen, significantly enhances B-cell activation, which in turn enhances the generation of antibodies directed against that antigen. The presence of C3dg in antigen complexes is also thought to help retain the antigen within the B-cell follicles of lymph nodes through interaction with CR2 on FDCs. This retention promotes prolonged antigen–B cell interaction, which further acts to enhance the humoral response to the complement-associated antigen—yet another example of an innate immune system outcome that enhances an adaptive immune response.

Clearance of Immune Complexes

Immune complexes consisting of matrices of antibodies and antigen can be generated during an immune reaction to an abundant antigen. These complexes, if not cleared, can be deposited in particular sites in the body of an animal (particularly in vessel walls, kidneys, joints, and eyes), resulting in a type III hypersensitivity (covered in chapter 16). Attachment of C3b to these complexes (through classical complement cascade) interrupts the antigen–antibody interactions, preventing complex growth and facilitating their dissociation. Integration of C3b into the complexes also allows them to be bound to the surface of erythrocytes through interaction with CR1. Once bound to erythrocytes, the immune complexes are not inappropriately deposited and can be safely removed by phagocytosis of the erythrocytes in the liver and spleen.

CLINICAL CORRELATION: FOLLOW-UP

Student Considerations

After reading this chapter, you should be able to list the outcomes of complement activation and reason why a deficiency in C3 would interfere with an animal's ability to control bacterial

infections. You should also be able to derive a possible explanation for the development of kidney disease in these Brittany dogs (Figure 4.9).

Possible Explanations

C3 is the most abundant complement protein. It is central to the classical, lectin, and alternative complement pathways and is also a prerequisite for the initiation of the common terminal membrane attack pathway. So, essentially, a deficiency in the C3 component renders the whole complement system defunct, which would result in deficiencies in direct bacterial killing by MAC, reduced bacterial phagocytosis, compromised acute inflammatory reactions, diminished activation and chemotaxis of leukocytes, and perhaps even reductions in humoral immune responses. All of these would directly compromise the dog's efficiency in mounting effective immune responses to invading bacteria, and thus it is easy to understand why an animal that is deficient in C3 would succumb to bacterial infection.

The renal disease that these Brittany dogs develop later in life is harder to explain. It is interesting to note that human patients with C3 deficiency develop a similar glomerulonephritis. The membrano-proliferative glomerulonephritis that both dogs and humans with C3 deficiency develop is thought to be the manifestation of an autoimmune-type disease. As you will discover in chapter 16, glomerulonephritis (literally, inflammation of the glomerulus) is one of the more common manifestations of a type III hypersensitivity, caused by antigen–antibody complexes that circulate through the blood and lodge in the maze of capillaries that form the glomerulus. Once in the glomeruli, these antigen–antibody complexes trigger inflammatory responses that damage the glomeruli. As you learned in this chapter, deposition of C3b on circulating immune complexes aids in their dissociation, immobilization, and removal (via binding to erythrocytes and phagocytic clearance in the liver and spleen). Without C3, im-

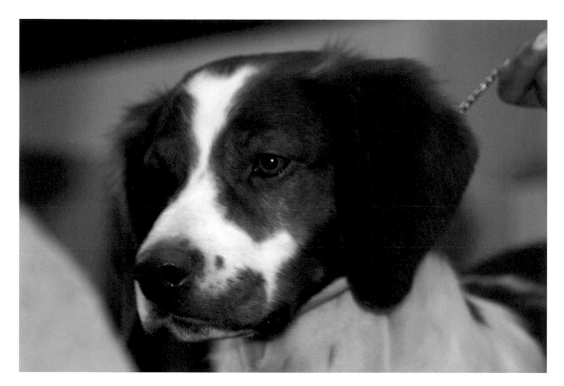

FIGURE 4.9. **A Brittany dog. Photograph by Lori Branham.**

mune complexes that develop during the multitude of adaptive responses in the lives of C3-deficient Brittany dogs lodge in glomeruli and incite inflammation. Over a period of years, the inflammation in the glomeruli results in their progressive dysfunction and the development of a membrano-proliferative glomerulonephritis and, eventually, renal failure. Thankfully, and presumably because of the immense selection pressure over eons of evolution, complete C3 deficiency in any animal species is considered to be extremely rare.

Robin M. Yates

Acute Inflammation

Chapter 5

10.5876_9781607322184.c005

CLINICAL CORRELATION: ACUTE BOVINE MASTITIS

Everyone has had experience with acute inflammation. It is characterized by hallmark features and usually indicates that an infection is present or that the tissue has had some physical or chemical damage. Dairy farmers deal with inflammation on a twice-daily basis in the form of mastitis in their milking herds (Figure 5.1).

Mastitis is inflammation of the mammary gland, which is almost always initiated by the infection of these high-performing glands by contagious or environmental bacteria. Economically, mastitis is one of the most important disease syndromes affecting the dairy industry. Clinical and subclinical mastitis results in lower milk production and poor milk quality and adversely affects the welfare of these animals.

Acute mastitis is the sudden dysfunction of the mammary gland, accompanied by swelling, heat, and obvious pain and discomfort for the cow. The milk expressed from the affected quarter often contains clots and debris and is unfit for consumption. A hallmark diagnostic feature of acute mastitis is the presence of leukocytes in the milk. Leukocytes, and indeed other somatic cells, can be detected using a cowside test called the California Mastitis Test (CMT). This test uses the agglutination of DNA, which forms a gel in the milk, as an indicator of the presence of leukocytes (see Figure 5.2). Nowadays, the CMT is gradually being replaced by automated cell counting. Sudden onset of clinical signs and a positive CMT or high leukocyte counts in the milk from a quarter are indicative of acute mastitis. They are handy diagnostic indicators, but what are the leukocytes doing there? How did they get there, and how did they know where to go?

LEARNING OBJECTIVES

After reading this chapter, you should be able to

- understand purposes of inflammation and its roles in immunity;
- describe the cardinal signs of acute inflammation and explain the basic underlying pathophysiological processes;
- list basic groups of mediators in acute inflammation and their origins and targets;
- describe the blood vessel changes that occur during acute inflammation;

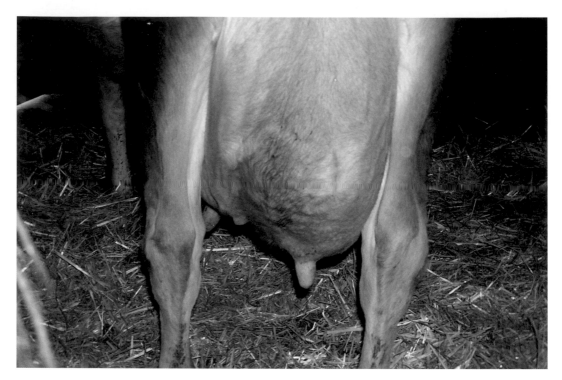

FIGURE 5.1. Acute bovine mastitis (photograph courtesy of Dr. Gordon Atkins, University of Calgary)

This photograph is of a four-year-old, mid–second-lactation Jersey cow with severe mastitis of the right hindquarter caused by *Staphylococcus aureus*.

- describe the steps of extravasation and chemotaxis of leukocytes in the acute inflammatory process;
- appreciate the diversity of inflammatory processes and timelines of leukocyte recruitment;
- describe the systemic clinical findings that may be associated with an acute inflammatory process;
- describe the systemic laboratory findings that may be associated with an acute inflammatory process.

PURPOSES OF ACUTE INFLAMMATION

The acute inflammation of a tissue is commonly viewed as an undesirable symptom of an injury or disease process. If this process serves only to provide discomfort and disfig-

urement, why is it inherent—in some form or another—to all species in the animal kingdom? As we discussed in chapter 3, sentinel cells such as tissue macrophages and DCs are dispersed throughout every tissue in the body. Although macrophages, by themselves, can phagocytose and destroy bacteria as well as clear cellular debris, in the face of major tissue damage or the introduction of a large microbial insult, they can be quickly overwhelmed. In these cases, macrophages need to enlist the aid of large numbers of other leukocytes. One of the most well equipped of these leukocytes is the neutrophil, but monocytes, eosinophils, and even certain lymphocytes can also be recruited to the affected tissue.

Neutrophils are armed with numerous powerful antimicrobial effector mechanisms to defend against major threats. But as you learned in chapter 2, neutrophils spend most of their

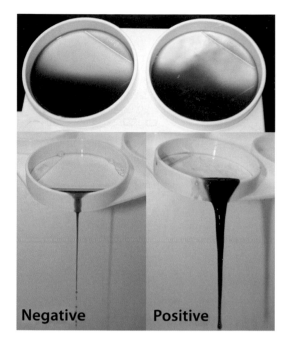

Negative   **Positive**

FIGURE 5.2. **California Mastitis Test (CMT)**

The CMT pictured was performed on milk expressed from a normal quarter of an udder (left) and a quarter of the same udder with severe acute mastitis (right). CMT reagent was added to both milk samples and mixed in a CMT paddle. The gelatinous material formed in the positive sample is leukocyte DNA, which can be assessed when the mixture is swirled (top) or poured out of the paddle (bottom).

lives inside the circulatory system. To be effective in infected or damaged tissues, neutrophils need to rapidly and accurately find infected and affected tissues, extravasate (get out of the circulatory system), and travel to the specific site of insult. In addition to cells, soluble components of the immune system (once again, mostly found in blood), such as complement proteins, acute phase proteins, and antibodies, need to gain access to affected tissue. Delivery of cellular and soluble immune components to the site of injury significantly enhances the local immune defenses, which act to eliminate microbes, trigger the adaptive immune system, and initiate tissue repair. The culmination of the influx of leukocytes and plasma proteins to the site of insult and the changes to the vasculature needed to facilitate the movement of these immune entities result in the cardinal signs associated with inflammation (Figure 5.3).

SIGNS OF ACUTE INFLAMMATION

The first known description of the signs associated with acute inflammation was found in an Egyptian papyrus dating back to 3000 BC. However, it was during the period of the Roman Empire when the encyclopedist Celsus documented the cardinal signs of inflammation in the Latin terminology that is still in use today:

1. *rubor* (redness);
2. *tumor* (swelling);
3. *calor* (heat);
4. *dolor* (pain);
5. *functio laesa* (loss of function; added to Celsus's list by the German pathologist Virchow in the late 1800s).

Many of these signs are consequences of the local vascular changes initiated by inflammation. Both rubor and calor arise from local vasodilation and increased blood flow to the affected area. It is important to point out that calor is due primarily to increased conduction of core body temperature to the periphery by increased blood flow to the area of inflammation (as a result of vasodilation) rather than local metabolic changes or pyrexia (fever). Tumor is primarily a result of increased permeability or leakiness of the local vasculature, leading to tissue edema. Dolor is attributed to the release of inflammatory mediators such as prostaglandins, neuropeptides, and cytokines by damaged tissue and activated immune cells. These mediators can act on pain receptors, resulting in hyperalgesia, although the physical and chemical trauma associated with tissue edema and antimicrobial functions of immune cells undoubtedly contribute. Functio laesa re-

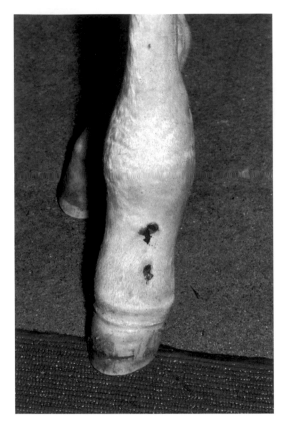

FIGURE 5.3. Inflammation of the fetlock of a foal (photograph courtesy of Dr. Michel Levy, University of Calgary)

This foal has a suppurative arthritis. There is diffuse, moderate swelling (tumor) of the fetlock and reddening of the skin (rubor). If you were to palpate it, it would feel warmer to the touch (calor) and would likely elicit a pain response (dolor). Clinically, the foal would present with an abnormal gait caused by loss of full function of the limb (functio laesa). Also note that distal to the fetlock are two puncture wounds oozing blood and suppurative material (pus).

sults from a culmination of tumor, dolor, and tissue damage, leading to general dysfunction and the instinctive behavior of the animal to protect the inflamed region.

Apart from dolor, which may provide a protective function for the inflamed area, the other cardinal signs have no obvious benefits and can be debilitating. So when is it appropriate for an inflammatory process to be initiated, and how is it triggered?

INITIATORS AND MEDIATORS OF ACUTE INFLAMMATION

The most common initiator of acute inflammation is the sentinel cell detection of microbial or parasitic products within host tissues. Recall from chapter 3 that the innate immune system is equipped with numerous PRRs that can recognize the conserved molecular motifs associated with microbes—the so-called PAMPs. Sentinel cells, such as macrophages, constitutively express PRRs that enable them to continually monitor the local tissue microenvironment for signs of microbial invasion. The detection of microbial products via PRRs leads to signaling cascades within the macrophages, which results in their activation. Once activated, the macrophages synthesize and release a slew of proinflammatory cytokines (such as IL-1β, IL-6, and TNF-α) that act as signals to other inflammatory cells and blood vessels in the area. Activated macrophages can also release chemokines such as CXCL8 (also known as IL-8). As you have learned, chemokines are chemotactic cytokines consisting of small proteins that can diffuse away from the secreting cell to set up a concentration gradient. Using this gradient, leukocytes, such as neutrophils, can move toward the particular site of insult by chemokine-directed chemotaxis.

Although microbial infections are the most commonly considered triggers of inflammation, many other tissue insults can initiate so-called sterile inflammation. These insults include trauma, physical and chemical injury, foreign bodies, or inappropriate products of adaptive immunity. Many of these insults result in the release of DAMPs, which, although endogenously derived, can also lead to the activation of macrophages.

Activation of macrophages with PAMPs, along with activation by DAMPs, indicates infection and tissue injury. Together, they combine to become a powerful stimulus to activate assembly of the inflammasome within macrophages, which dramatically enhances the release of IL-1β and IL-18, both potent proinflammatory cytokines. The macrophage-derived proinflammatory cytokines (IL-1β, IL-6, and TNF-α) can act directly on endothelial cells in local vasculature and can additionally act on neighboring immune cells, often prompting them to also release proinflammatory mediators.

One cell in particular that can rapidly amplify proinflammatory signals in response to the cytokines produced by macrophages is the mast cell. As mentioned in chapter 2, mast cells are typically situated near blood vessels and nerves, and contain numerous cytoplasmic granules rich in histamine and serotonin, both vasoactive compounds. Mast cells and histamine are commonly associated with type I hypersensitivities (allergies) in response to an inappropriate humoral response to allergens and are discussed in depth in chapter 16. Aside from unwanted degranulation in allergies, however, mast-cell degranulation in response to proinflammatory cytokines such as IL-1 acts to rapidly facilitate the changes to local vasculature needed for inflammation. In addition to macrophage products, mast cells can be directly induced to degranulate by surface-bound IgE (a specific antibody isotype associated with allergies) after the detection of specific antigens. Furthermore, products of complement activation (C3a and C5a), physical or chemical trauma, and even extreme temperatures can induce mast-cell degranulation.

Another group of important mediators of acute inflammation is the eicosanoids—in particular, leukotrienes and prostaglandins. Unlike cytokines, which are proteins, the eicosanoids are oxidized derivatives of fatty acids. These compounds typically have a short half-life and thus act in an autocrine or paracrine capacity in an inflamed tissue. Within minutes of detecting an inflammatory stimulus (e.g., cytokines or trauma), both macrophages and mast cells synthesize leukotrienes and prostaglandins from the normal cellular diacylglycerols or phospholipids found in cellular or nuclear membranes. The first step is the liberation of a polyunsaturated 20-carbon fatty acid (called arachidonic acid) from diacylglycerols or phospholipids (Figure 5.4), which is mediated by phospholipases (phospholipase C or phospholipase A_2, respectively). Although leukotrienes and prostaglandins derive from this common precursor and have overlapping functions, it is important to differentiate between the two classes of molecules because of their distinct contributions to clinically important situations.

The enzyme lipoxygenase uses the freed arachidonic acid to synthesize leukotrienes. There are several immunologically important leukotrienes, including leukotriene B_4 and leukotriene D_4. These leukotrienes act locally as powerful chemoattractants for neutrophils (B_4) and effect changes in the vascular endothelium (B_4 and D_4).

Prostaglandins are synthesized from the arachidonic acid pool by cyclooxygenase (COX) enzymes. The two major COX isoforms, COX-1 and COX-2, are expressed at different levels in different tissues. Although COX-1 is needed to synthesize prostaglandins with homeostatic roles, COX-2 is responsible primarily for prostaglandin synthesis in inflammation. These enzymes become critically important in the pharmacological management of inflammation because they are the target of the nonsteroidal anti-inflammatory drugs (NSAIDs) commonly used in veterinary medicine (e.g., meloxicam [Metacam®]; phenylbutazone, or "bute"; and carprofen [Rimadyl®]). The major prostaglandin involved in inflammation is prostaglandin E_2. Prostaglandin E_2 is synthesized by both macrophages and mast cells and acts on local vasculature and endothelium.

Collectively, in response to local noxious or microbial stimuli, macrophages, in concert with other immune cells such as mast cells, can rapidly release proinflammatory cytokines and other mediators such as histamine. These

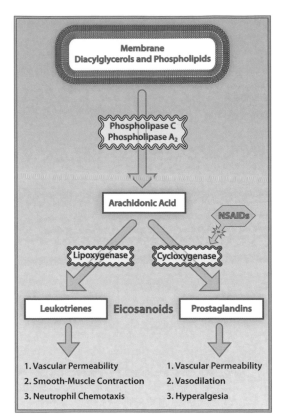

FIGURE 5.4. Eicosanoid synthesis

Leukotrienes, and prostaglandins are synthesized from arachidonic acid released from membrane lipids. Pools of arachidonic acid can be acted on by lipoxygenase or cycloxygenase enzymes to produce a variety of leukotrienes and prostaglandins, respectively. Cycloxygenases can be inhibited by NSAIDs, which decrease prostaglandin synthesis and prostaglandin-induced inflammatory sequelae.

mediators can act on local vasculature to initiate the vascular changes needed for the infiltration of cellular and plasma-derived immune mediators (see Table 5.1).

VASCULAR CHANGES IN ACUTE INFLAMMATION

Three main changes to local blood vessels occur in response to inflammatory mediators:

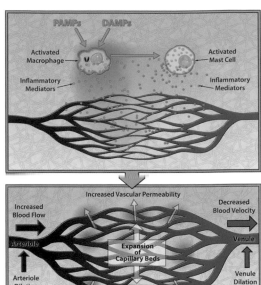

FIGURE 5.5. Vascular changes in acute inflammation

This figure shows the major changes to vasculature in response to inflammatory signals detected within a tissue. In brief, indicators of infection or trauma can be detected by sentinel cells, such as macrophages, resulting in the release of inflammatory mediators, which is often amplified by neighboring mast cells. These inflammatory mediators act on local vasculature to effect vasodilation, expansion of capillary beds, increased vascular permeability, and decreased blood velocity in the postcapillary venules.

1. vasodilation and local stasis of blood flow;

2. increased vascular permeability;

3. expression of cell-adhesion molecules on vascular endothelium.

Vasodilation occurs through the action of inflammatory mediators on the arteriole and the postcapillary venule smooth muscle. Decreasing the tone of the periarteriolar musculature acts to widen the lumen of the vessels, which in turn opens new capillary beds in the affected tissue (Figure 5.5). As mentioned earlier, these expanded capillary beds contribute

TABLE 5.1. A summary of the major mediators of inflammation

Inflammatory mediator	Primary source	Inflammatory action
CYTOKINES AND CHEMOKINES		
IL-1β, IL-6, and TNF-α	Macrophages	Leukocyte and endothelial activation; systemic reactions
CXCL8 (IL-8)	Leukocytes	Leukocyte activation and chemotaxis
PLASMA PROTEINS		
C3a	Complement activation	Mast-cell degranulation; smooth-muscle contraction
C5a	Complement activation	Leukocyte chemotaxis; mast-cell degranulation; smooth-muscle contraction; vascular permeability
Bradykinin	Kinin–kallikrein system	Vasodilation; vascular permeability; pain
VASOACTIVE AMINES		
Histamine	Mast-cell degranulation	Vascular permeability; smooth-muscle contraction
Serotonin (5-hydroxytryptamine)	Mast-cell degranulation	Vascular permeability; smooth-muscle contraction
EICOSANOIDS		
Leukotriene B4	Leukocytes	Leukocyte activation and chemotaxis; vascular permeability
Leukotrienes B4, D4, and E4	Leukocytes (particularly mast cells)	Smooth-muscle contraction; vascular permeability
Prostaglandin E2	Leukocytes (particularly mast cells)	Vasodilation; vascular permeability; pain

to both rubor and calor by increasing the volume of blood in the area. By widening the venules, vasodilation also acts to slow the velocity of the blood in these postcapillary vessels, akin to water current in a river—the wider and deeper the river is, the slower and less turbulent the water flow. Coupled with the "leakiness" of endothelium, vasodilation contributes to the local stasis of blood flow. Slower velocity or stasis of blood flow is important to decrease the shear force on the leukocytes during the process of extravasation, which we discuss in depth later.

Increased vascular permeability or leakiness is another important vascular change associated with inflammation. It permits the movement of fluid and plasma proteins—including complement, antibodies, and acute phase proteins (discussed later in this chapter)—into the affected interstitial tissue. The protein-rich fluid that escapes from vasculature is known as exudate. As mentioned earlier, vascular permeabil-

ity also contributes to the local stasis of blood flow; akin to the flow of water in a pipe with numerous holes in it, the more water that leaks out, the slower the flow of water in the pipe.

In healthy tissue, endothelial cells lining the microvasculature typically prevent the movement of protein-rich fluid out of the blood vessels. They do this by creating a continuous barrier on the inside of vessels through intercellular tight junctions, which is critical for the maintenance of fluid homeostasis. However, within minutes of the detection of infectious or noxious stimuli by sentinel cells, inflammatory mediators can act on endothelial cells (typically in postcapillary venules) and trigger conformational changes in these cells, leading to the breakdown of the endothelial barrier (Figure 5.6A–D). Mediators such as histamine and IL-1 stimulate endothelial cells to contract or rearrange their cytoskeletons, which decreases their surface areas, creating gaps between endothelial cells and allowing protein-rich fluid

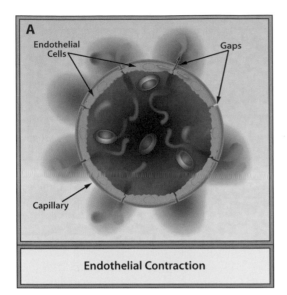

Endothelial Contraction

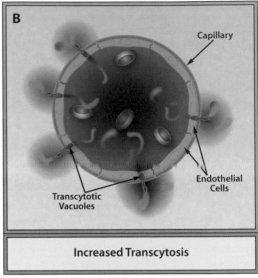

Increased Transcytosis

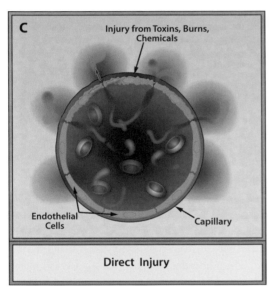

Direct Injury

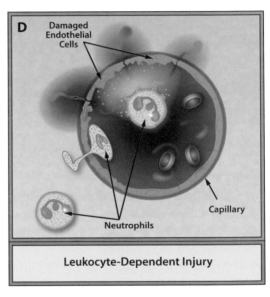

Leukocyte-Dependent Injury

FIGURE 5.6A–D. Mechanisms that increase vascular permeability during inflammation

Four mechanisms are thought to contribute to the increase in vascular permeability during inflammation: endothelial contraction (panel A), active transcytosis (panel B), direct physical or chemical injury to the vasculature (panel C), and injury to the vasculature after leukocyte extravasation or activation (panel D).

(exudate) to leak out of these vessels and into the surrounding tissue.

Another mechanism by which increased vascular permeability is thought to be induced in inflammation is through the upregulation of transcytosis in venule endothelial cells. Trans-cytosis is the active transport of fluid and macromolecules across the cytoplasm through a series of separate or interconnected cytoplasmic vesicles. These vesicles effectively form tunnels or channels through the cells, allowing protein-rich fluid to pass directly through the activated endothelial barrier. Finally, aside from purposeful changes to endothelial cells in postcapillary venules induced by inflammatory mediators, inadvertent injury to vasculature can also contribute to vascular permeability after injury or inflammation. Injury can include direct physical or chemical injury to vascular beds by the inciting insult (e.g., a heat or chemical burn) or collateral damage associated with leukocyte extravasation and the subsequent antimicrobial effector function.

In addition to promoting vascular permeability, the activation of vascular endothelium by cytokines (such as IL-1 and TNF-α) induces the expression of cell-adhesion molecules. These cell-adhesion molecules are displayed in high numbers on the lumenal membranes of the endothelial cells that line postcapillary venules, where they act to snag circulating leukocytes. This process serves to slow and tether useful leukocytes and also to signal to them that a threat is in the vicinity and that they should extravasate.

Overall, the changes to vasculature in the vicinity of a detected proinflammatory threat act to deliver more blood to the vasculature beds in the area (vasodilation); slow the velocity of the blood flow (vasodilation and vascular permeability); allow protein-rich fluid into the tissue (vascular permeability); and select, tether, and concentrate circulating leukocytes (cell-adhesion molecule expression). Vascular changes are important steps in the early process of inflammation and account for many of the cardinal signs (rubor, calor, and tumor), but they are just the beginning of the inflammatory process.

LEUKOCYTE RECRUITMENT

Leukocyte Extravasation

As mentioned earlier, one of the major purposes of inflammation is to recruit additional leukocytes to the site of a detected threat. In acute inflammation, neutrophils—well equipped with an antimicrobial arsenal—are usually the first to respond. Unlike macrophages, however, before inflammation, neutrophils appear almost exclusively in the blood. To be useful, neutrophils need to find the general area of inflamed tissue, exit the circulation, and migrate within the tissue to the specific locale of insult. They achieve this in four stages of extravasation (Figure 5.7):

1. tethering (margination) and rolling;
2. firm adhesion (pavementing) and crawling;
3. transmigration (diapedesis);
4. chemotaxis through tissue.

Even though vascular changes help to slow the blood flow in an inflamed region, normal neutrophil velocity in the circulation, coupled with the shear forces on stationary objects within blood vessels, makes the task of extravasation difficult. Tethering and rolling of neutrophils on activated endothelium are necessary to marginalize and slow down the otherwise fast-moving cells. As mentioned earlier, IL-1 and TNF-α activate vascular endothelial cells in venules to express and display cell-adhesion molecules. An important family of cell-adhesion molecules is the selectins, named because they function as selective lectins (recall that lectins are carbohydrate-binding proteins). Selectins are expressed on activated endothelium, where they function to marginalize and slow down circulating leukocytes. E-selectin binds to sialylated Lewis X–modified glycoproteins that are displayed on the surface of circulating neutrophils and eosinophils. P-selectin, which is also is displayed on activated endothelium, binds platelet selectin glycoprotein ligand 1, which is a glycoprotein found on all circulating leukocytes. The interactions between the selectins on activated endothelia and their glycoprotein ligands on leukocytes are relatively low affinity. Through numerous low-affinity selectin and ligand interactions, however, leukocytes can loosely adhere to activated endothelium, causing them to be marginalized within the vasculature and roll along

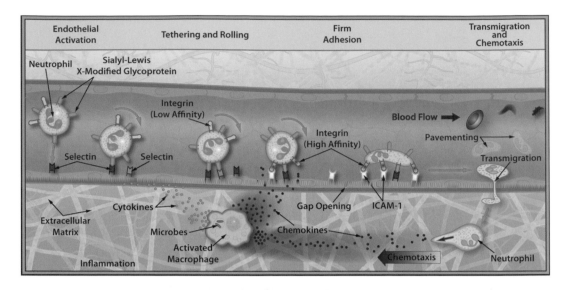

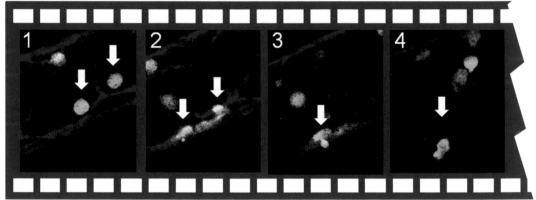

FIGURE 5.7. **Leukocyte extravasation (video courtesy of Dr. Paul Kubes, University of Calgary)**

Diagram (top) and video micrograph (bottom) showing the four stages of leukocyte extravasation. The bottom panel is a sequential montage taken from a video micrograph of neutrophils extravasating from a postcapillary venule in the cremaster muscle of a mouse after experimental induction of local acute inflammation. Endothelial cells and their tight junctions are highlighted in red. Neutrophils are green. From left to right, arrows indicate neutrophils undergoing (1) tethering and rolling, (2) firm adhesion, (3) transmigration, and (4) chemotaxis. The video was taken using a mulitphoton confocal microscope.

the endothelial surface. Through this process involving multiple weak interactions with passing leukocytes, the endothelium slows but does not stop the cells in the high-shear environment of the blood vessel.

Being tethered and rolled gives the leukocyte time to detect local proinflammatory chemokines at the endothelial surface. The detection of chemokines, such as CXCL8, further slows the neutrophils and induces conformational changes in a second group of neutrophil proteins called integrins. These structural changes switch the integrins from low- to high-affinity receptors. Lymphocyte function–associated antigen 1 (LFA-1) is one such integrin found on the surface of lymphocytes, monocytes, and neutrophils. LFA-1 binds to intercellular adhesion molecule 1 (ICAM-1), which is another cell-adhesion molecule that endothelial cells express in response to proinflammatory mediators. In its low-affinity state, LFA-1 on neutrophils does not bind endothelial ICAM-1, but the conformational switch to its high-affinity state quickly enables LFA-1 to bind ICAM-1 with great strength, allowing the rolling neutrophil—if given the right chemokine stimulus—to slow its rolling down to a complete stop and to firmly adhere to the activated endothelium. Once stopped, the shear force on the adhered neutrophil causes it to spread out from a spherical shape to a flattened morphology. This stage of firm adhesion is also referred to by pathologists as pavementing, because the local endothelium starts to resemble a tiled pavement as more neutrophils adhere and flatten out. With the advent of sophisticated microscopic techniques, we now know that adhered neutrophils are not stationary on the endothelium but crawl in their flattened state to try to find a suitable area to transmigrate.

The importance of the ability of neutrophils to firmly adhere to the endothelium is demonstrated by the clinical manifestations of bovine leukocyte adhesion deficiency (BLAD). BLAD is an autosomal recessive disease that affects Holstein cattle as a result of a mutation in the gene that encodes β_2-integrin (CD18). An animal that is homozygous for this mutation has impaired expression of LFA-1 on its neutrophils. Because LFA-1 is required to form a firm adhesion with activated endothelium (through interaction with ICAM-1), tethered and rolling neutrophils cannot stably adhere to the endothelium and are thus unable to extravasate. Without the ability to mobilize its first responders to a site of inflammation, the animal suffers frequent and recurrent bacterial infections that result in premature death.

Transmigration, commonly referred to as diapedesis, is the movement of leukocytes from the lumen of the blood vessel through the vessel wall and into the interstitium. It typically occurs in the thin-walled postcapillary venules; however, transmigrating neutrophils must still penetrate the endothelial barrier and the underlying basement membrane. Although neutrophils have been reported to exit the vessel by moving through intact endothelial cells, adhered neutrophils usually crawl to the junctions between these cells to transmigrate. Here neutrophils, in cooperation with the endothelial cells, break down the tight junctions of the endothelium, creating small gaps between the endothelial cells. The neutrophils then attempt to squeeze through these gaps and digest the underlying basement membrane through localized secretion of collagenases. Using another series of cell-adhesion molecules, the leading edge of each neutrophil adheres to the extracellular matrix, allowing the neutrophils to pull themselves out of the vasculature. It is not surprising that by breaching the endothelial and basement membrane barriers, the process of transmigration additionally increases the permeability (leakiness) of the vessel. Microscopic studies have also shown that the hole left by transmigrating neutrophils is commonly used by other transmigrating leukocytes, increasing the efficiency of extravasation. Now out of the circulation, the neutrophils must migrate to the specific location of the potential threat.

The recruitment of leukocytes to a specific site of insult relies on the establishment of chemical gradients of chemoattractants. These chemoattractants can be endogenously derived from activated macrophages and other immune processes or can be exogenously derived microbial products diffusing away from a site of infection. As mentioned earlier, sentinel cells such as macrophages, once activated by PAMPs, DAMPs, or both, produce proinflammatory mediators. These mediators include chemoattractants, for example lipid-derived mediators such as leukotriene B_4 and chemokines such as CXCL8. These endogenous chemoattractants diffuse away from activated macrophages at the site of insult, setting up a concentration gradient. Another powerful endogenous

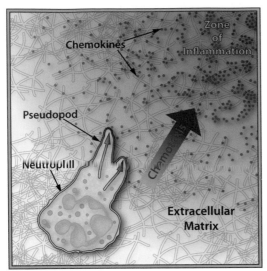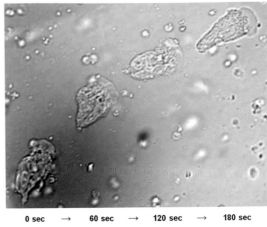

0 sec → 60 sec → 120 sec → 180 sec

FIGURE 5.8. Leukocyte chemotaxis (photograph courtesy of Dr. Paul Kubes, University of Calgary)

Diagram (left) and video micrograph (right) showing leukocyte chemotaxis up a chemoattractant gradient. The micrograph is a sequential montage taken from a video of an activated neutrophil migrating up a concentration gradient of the chemoattractant of N-formylmethionine–containing peptide in a petri dish. Note the neutrophil morphology, particularly the leading edge and trailing tail between which the neutrophil can detect minute differences in concentration of the chemoattractant. The four sequential photos are taken approximately 60 seconds apart using a phase-contrast microscope.

chemoattractant is a small protein by-product of complement activation, C5a. Recall from chapter 4 that following classical, alternative, or lectin pathways of complement activation, C5 is cleaved by the C5 convertases to produce a large C5b fragment (which is involved in initiation of the MAC) and a small, often forgotten C5a fragment. C5a diffuses away from the site of complement activation and establishes a chemoattractant gradient around complement-activating surfaces.

Exogenously derived chemoattractants (such as microbial products—PAMPs) can also be used by neutrophils to navigate toward a nidus of infection. One particular chemotactic PAMP is N-formylmethionine–containing peptides. Because N-formylmethionine is common in proteins of bacterial origin (but not common in host proteins), a neutrophil that migrates up a gradient of N-formylmethionine peptides should be moving toward its target. How,

though, does the neutrophil detect a chemotactic gradient and move in the right direction?

When clinicians think of neutrophils, they usually picture a snowball-shaped cell with a segmented nucleus in blood smears. However, once out of the circulation, the neutrophil can take on an amoeboid-like morphology with an extending pseudopod leading edge and a trailing tail (Figure 5.8). Using receptors for chemoattractants dispersed on its plasma membrane, the neutrophil extends its pseudopod in the region of the greatest chemotactic receptor activation and then pulls the rest of itself toward the stimulus. Clearly, these migrating leukocytes can actually detect the very small difference in concentration of a chemoattractant between its leading edge and trailing tail (some 8–12 μm apart). During the journey to the site of injury or infection, stimulated by local proinflammatory mediators, the neutrophil activates, making it much more efficient at

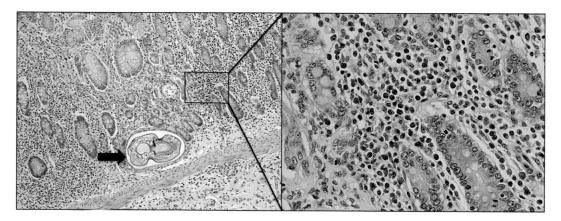

FIGURE 5.9. Eosinophilic inflammation

Histopathological section of the intestinal mucosa of a horse with a strongyle infection (arrow) showing an acute inflammatory reaction with recruitment eosinophils. Note that a high proportion of the cells have the bright red cytoplasmic granules characteristic of eosinophils.

locating, ingesting, and destroying pathogens (covered in chapter 6).

Once at the site of inflammation, the neutrophil is short-lived; thus, a constant stream of new neutrophils needs to be recruited. In many bacterial infections, the neutrophils infiltrate and die in such large numbers that they visibly manifest as pus or suppuration.

Diversity and Timeline of Leukocyte Recruitment

Although neutrophils are the most common early cells in many acute inflammatory conditions, other leukocytes (such as monocytes, eosinophils, and lymphocytes) can also be recruited to the site of inflammation. The mechanisms of extravasation and chemotaxis for these other leukocytes are similar to those described earlier for neutrophils. Which leukocytes are recruited and the timing of their recruitment are dependent on the type and extent of the tissue insult. Coordination of the type and timing of leukocyte recruitment to an inflammatory site is achieved through a complex combination of chemotactic molecules and cytokines released in the area, the types of adhesion molecules displayed on the endothelium, and the types of adhesion molecules and chemokine receptors on the surface of the circulating leukocytes. For instance, acute inflammation associated with parasitic infections (such as strongyle infection in horses) is associated primarily with eosinophil recruitment (recall from chapter 2 that eosinophils are best equipped to fight helminthic infections; Figure 5.9). The recruitment of eosinophils is mediated by release of the chemokine CCL11 (also called eotaxin), which promotes the extravasation and chemotaxis of eosinophils (as opposed to CXCL8, which attracts primarily neutrophils).

Circulating monocytes are a common second responder in acute inflammation, with the majority being recruited one to two days after the initial insult, as the neutrophil recruitment wanes. As soon as they extravasate, these monocytes mature into macrophages, which further activate as they migrate toward the site of inflammation. As mentioned in chapter 2, macrophages are moderately proficient at killing microbes, but they also have the ability to phagocytose and break down debris, as well as present antigen. Hence, these new macrophages start the task of cleaning up the dead neutrophils,

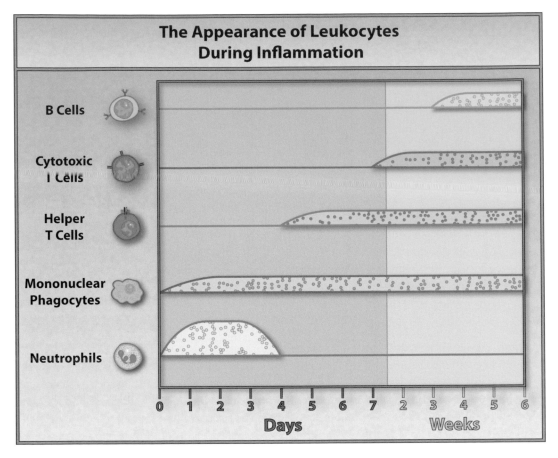

FIGURE 5.10. Phases of leukocyte recruitment in persisting inflammation

Although neutrophils are a common first responder in acutely inflamed tissue, mononuclear cells and lymphocytes are often recruited in later stages of inflammation. This figure shows the phases of leukocyte recruitment in a typical site of inflammation that persists over several weeks.

debris, and remaining microbes, which is not only important in the fight against infection, but a necessary step in the resolution of inflammation, wound healing, and tissue repair.

In most instances, local acute inflammation is self-limiting and quickly resolves without further sequelae. However, infection with a bona fide pathogen that is adapted to resist antimicrobial mechanisms of the innate immune system may cause persistent inflammation. In these instances, the adaptive immune system is brought into play, and the acute inflammation may evolve into chronic inflammation. Chronic inflammatory processes are very diverse and

are dependent on the pathogen and tissue involved and the nature of the adaptive immune response (e.g., Th1 vs. Th2 responses; covered in later chapters). Invariably, the neutrophil plays a diminished role in chronic inflammation, but macrophages, Th cells, Tc cells, and even B cells play major roles (Figure 5.10).

SYSTEMIC EFFECTS OF ACUTE INFLAMMATION

Aside from the local effects of acute inflammation (rubor, tumor, calor, dolor, and functio laesa), significant localized inflammation or

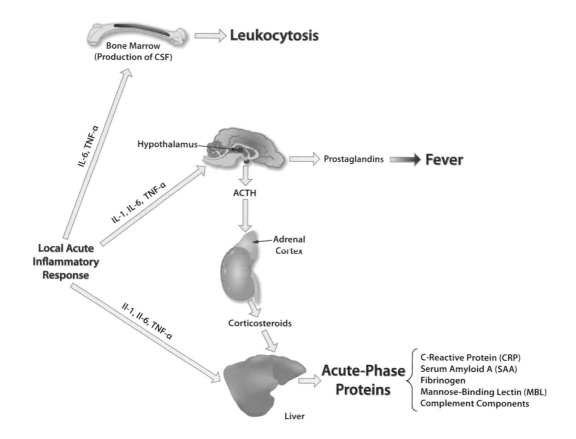

Bone Marrow (Production of CSF) → **Leukocytosis**

IL-6, TNF-α

Hypothalamus

IL-1, IL-6, TNF-α

Prostaglandins ⟹ **Fever**

ACTH

Local Acute Inflammatory Response

Adrenal Cortex

IL-1, IL-6, TNF-α

Corticosteroids

Acute-Phase Proteins

C-Reactive Protein (CRP)
Serum Amyloid A (SAA)
Fibrinogen
Mannose-Binding Lectin (MBL)
Complement Components

Liver

FIGURE 5.11. **Systemic effects of acute inflammation**

Certain proinflammatory cytokines generated at the site of acute inflammation can be distributed throughout the body of an animal, resulting in systemic inflammatory responses involving many organs. ACTH = adrenocorticotropic hormone; CSF = colony-stimulating factors.

disseminated acute inflammation can have systemic effects on the animal that may be clinically apparent. These effects become important indicators of an acute inflammatory process in tissues or organs not immediately visible in a clinical examination (e.g., pyothorax or prostatitis). In these situations, it is common for animals to be presented for these systemic symptoms rather than for the inflamed tissue itself.

Systemic effects of acute inflammation include

1. loss of appetite (anorexia);
2. altered sleep patterns (increased slow-wave sleep);
3. lethargy;
4. muscular wasting (cachexia);
5. hemodynamic changes (shock);
6. fever (pyrexia);
7. leukocytosis (commonly neutrophilia);
8. metabolic acidosis (lowered blood pH);
9. alterations to acute phase proteins.

The majority of the systemic effects of acute inflammation are mediated by the systemic release of TNF-α, IL-1, and to a lesser extent IL-6 by activated leukocytes at the site of inflammation (Figure 5.11). These proinflammatory cytokines can rapidly disseminate throughout the body and mediate responses in many organs, including the hypothalamus, liver, and bone marrow. Generally speaking, many of these systemic effects serve to conserve energy and mobilize resources (particularly protein) to aid in the resource-expensive process of inflammation. These systemic effects include anorexia, altered sleep patterns, lethargy, and cachexia (which contributes to metabolic acidosis)—most of which are directed by TNF-α. Other systemic effects, however, perform specific functions in the acute inflammatory process.

Fever (pyrexia) is the elevation of the core body temperature as a result of a higher-than-normal thermoregulatory set point within the anterior hypothalamus. This set point is raised (typically between 1° and 5°C [~2° and 9°F]) above the normal body temperature of the animal in response to pyrogens. *Pyrogen* is a term used for any substance that induces fever and can be exogenously or endogenously derived. Immunologically speaking, exogenous pyrogens (typically PAMPs or DAMPs such as LPS and adenosine) can induce leukocytes to produce endogenous pyrogens, which are proinflammatory cytokines such as TNF-α and IL-1 (Figure 5.12). These endogenous pyrogens can be released into the circulation to act on the vascular endothelial and perivascular cells of the anterior hypothalamus. Here, they can stimulate the synthesis of prostaglandins (particularly prostaglandin E_2), which will then act on neurons in the preoptic nucleus involved in thermoregulation. Nonsteroidal anti-inflammatory drugs (such as meloxicam) are often antipyretic as well as anti-inflammatory because they block cycloxygenase enzymes, thus reducing the production of prostaglandins at the site of inflammation (anti-inflammatory) as well as in the anterior hypothalamus (antipyretic).

Fever in response to acute inflammation is well accepted, but what are the functions of fever? Surprisingly, it is poorly understood. There are many theories, but no one theory can explain the benefits of fever to everyone's satisfaction (Figure 5.13). Nevertheless, fever is extraordinarily conserved (even reptiles display fever in response to inflammation), and thus it presumably offers some survival advantage to the host.

Leukocytosis is the increased number of leukocytes circulating in the blood. Leukocytosis in response to acute inflammation is primarily a neutrophilia (increased numbers of circulating neutrophils), which is due to the increased release of neutrophils from the bone marrow in response to IL-1 and TNF-α that provides greater numbers of these short-lived leukocytes so that more can extravasate and contribute to the immune defense at the site of inflammation. Prolonged release of neutrophils from the bone marrow will deplete its store of the mature cells, prompting increased synthesis of CSFs such as granulocyte CSF (products of inflammation such as C3a also lead to elevations in G-CSF). This increased synthesis in turn enhances granulocyte differentiation from myeloid precursor cells, and the release of the less mature band neutrophils. As mentioned in chapter 2, band neutrophils can be identified by their unsegmented band nuclei. Clinically, this release of less mature band neutrophils is referred to as a neutrophilia with a left shift (more circulating neutrophils that are on average less mature) and is commonly associated with acute inflammation. It is one of the most important clues a veterinarian has in gauging whether the animal's clinical signs stem from an inflammatory process (especially if the site of inflammation is not immediately apparent). The degrees of neutrophilia and left shift are also important diagnostic indicators of the severity of the inflammatory response occurring in the animal (Figure 5.14).

Another common laboratory finding in acute inflammation is the change to the acute phase protein (APP) profile of the serum. APPs are serum proteins whose abundance is altered in response to an acute inflammatory process. They can be divided into positive and negative APPs, with serum levels of positive APPs increasing, and those for negative APPs

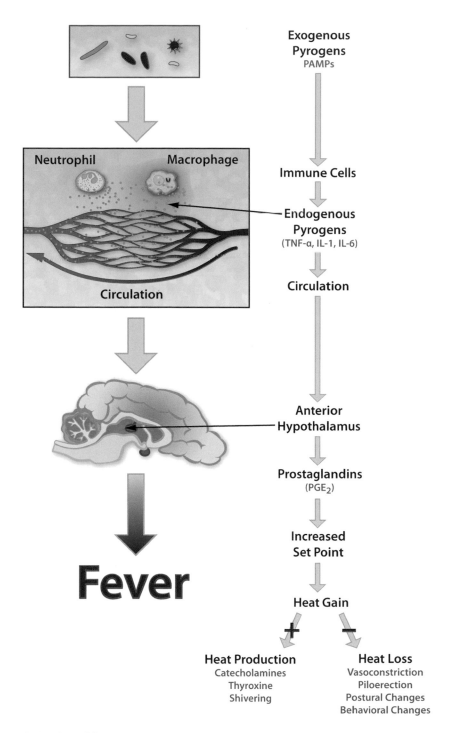

FIGURE 5.12. Induction of fever

Exogenous and endogenous pyrogens stimulate the release of prostaglandins (prostaglandin E$_2$) in the anterior hypothalamus that act on the thermoregulatory neurons that control the body's temperature set point. Increasing the set point promotes metabolic and behavioral changes in the animal that serve to increase heat production and minimize heat loss.

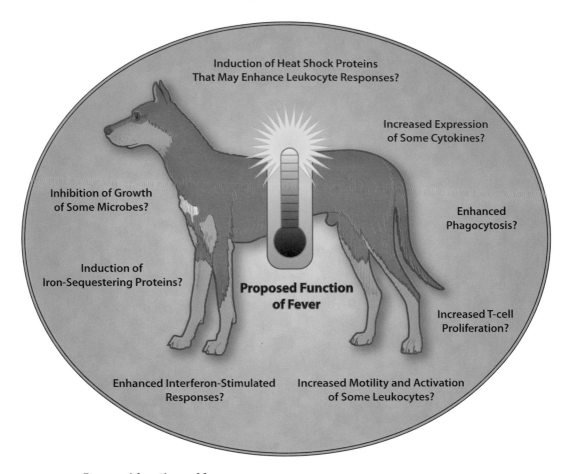

FIGURE 5.13. **Proposed functions of fever**

The true function of fever is nebulous. Over the years, numerous reports have shown immunological benefits of fever to the host animal. This diagram attempts to summarize these possible benefits of fever.

decreasing, in response to acute inflammation. Positive and negative APPs in various species and their relative association with acute inflammation can be found in Table 5.2. APPs are named as such because they are indicative of an inflammatory process taking place in the animal, not necessarily because they have common functions or are proinflammatory. In fact, the reported actions of different positive APPs include a wide range of homeostatic, proinflammatory, and anti-inflammatory actions. APP concentrations rise very quickly in the serum of animals with inflammation (peaking within twenty-four to forty-eight hours of onset of inflammation) and can reach levels ten to one hundred times their normal serum concentrations. Veterinarians exploit this feature by using increased APP concentrations as an indicator of inflammation, well before classic blood leukocyte concentration changes (such as neutrophilia). The use of APPs in diagnostic medicine has received a great deal of attention in recent years as an aid in the diagnosis of a broad range of diseases, including bovine respiratory syncytial virus infections, prostate cancer, bronchopneumonia, multiple myeloma, mastitis, *Streptococcus suis* infection, starvation, and lymphoid neoplasia.

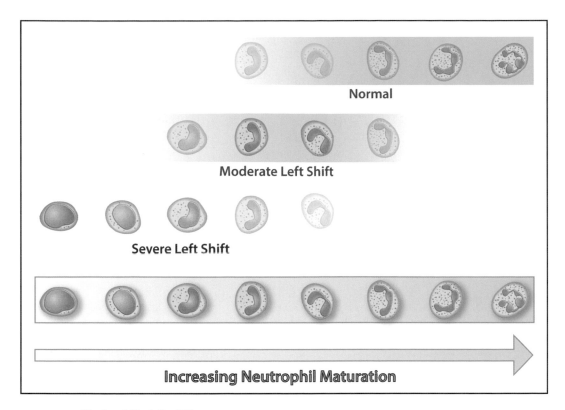

FIGURE 5.14. Neutrophilia left shift

As bone marrow stores of mature neutrophils diminish during the course of acute inflammation, less mature neutrophils will be released into circulation, which is termed a left shift of the population of circulating neutrophils. This figure shows the range of maturation in states of normal, left-shifted, and severely left-shifted neutrophil populations.

Many of the positive APPs are produced by the liver in response to cytokines such as IL-6, although the gastrointestinal tract, kidney, heart, adipocytes, and even leukocytes themselves have been shown to synthesize various APPs. One of the more prominent positive APPs in dogs, rabbits, pigs, and primates is C-reactive protein (CRP). CRP is a pentameric protein produced by hepatocytes and adipocytes in response to IL-6. It contains domains that can bind phosphocholine as well as certain polysaccharides and glycolipids that are commonly found on the surface of bacteria, parasites, and damaged cells. Other domains can bind certain Fc (antibody) receptors on macrophages (enhancing the phagocytosis of microbes and dead cells) or can bind C1q (initiating complement activation). Thus, CRP acts as a secreted PRR that enhances the clearance of microbes and damaged host cells during periods of acute inflammation. Numerous other pro- and anti-inflammatory roles of CRP have been reported, including the induction of various cytokines, attenuation of neutrophil chemotaxis and degranulation, and promotion of tissue repair.

CLINICAL CORRELATION: FOLLOW-UP

As we discussed at the start of this chapter, acute mastitis is an acute inflammatory reaction in the mammary gland, leading to its dysfunction (Figure 5.15). Lactating dairy herds are highly susceptible to mastitis, which is commonly initiated by contagious or environmental

TABLE 5.2. Acute-phase proteins in domestic species

APP	Immunologic function	Species variability
C-reactive protein (CRP)	Binds to bacteria Promotes complement binding and opsonization Induces cytokine production Modulates monocytes and macrophages	Major APP in dog and pig (increases 10 to 100 times) Not seen in cats
Serum amyloid A	Chemotactically recruits leukocytes Downregulates inflammatory response Has an inhibitory effect on fever, oxidative burst of neutrophils, and immune response Involved in lipid metabolism and transport (e.g., cholesterol from dying cells) Plays a pathological role in systemic (reactive) amyloidosis	Major APP in dogs, cats, cattle, and pigs (increases 10–100 times)
Haptoglobin	Binds hemoglobin; reduces tissue toxicity and sequesters iron from microbe Inhibits granulocyte chemotaxis and phagocytosis	Major APP in pigs, cattle, and sheep (increases 10–100 times) Moderate APP in dogs and cats (increases 2–3 times)
Alpha-1-acid glycoprotein	Antineutrophil and anticomplement activity Increases macrophage IL-1R antagonist secretion	Major APP in cats (increases 10–100 times) Increases in feline infectious peritonitis and inflammatory peritonitis in cats Moderate APP in dogs (increases 2–3 times) Minor APP in cattle
Ceruloplasmin	Transports copper for wound healing, collagen formation, and maturation Antioxidant	Moderate APP in dogs (increases 2–3 times) Minor APP in cattle
Hepcidin	Sequesters iron in anemia of chronic disease	
Fibrinogen	Coagulation	Important indicator of acute inflammation in horses and cattle
Albumin (negative)	Decreases inflammation	
Transferrin (negative)	Iron binding, so reduced concentration sequesters iron from bacterial use	

bacteria. Hallmark characteristics of acute mastitis include redness, heat, swelling and pain in the udder, and the presence of leukocytes in the milk.

Student Considerations

After learning about the onset and development of acute inflammation, you should be able to describe the sequence of events that leads to acute mastitis and outline the key clinical and laboratory findings that would aid a veterinarian in his or her diagnosis.

Possible Explanations

High-performing mammary glands such as those of a lactating dairy cow are highly susceptible to microbial infection with contagious or environmental bacteria. These bacteria can pass through the streak canal, particularly after milking, and proliferate in the gland. The proliferating microbes release PAMPs (such as endotoxin in the case of coliform mastitis), which are detected by sentinel cells (such as macrophages) resident in the gland's tissue. These cells release proinflammatory cytokines, including TNF-α, IL-1, and IL-6, and other mediators such as pros-

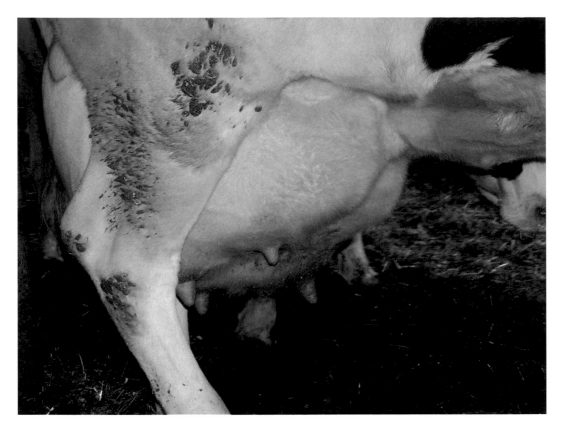

FIGURE 5.15. Acute bovine mastitis (photograph courtesy of Dr. Gordon Atkins, University of Calgary)

This photograph is of a five-year-old, mid–third-lactation Holstein cow with severe mastitis of the left front quarter caused by *Klebsiella* bacteria.

taglandins and leukotrienes that, together with mediators from other cell types such as histamine, result in changes to the local vasculature. These changes allow serum proteins containing complement and antibodies into the tissue and also promote the tethering and adhesion of circulating neutrophils. Sensing chemokines emanating from within the tissue, the tethered and rolling neutrophils extravasate and migrate up a proinflammatory chemoattractant gradient. Here, they can bolster the local macrophage defense against the invading microbes by using their potent antimicrobial effector mechanisms. The details of these mechanisms are discussed in the next chapter.

Clinically, these changes manifest in a mammary quarter that is swollen, red, and hot to the touch. When a milk sample is taken, increased numbers of infiltrated neutrophils along with sloughed epithelial cells can be detected by milk smear, CMT, or automated cell counting. The cow may be febrile and show signs of lethargy, anorexia, and altered behavior resulting from the systemic release of TNF-α and IL-1. Blood samples would reveal a neutrophilia with left shift and, if measured, increased serum concentrations of APPs, including haptoglobin and serum amyloid A (the major APPs in cattle).

To the dairy farmer, acute mastitis signifies a loss of income and considerable effort and time lost in both individual treatment (often intragland antibiotic preparations) and herd prevention. To the cow, acute mastitis is painful and uncomfortable and is often accompanied by systemic ill thrift. Nonetheless, as illustrated by deficiencies such as bovine leukocyte adhesion deficiency, acute inflammation is a fundamentally important process of the innate and adaptive immune systems and is essential for the survival of animals in this microbe-rich world.

Innate Cellular Effector Mechanisms

Chapter 6

10.5876_9781607322184.c006

CLINICAL CORRELATION: RATTLES IN FOALS

A veterinarian is called out to examine a four-month-old thoroughbred filly that the owners report as having "rattling breath" and "being off feed." Unfortunately, the filly dies before the veterinarian arrives. On postmortem of the foal, the veterinarian discovers tuberculosis-like granulomas throughout the lungs and tentatively attributes the filly's death to pneumonia caused by a disease known as *rattles* (Figure 6.1).

Rattles, so named because of its presenting sign of rattly breathing, is a severe form of bacterial pneumonia that commonly affects foals. It is caused by the Gram-positive bacterium *Rhodococcus equi,* which is related to *Mycobacterium tuberculosis* (the etiological agent of tuberculosis). *R. equi* is found in soil and is endemic on certain horse farms. The majority of cases occur in hot, dry summers when conditions are dusty. It is thought that foals inhale the bacteria in the dust, which are then deposited in terminal bronchi and alveoli. Here the *R. equi* microbes are engulfed by resident alveolar macrophages. These specialized macrophages are the primary immune cells defending these respiratory surfaces. They are extremely proficient at recognizing and phagocytosing inhaled debris and microbes and very effective at killing them. *R. equi* bacteria, however, are not typically killed by alveolar macrophages in foals. In fact, they can thrive within the macrophage. Macrophages infected with *R. equi* quickly recruit other immune cells through the release of proinflammatory cytokines, eventually forming granulomas. How is the macrophage able to kill most microbes easily but unable to kill *R. equi*?

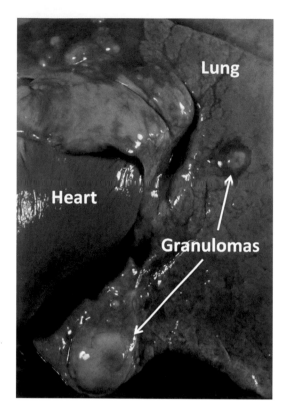

FIGURE 6.1. Lung granulomas found at necropsy in a five-month-old foal infected with *Rhodococcus equi* (photograph courtesy of Dr. Rachel Peters, Takeda Pharmaceuticals)

LEARNING OBJECTIVES

After reading this chapter, you should be able to

- explain in general terms the effector mechanisms of the innate immune system;
- identify which innate immune effectors are most efficient at controlling
  - » small extracellular threats, such as bacteria,
  - » large extracellular threats, such as multicellular parasites,
  - » intracellular infections, such as viruses;
- list the major professional phagocytes and describe how they recognize, ingest, and kill target microbes;
- describe the process of phagosomal maturation and list attributes of the phagolyso-

some that mediates the killing and digestion of microbes;

- describe the process of degranulation of neutrophils and eosinophils and list the major products released by these cells;
- describe the formation and composition of NETs and explain their proposed function;
- explain in general terms the recognition of target cells by NK cells;
- explain how NK cells kill target cells;
- explain the augmentation of the innate effector mechanisms by the adaptive immune system.

CLASSIFICATION OF INNATE CELLULAR EFFECTOR MECHANISMS

Thus far, you have learned that innate immune cells can recognize microbes and parasites, alert neighboring cells, and coordinate recruitment of specific innate immune cells to a site of infection. But what do these cells do when they get there, and how do they control infection? The mechanisms of microbial killing are as diverse as the microbial threats to an animal. These mechanisms depend on the type of infection (particularly location and physical size of the invader) and which innate immune cell responds to the infection.

Generally, the killing mechanisms can be categorized as

1. phagocytosis by phagocytes and killing of microbes within the phagosome;
2. release of antimicrobial products to kill extracellular microbes and parasites;
3. targeted destruction of infected host cells by NK cell–mediated cytotoxicity.

Together, these mechanisms can defend against pathogens large or small, intracellular or extracellular, often without any help from the adaptive immune system. The response to a given infection may use effector mechanisms in just one, two, or all three of these categories.

Although these cellular effector mechanisms are considered part of the innate immune system (because they can be immediately deployed without previous exposure to the threat), these mechanisms also play an important role in the elimination of infection after an adaptive immune response has been mounted. In many cases, adaptive immune responses (such as the production of antibodies) specifically act to enhance the efficiency of these innate cellular effector mechanisms.

PHAGOCYTES AND PHAGOCYTOSIS

As mentioned in chapter 2, both macrophages and neutrophils (and to a lesser extent DCs) have the ability to engulf small particles by a process called *phagocytosis.* In fact, these cells are so adept at "eating" particles that they are often collectively referred to as *professional phagocytes* (i.e., professional eating cells). Once these phagocytes have phagocytosed microbes and other material, they can kill and digest the phagocytosed products within an intracellular vacuole called a *phagolysosome,* which allows the cell to kill microbes, using high concentrations of toxic compounds and enzymes, while minimizing collateral damage to neighboring host cells.

The process of microbial killing via phagocytosis can be broken down into three stages:

1. recognition and adhesion of particles on the plasma membrane of the phagocyte;

2. membrane and cytoskeletal reorganization to mediate particle engulfment and the creation of a phagosome;

3. maturation of the phagosome to a microbicidal and degradative phagolysosome.

Phagocytosis Part I: Recognition and Adhesion of Particles on the Plasma Membrane of the Phagocyte

The recognition and adhesion of particles destined for phagocytosis involve both specialized PRRs and opsonic receptors on the surface of the phagocyte. As you recall from chapter 4, PRRs are immune receptors that can recognize certain evolutionarily conserved molecular patterns that are unique to foreign material such as microbes (PAMPs) but are absent in normal healthy host tissue. In many circumstances, ligation of these PRRs (e.g., by TLRs) leads to proinflammatory signaling and activation of the cell. In addition to proinflammatory PRRs, phagocytes express phagocytic PRRs. These receptors bind to PAMPs displayed on the surface of microbes and instigate phagocytosis.

Table 6.1 lists several known PRRs that can initiate phagocytosis. As covered in chapter 3, the best-characterized phagocytic PRR is the mannose receptor (MR, CD206). This receptor is found on the surface of macrophages and binds terminal sugar residues on proteins that are common on the surface of microbes (but absent on healthy host tissues). When microbes come into contact with the membrane of phagocytes, the MR (along with other phagocytic PRRs) binds to molecules on the microbe's surface. The ligated receptors then initiate intracellular signaling pathways that coordinate phagocytosis of the microbe. Thus, through phagocytic PRR, phagocytes can directly recognize and selectively engulf foreign particles but leave normal healthy host cells alone. Similar receptors, however, can recognize molecules on the surface of host cells that have been damaged or have gone through apoptosis (such as phosphatidyl serine). These receptors facilitate phagocytosis of dead and dying host cells (a process often referred to as *efferocytosis*), which is necessary for homeostasis, wound repair, and removal of cells that have been killed by an intracellular infection such as a virus. These receptors, some of which are listed in Table 6.1, permit professional phagocytes to recognize a wide range of particles from microbes to apoptotic host cells and to stimulate their phagocytosis.

Although macrophages and neutrophils can autonomously recognize and phagocytose foreign objects using their phagocytic PRRs, this

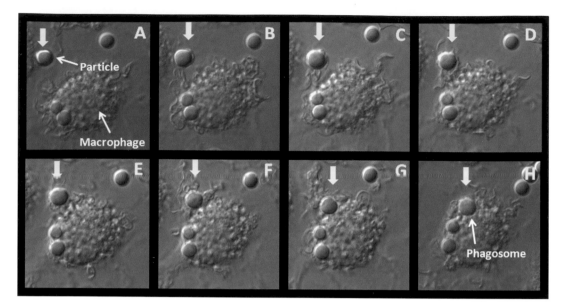

FIGURE 6.2A–H. **Phagocytosis of an IgG-opsonized particle (yellow arrow) by a tissue macrophage (images acquired at the Live Cell Imaging Facility, University of Calgary)**

This series of micrographs was taken over a period of 30 minutes and illustrate the three stages of phagocytosis: recognition and adhesion of particles on the plasma membrane of the phagocyte (panels A–B), membrane and cytoskeletal reorganization to mediate particle engulfment and creation of a phagosome (panels C–E), and maturation of the early phagosome that will eventually become a microbicidal and degradative phagolysosome (panels F–H).

process is dramatically enhanced by a process known as opsonization. Opsonization is the process whereby particles destined for phagocytosis are coated with a protein-binding enhancer known as an opsonin (derived from the Greek *opson,* which is a condiment such as relish that is added to food to make it more tasty, hence *opsonin*). Mammals have two major opsonins—complement (specifically C3b) and antibodies (particularly certain IgG isotypes). C-reactive protein (the major acute-phase protein in many animal species) can also act as an opsonin. These proteins are found in the serum and can bind to microbes. C3b covalently binds to microbes after initiation of the complement cascade (recall from chapter 4). IgG noncovalently, but very specifically, binds to antigens on the surface of microbes after a humoral immune response (covered in chapter 12). These

molecules essentially tag the microbe for phagocytosis (making it more tasty to phagocytes). Phagocytes can strongly adhere to microbes coated with the C3b and IgG opsonins through receptors for C3b (CR1 and CR3) and receptors that recognize the constant or Fc portion of IgG (Fcγ receptors) (Table 6.1). These receptors also provide a powerful stimulus to initiate phagocytosis of the bound, opsonized microbes (Figure 6.2). Phagocytosis of opsonized particles occurs with much greater efficiency than phagocytosis initiated through phagocytic PRRs alone (see Figure 6.3). Hence, although phagocytosis by macrophages and neutrophils is considered an innate immune response, the production of certain antibodies after the stimulation of an adaptive immune response acts to significantly enhance this innate effector process.

TABLE 6.1. Examples of pattern recognition and opsonic phagocytic receptors that can be found on professional phagocytes

Phagocytic receptor type	Receptor example	Ligand	Major target
Direct PRR	MR (CD206)	Terminal mannose and fucose residues	Bacteria, fungi, viruses
Direct PRR	Dectin-1	β-glucan residues	Fungi
Direct PRR	Scavenger receptor A I	Polyanionic ligands (e.g., LPS)	Diverse (e.g., foreign) particles, microbes, and lipoproteins
Direct PRR	Phosphatidyl serine receptor	Phosphatidyl serine	Apoptotic cells
Opsonic receptor	CR 3 (CD11b–CD18)	C3b	Any surface labeled with C3b
Opsonic receptor	Fcγ receptor 1 (CD64)	Fc portion of IgG	Any IgG-bound surface

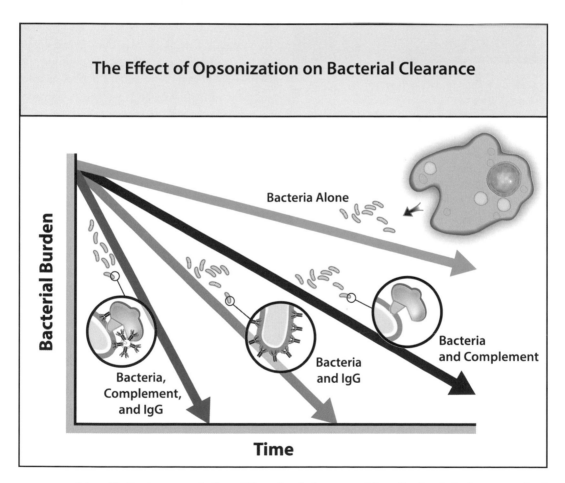

FIGURE 6.3. A hypothetical representation of the rate of clearance of invading bacteria from an animal in the presence or absence of opsonization

Bacteria alone could eventually be cleared from the body by phagocytosis via the direct recognition by phagocytic PRRs (e.g., MR). However, the rate of clearance would be enhanced with the addition of the complement- and Ig-based opsonins through more efficient bacterial recognition by phagocytic cells.

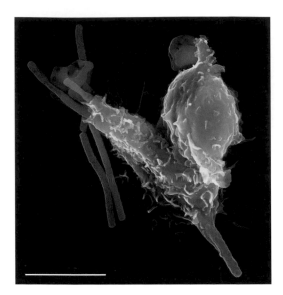

FIGURE 6.4. Phagocytosis of bacteria by neutrophils

Neutrophil (yellow) in the process of engulfing anthrax bacteria (orange) via phagocytosis. This image was taken by Volker Brinkman using a scanning electron microscope (reprinted from Brinkman, 2005, *PLoS Pathogens* 1[3]: cover).

Phagocytosis Part II: Membrane and Cytoskeletal Reorganization to Mediate Particle Engulfment and the Creation of a Phagosome

The actual process of phagocytosis refers to the physical engulfment of particles bound to the plasma membrane, resulting in their being trapped in an intracellular vacuole called a phagosome. Macrophages and neutrophils can easily phagocytose irregularly shaped particles and particles as much as 5 μm in diameter (about half the size of the phagocytes themselves; Figure 6.4). Moreover, macrophages and neutrophils can engulf numerous particles within minutes, and it is not uncommon to see these cells laden with upward of twenty microbes. Obviously, this level of phagocytosis requires significant alteration of the cytoskeleton and membrane of the phagocyte.

Recognition of the particle by phagocytic receptors on the surface of the phagocytes results in tight adhesion of the particle to the plasma membrane and also serves to cluster the receptors together. This process of receptor clustering is often enough to initiate regional signals that orchestrate the cytoskeletal rearrangement necessary for the engulfment of the particle at the plasma membrane. Several models of phagocytosis exist, depending on the size of the particle and the type of phagocytic receptors engaged, but this process essentially results in involution of the plasma membrane to which the particle is bound (Figure 6.5). This inversion creates an inward-facing pouch of plasma membrane that is eventually pinched off, resealing the plasma membrane and creating a cytoplasmic vacuole (sac) containing the particle. This vacuole is called the phagosome, and for the first few seconds after being formed, it contains only the particle and the extracellular fluid that was brought in with it—but all of this changes rapidly.

Phagocytosis Part III: Maturation of the Phagosome into a Microbicidal and Degradative Phagolysosome

The interior of the phagosome—potentially containing living microbes—quickly evolves from an innocuous environment with a neutral pH to an acidic, oxidative, degradative, antimicrobial chamber. This cellular process is aptly named *phagosomal maturation* (Figure 6.6). For it to occur, the newly formed phagosome begins to fuse with endosomes and lysosomes within the cytoplasm of the phagocyte. Initially, the phagosome preferentially fuses with the relatively immature early endosomes; however, over a period of several minutes, the maturing phagosome starts to fuse with late endosomes and eventually with fully formed lysosomes. In neutrophils, the azurophilic granules—which are essentially modified lysosomes that are densely packed with high concentrations of antimicrobial proteins—also fuse with the phagosome. This process of fusion between the phagosome and the endosomal and

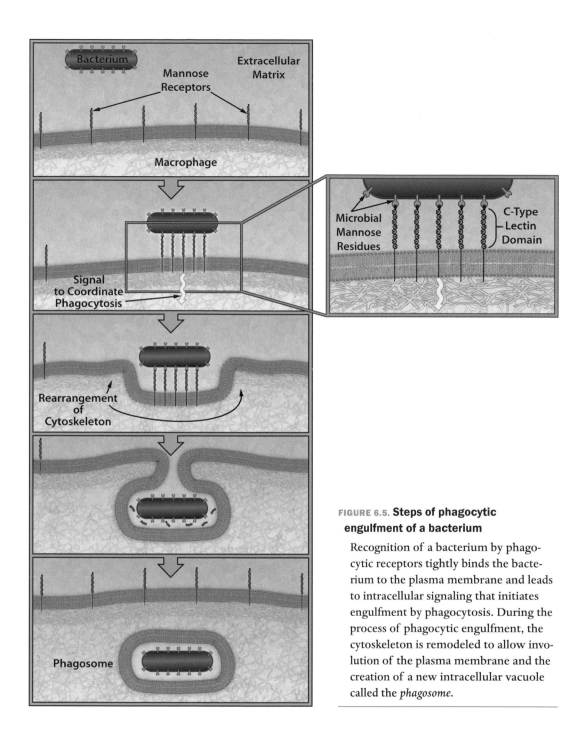

FIGURE 6.5. Steps of phagocytic engulfment of a bacterium

Recognition of a bacterium by phagocytic receptors tightly binds the bacterium to the plasma membrane and leads to intracellular signaling that initiates engulfment by phagocytosis. During the process of phagocytic engulfment, the cytoskeleton is remodeled to allow involution of the plasma membrane and the creation of a new intracellular vacuole called the *phagosome*.

lysosomal compartments results in the delivery of hydrolytic enzymes and other antimicrobial molecules (such as antimicrobial peptides) to the phagosome. The phagosome also starts to accumulate complexes in its membrane that actively pump protons into its interior, making it acidic (around pH 4–5). This acid not only serves to help kill any microbes directly but also activates many of the antimicrobial enzymes that have been delivered to the phagosome.

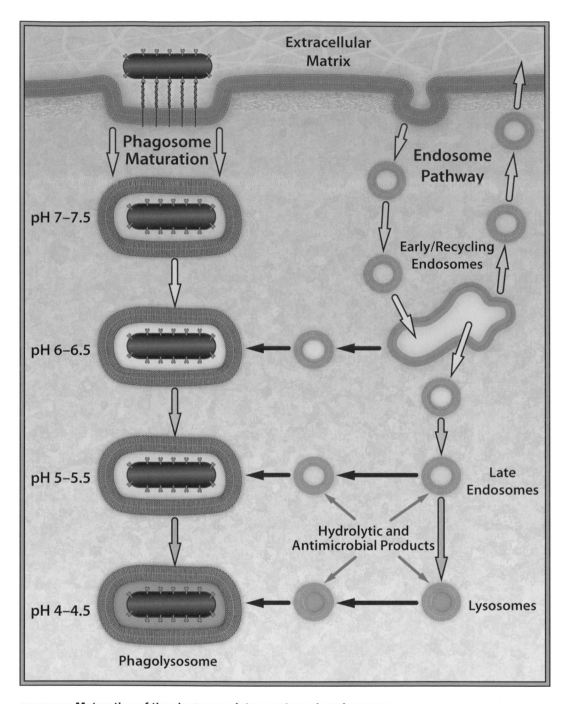

FIGURE 6.6. Maturation of the phagosome into a mature phagolysosome

After phagocytosis of a microbe, proton pumps are quickly assembled on the phagosomal membrane, which serve to acidify its interior. In addition, endosomal and lysosomal compartments containing hydrolytic enxymes and antimicrobial products progressively fuse with the nascent phagosome during its maturation. These events rapidly remodel the newly formed vacuole into an acidic, digestive, antimicrobial phagolysosome.

After extensive fusion with endosomes and lysosomes, the mature phagosome is considered a hybrid vacuole called a phagolysosome.

Another extremely effective strategy used by the phagosome to kill ingested microbes is the generation of reactive oxygen species, often referred to as the oxidative or respiratory burst. This strategy is achieved by a multisubunit complex called NADPH oxidase that is assembled on the phagosomal membrane. This complex transfers unpaired electrons from NADPH to molecular oxygen (O_2), generating the free radical superoxide (O_2-) within the phagosome (Figure 6.7). Having an unpaired electron, superoxide is extremely reactive (and damaging) to molecules in its vicinity. If it does not react with an organic compound, it typically reacts with hydrogen ions and water to produce hydrogen peroxide (H_2O_2) in a chemical reaction called *dismutation*. Although hydrogen peroxide is not a free radical per se, it is a powerful oxidant—particularly at a low pH, as in the phagosome. In the phagosome, hydrogen peroxide can be further converted into hydroxyl radicals (OH-), particularly in the presence of ferrous ions. Similar to superoxide, these free radicals are extremely damaging to virtually all macromolecules within the phagosome. However, these reactions do not necessarily stop here.

Neutrophils make a heme-containing enzyme called myeloperoxidase (MPO) in large amounts and store it in their granules. (An interesting fact is that the heme group in MPO has a green hue. It is this pigment that gives pus, which is made up of dead neutrophils, its green tinge.) When these granules fuse with the phagosome, MPO can combine hydrogen peroxide with a chloride ion to make the hypochlorite ion (ClO-). (ClO- is the active ingredient in bleach, a powerful disinfectant.)

Hence, the oxidative burst in phagosomes generates numerous reactive oxygen species, which serve to kill phagocytosed microbes through oxidation. Humans and mice deficient in parts of the NADPH oxidase complex cannot generate an oxidative burst in phagocytes and thus suffer recurrent bacterial infections in a condition called chronic granulomatous disease. Although no naturally occurring NADPH oxidase deficiencies have been reported in veterinary species, they undoubtedly exist but go undiagnosed.

The phagosome can also produce another oxidative radical group called the reactive nitrogen intermediates (RNI). Using the amino acid arginine as a substrate, inducible nitric oxide synthase (iNOS) produces the RNI nitric oxide (NO). Nitric oxide is produced by many cells as an important signaling molecule, but at the high concentrations generated in the phagosomes of activated phagocytes (activation increases expression of iNOS—hence *inducible* nitric oxide synthase), the nitric oxide free radical is antimicrobial, reacting with DNA and microbial enzymes. Nitric oxide can also combine with superoxide to produce a highly unstable isomer of nitrate called *peroxynitrite.* Peroxynitrite and its downstream products are extremely damaging to the lipids, DNA, and protein contained within the phagosome.

Aside from a low pH and the production of oxidative compounds, fusion with lysosomes and granules delivers a variety of digestive enzymes and antimicrobial peptides to the phagosome. Because lysosomes function as the garbage disposal system of the cell, they contain numerous acid hydrolases that can break down a variety of macromolecules, including lipids, carbohydrates, proteins, and nucleic acids. Within their phagosomes, macrophages use these enzymes to digest and recycle components of quiescent cells and debris in their normal homeostatic tasks. These enzymes, though, also serve to help kill and digest phagocytosed microbes during infection. One extremely important set of hydrolases delivered to the phagosome is the proteases. As you will learn in chapter 8, these enzymes function in the phagosomes of macrophages and DCs to break down protein antigens into small pieces that can be recognized by T cells. This process

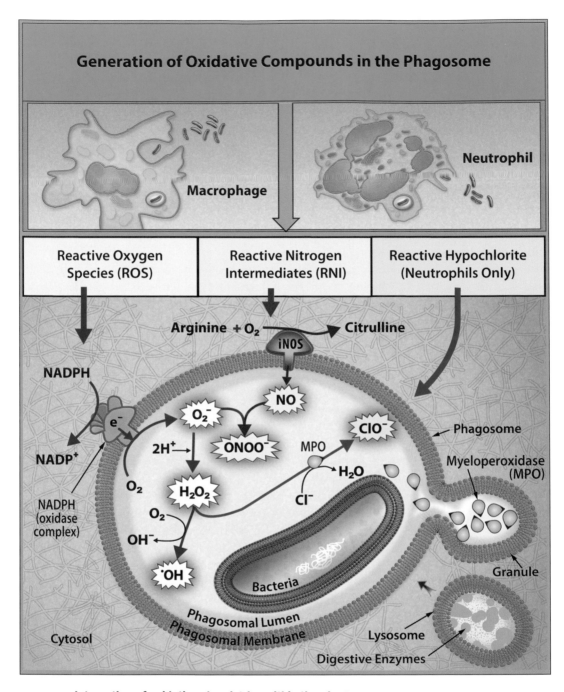

FIGURE 6.7. Interaction of oxidative chemistries within the phagosome

Superoxide (O_2^-), hydrogen peroxide (H_2O_2), hydroxyl radicals (OH-), nitric oxide (NO), peroxynitrite (ONOO-), and hypochlorite ion (ClO-), although not all free radicals, can all damage biologically important molecules within the phagosome.

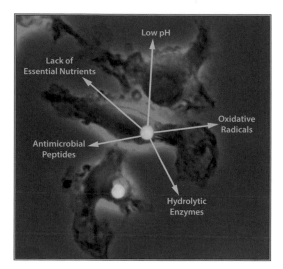

FIGURE 6.8. The environment within the phagolysosome

After minutes to hours, the newly formed phagosome is matured into an acidic, oxidative, digestive, antimicrobial compartment. Micrograph shows three tissue macrophages, two of which have phagocytosed IgG-opsonized particles (green). Nuclei are stained blue.

is called antigen processing and is essential for the development of T-cell–mediated adaptive immunity.

Hence, professional phagocytes, such as macrophages and neutrophils, can recognize microbes (especially ones that have been opsonized), engulf them by the process of phagocytosis, entrap them in an intracellular vacuole called a phagosome, and then proceed to pump acid, toxic chemicals, and digestive enzymes into the compartment (Figure 6.8). By carefully selecting what to phagocytose and by containing the majority of the cytotoxic components used to kill internalized microbes, phagocytosis is a relatively precise antimicrobial effector mechanism that limits collateral damage to neighboring host cells. But what happens if the invading threat is too big to phagocytose (such as a worm), or there are just too many threats to handle?

EXTRACELLULAR INNATE EFFECTOR MECHANISMS

Degranulation by Neutrophils and Eosinophils

To defend against threats that are too big or too numerous to phagocytose, neutrophils and eosinophils can release their arsenals of granules into the extracellular space in a process called degranulation. Unlike mast-cell degranulation, which releases mostly vasoactive amines such as histamine, degranulation by neutrophils and eosinophils releases cytotoxic and degradative proteins and peptides. Although the aim is to kill the foreign invader, a high amount of collateral damage occurs to the host tissue.

In the face of significant proinflammatory stimulation and the presence of high levels of microbial products, neutrophils can induce degranulation by fusing certain granules to the cells' plasma membranes. All of the granule products are then released into the extracellular space (many of these products are the same as those delivered to the controlled environment within the phagosome after phagocytosis). These products include numerous proteases (many of which degrade connective tissue), MPO, and antimicrobial peptides (such as defensins and cathelicidins). In addition to the release of these granule components, NADPH oxidase can form on the plasma membrane of the neutrophil and generate superoxide in the extracellular space. The very same dismutation reactions that occur in the phagosome can thus occur in the extracellular space. Hence, the outwardly directed respiratory burst also generates hydrogen peroxide, hydroxyl radicals, and (because MPO is released by degranulation) hypochlorite ion (ClO-). Although some of these products released by neutrophils are somewhat selective toward microbes (such as defensins), most (including proteinases, oxidative radicals, etc.) are just as toxic to host cells as the targeted microbes. Excessive degranulation by neutrophils can be life threatening to an animal and is common in acute lung injury and septic shock.

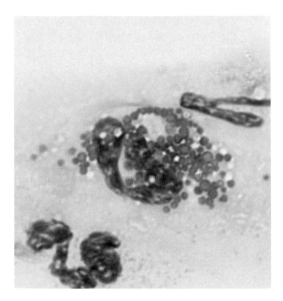

FIGURE 6.9. A canine eosinophil in the process of degranulation

Note the release of the red granules from the eosinophil's cytoplasm.

Eosinophils, as mentioned in chapter 3, are specialist antiparasite leukocytes. Although they often play roles in defending against certain bacterial and viral threats, they are best equipped to fight multicellular parasites—those that are too big to phagocytose. As such, in an acute inflammatory response to parasites, the eosinophils are often the major recruited leukocyte. After activation by proinflammatory stimuli, eosinophils can release their cytotoxic granule contents into the surrounding area via degranulation. Eosinophil granules contain several cytotoxic proteins, including major basic protein (a cytotoxin with antihelminthic properties), eosinophil cationic protein (a pore-forming protein that punches holes in cell membranes; it is also reported to be a ribonuclease that digests RNA), eosinophil-derived neurotoxin (ribonuclease that has antiviral properties), and eosinophil peroxidase (facilitates oxidative damage by generation of hydrogen peroxide). As with neutrophils, eosinophils can also assemble NADPH oxidase on their plasma membrane and generate extracellular superoxide and hydrogen peroxide during a respiratory burst. Products released by activated eosinophils, although antiparasitic, are also extremely damaging to bystander host cells. Eosinophil degranulation also triggers mast-cell degranulation and is commonly associated with allergies.

Release of Neutrophil Extracellular Traps

More recently, researchers have discovered that, when faced with high levels of proinflammatory stimulus, neutrophils can extrude a sticky, meshlike substance into the extracellular space to which bacteria and yeast stick and are killed. These substances are named neutrophil extracellular traps (NETs). With the use of NETs, neutrophils can efficiently trap and kill many microbes while minimizing collateral damage to host tissue. NETs are formed in the final stages of active neutrophil death, in the presence of cytokines such as IL-8 and PAMPs such as LPS in inflamed tissue. The fibers of the NETs are actually strands of the neutrophils' own DNA. Both nuclear and granule membranes break down during the process of NET release, allowing antimicrobial granule proteins (such as elastase, defensins, and MPO), along with nuclear histones (which surprisingly also have antimicrobial properties), to stick to the negatively charged DNA fibers. Decorated with antimicrobial proteins, these sticky networks of DNA fibers can not only trap bacteria and yeast, but also kill them directly (Figure 6.10). NET formation has also been shown to occur in the blood, particularly in the capillaries of the lung and in liver sinusoids during periods of sepsis. Although these NETs may function to ensnare microbes in the blood, they may have detrimental consequences to the animal. Not surprisingly, the breakdown of the nucleus and the extrusion of DNA during NET formation results in death of the short-lived neutrophil.

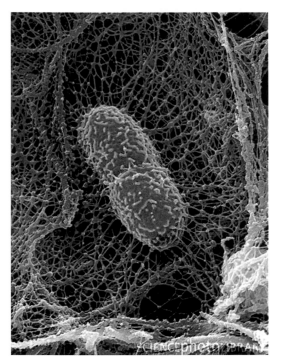

FIGURE 6.10. NETs

This is a scanning electron microscope image of a bacterium (*Klebsiella pneumoniae*) ensnared in a NET in an infected lung of a mouse. The image has been pseudocolored to differentiate the bacterium (pink) and the NET (green and white). Image from "The tangled NETs of the immune system." © Klaus Wilhelm, 2011. Originally published in *MaxPlanckReasearch* 1:11, 72–78.

NATURAL KILLER CELL– MEDIATED CYTOTOXICITY

Although phagocytes and granulocytes can identify and destroy extracellular threats, threats that exist within host cells (such as virus and certain bacteria and parasites) are generally hidden from the majority of innate effectors. Identifying potentially infected host cells, without prior exposure to the infective agent, is the specialty of NK cells. As covered in chapter 2, NK cells are actually lymphocytes. Unlike most T and B cells, however, they do not possess the receptor diversity generated by recombination of their chromosomal DNA. Instead, NK cells use families of conserved surface receptors that recognize sick and stressed host cells, as well as those cells that are not correctly displaying their self-markers because they are most likely harboring infectious agents (such as viruses) or are possibly transformed (neoplastic) cells. In response, NK cells can kill infected host cells, helping to contain intracellular infectious agents while the Tc lymphocyte arm of the adaptive immune system prepares an antigen-specific response.

Recognition of Target Cells

The exact mechanisms by which NK cells recognize potentially infected or transformed host cells are largely unknown. Generally, the killing of a particular host cell relies on the balance of the activating and inhibitory signals from the surface receptors of the NK cells that make contact with the host cell. These surface receptors belong to two structural families: the killer lectin-like receptors (KLRs; receptors that resemble the C-type lectins such as the MR) and the killer cell immunoglobulin-like receptors (KIRs; receptors with domains that share homology with parts of Igs). To make things more confusing, activating and inhibitory receptors belong to both families of receptors.

ACTIVATING STIMULUS

Receptors that provide activating stimulus in NK cells sense a variety of ligands that indicate abnormality on the surfaces of the target cells. In some cases, NK cell–activating receptors can directly detect conserved viral proteins on the surface of infected cells. Infection with certain members of the herpes virus family, for instance, can be directly detected by NK cells through this type of receptor. Aside from these specific examples, most activating receptors are thought to detect ill-defined ligands that indicate an altered cellular state, which may arise through infection with viruses, intracellular bacteria or parasites, or a state of malignancy. These activating ligands are derived from alterations to surface glycoproteins induced by metabolic stress or altered posttranslational modification of normal surface proteins. Metabolic stress and altered protein processing are commonly found in virally infected cells (whose synthesis machinery has been hijacked by viruses). Transformed cells, which are replicating at an abnormal rate, also show metabolic stress and altered protein expression.

INHIBITORY STIMULUS

Even if host cells display surface ligands that indicate ill thrift, these cells are not killed by NK cells if the cells are also displaying normal self-markers. This sort of inhibition is achieved through inhibitory receptors on the NK cell that detect the normal expression of major histocompatibility complex class I (MHC I) molecules on host cells. MHC I molecules are usually expressed on every nucleated cell, and because they differ between individual animals, they constitute an important marker to differentiate self cells from non-self cells. They are also a critical element in the adaptive immune response to intracellular infections because they display samples of proteins that are present within the cell's cytoplasm and "show" them to Tc cells. The details on MHC molecules are covered in chapter 8. The presence of normal levels of MHC I on the surface of target cells indicates that, although they might be slightly altered, these cells are behaving relatively normally. This indication triggers inhibitory signals that override the activating stimulus, thus preventing activation of the NK-cell killing mechanism. However, altered levels or unrecognizable MHC I expression indicate that the host cell's metabolism has significantly changed or that there is covert inhibition of MHC I expression. Purposeful downregulation of the surface expression of MHC I is a common strategy used by many viruses to hide from Tc cells. Many transformed neoplastic cells also have decreased levels of MHC I on their plasma membranes. Hence, decreased levels of MHC I, or unrecognizable MHC I, do not trigger inhibitory signaling within the NK cell, and activating receptors can fully activate the NK-cell killing mechanism (Figure 6.11).

Targeted Degranulation by Natural Killer Cells

The major mechanism by which NK cells kill their target cells is very similar to that used by Tc cells (covered in chapter 10). Once an NK cell detects a host cell that triggers its activating receptors without triggering its inhibitory receptors, changes occur within the NK cell that allow it to kill the target cell with great precision. NK cells possess cytoplasmic granules termed *lytic granules*. These lytic granules contain cytotoxic molecules that can kill target cells after degranulation. Unlike degranulation by neutrophils and eosinophils, which results in widespread collateral damage, NK-cell degranulation is restricted to killing target cells, but not neighboring normal cells. NK cells do this by forming a tight area of adhesion with the target cell through which degranulation can occur without the cytotoxic components leaking into the surrounding tissue. This adhesion complex, termed an *NK immunological synapse,* consists of a collection of adhesion molecules carefully arranged into a ring by the NK cytoskeleton (Figure 6.12). This ring—almost like a suction cup—acts to "dock" NK cells onto target cells and form a tight seal within which granule components may be released into the target cell while being fully contained between both cells. Figure 6.12 shows the NK immunological synapse between an activated NK cell and a target cell and the beginning of the polarized degranulation.

Degranulation within the NK immunological synapse releases cytotoxic molecules that can act on the target cell. Two of these cytotoxic molecules are the proteins perforin and granzyme. When released into the NK immunological synapse, perforin inserts itself into the plasma membrane of the target cells

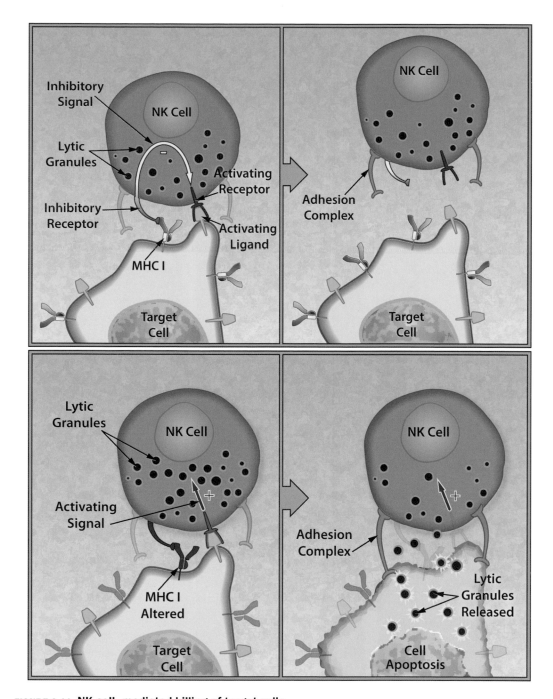

FIGURE 6.11. NK cell–mediated killing of target cells

Activation of the cytotoxic function of NK cells requires the presence of activating ligands and the absence of inhibitory ligands on the target cell surface. The top panel depicts inhibition of NK killing through recognition of normal MHC I on the surface of the target cell. Despite displaying activating ligands, the host cell is spared by the NK cell. The lower panel depicts a target cell displaying both an activating ligand and altered MHC I expression, which triggers the NK-cell killing mechanism, resulting in the death of the host cell via forced apoptosis.

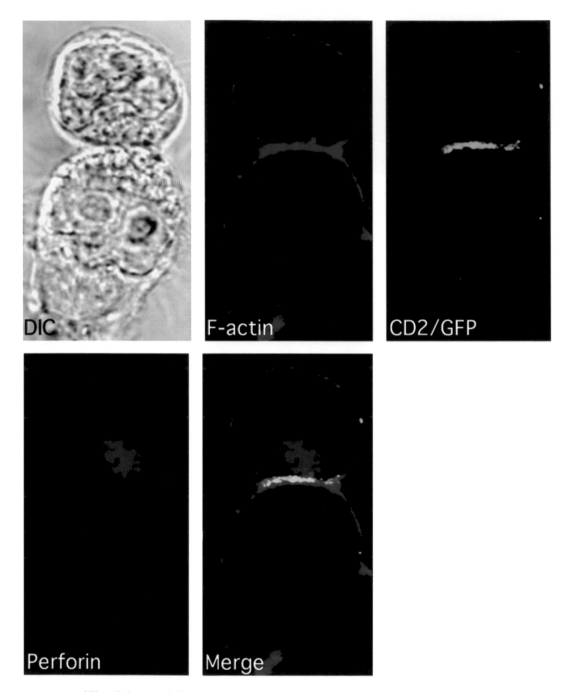

FIGURE 6.12. NK cell degranulation

NK cells carefully degranulate into an NK immunological synapse (NKIS) formed with the target cell. This series of micrographs depicts the NKIS between the NK cell (top) and the target cell (bottom). The actin cytoskeleton (blue) and adhesion molecule CD2 (green) form a ring through which the perforin (red) and granzyme can be delivered to the target cell. (From Orange et al., "The Mature Natural Activating Killer Cell Immunologic Synapse Is Formed in Distinct Stages," *PNAS* 100 (24): fig. 1, © 2003, National Academy of Sciences, USA)

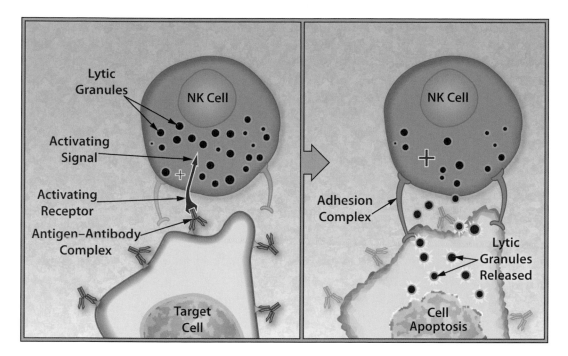

FIGURE 6.13. Antibody-dependent, cell-mediated cytotoxicity

NK cells can recognize surface-bound antibodies (such as IgG) through the receptors that recognize the Fc portion of the antibody (Fc receptors), thus providing a powerful activating stimulus to initiate the NK cell's cytotoxic function.

(perforating the membrane, as its name suggests), forming pores. Granzymes are a family of serine proteases that can gain access to the target cell's cytoplasm via the pores created by perforin. Here granzymes can act on caspases, activating pathways that force the target cell to go through apoptosis and die. The NK cell is resistant to its own perforin and granzymes and, thus, after the directed apoptosis of the target cell, it can disengage and seek another abnormal cell for destruction.

Antibody-Dependent Cell-Mediated Cytotoxicity

As with many innate effector mechanisms, NK cell–mediated cytotoxicity does not simply serve to contain infection between exposure and the more specific yet slow-reacting adaptive immune response. It also acts in an enhanced capacity after the induction of adaptive immunity. Specifically, akin to opsonization for phagocytosis, antibody-dependent cell cytotoxicity is a process through which the humoral immune system can augment NK cell–mediated cytotoxicity. After the production and binding of antibodies to cell-associated viral or neoplasm-associated antigens on the surface of abnormal cells, NK cells can more readily identify these antibody-coated cells as targets. Recognition of antibodies on the surface of a cell is achieved through the Fc receptors on the NK cell, which serve to provide a very powerful activating stimulus to initiate the NK cell's cytotoxic function (Figure 6.13).

CLINICAL CORRELATION: FOLLOW-UP

Student Considerations

After reading through this material, you should be able to list the ways in which macro-

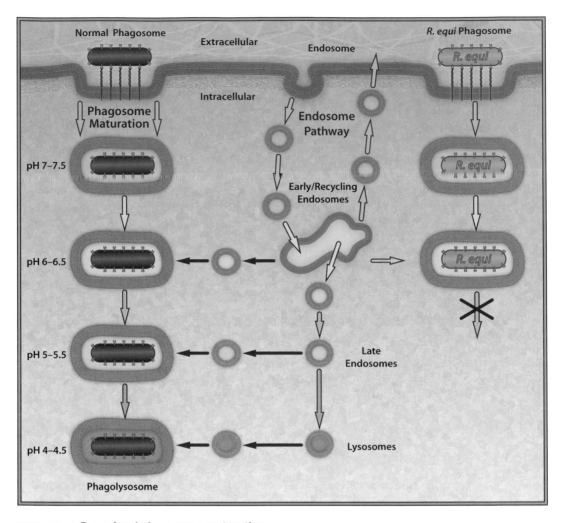

FIGURE 6.14. *R. equi* **and phagosome maturation**

The *R. equi* bacterium actively arrests the maturation of the phagosome. The arrested phagosome fails to fully acidify or fuse with the hydrolytic lysosomes, allowing the bacterium to survive within the macrophage.

phages are able to kill ingested microbes. You should also be able to think of several points in that arsenal at which *R. equi* is able to hijack this machinery and avoid destruction.

Possible Explanation

R. equi is a well-adapted pathogen that has evolved several means for circumventing host immune responses. One of these is the abil-

ity of the bacterium to avoid being destroyed by the macrophage after its phagocytosis in the pulmonary alveolus. *R. equi* is thought to achieve this by blocking the maturation of the phagosome that is created around these bacteria. Without phagosomal maturation, the interior does not acidify, and lysosomal products (such as digestive enzymes and antimicrobial products) are not delivered to the phagosome. The *R. equi* bacterium also has the ability to prevent the assembly of the NADPH oxidase complex on the membrane of the phagosome, which reduces the oxidative stress placed on the bacterium. It is thought that the phagosomes containing *R. equi* bacteria maintain some fusion capability with early and recycling endosomes, which can bring nutrients to the inhabiting microbe. Hence, the bacterium survives and replicates within this intracellular niche and for the most part is protected from the majority of immune effectors. The exact mechanism by which *R. equi* arrests phagosomal maturation is still debated, but certain lipid and protein products produced by the bacterium have been implicated in this pathogenic feature.

The infected macrophage, detecting the presence of the microbe through PRRs such as the TLRs, releases proinflammatory cytokines and chemokines into the surroundings, which recruits other mononuclear cells, thus creating a local inflammatory reaction. If not given the correct stimulus, these monocytes-turned-macrophages cannot kill the *R. equi* bacteria either but instead become infected themselves, further recruiting other immune cells, and so on, which eventually creates a chronic focal immune reaction and the formation of a granuloma.

An interesting fact is that the macrophage does have the ability to kill *R. equi* within its phagosomes, but it cannot do it alone. It needs to be activated by the correct cytokines that can be provided by the Th1 cells of the adaptive immune system (covered in subsequent chapters). Foals are particularly susceptible to *R. equi* because they do not generate a strong Th1 cell response. Adult horses, however, do generate a robust Th1-type adaptive immune response to *R. equi* and therefore rarely develop rattles.

Gerald N. Callahan

Cells and Organs of the Adaptive Immune System

Chapter 7

10.5876_9781607322184.c007

CLINICAL CORRELATION: FELINE LYMPHADENOPATHY

A five-year-old intact male cat presents at a small-animal clinic. The owner states the cat is lethargic and will not eat or drink. A quick examination of the cat reveals that the animal has a fever (>40°C, 104°F) and swollen superficial cervical and mandibular lymph nodes. Lymphadenopathy (especially swollen lymph nodes) is a common presenting symptom for several diseases of cats (see Table 7.1).

With cats, it seems obvious why neoplastic diseases of lymphocytes might lead to swollen nodes: uncontrolled proliferation of lymphocytes. For the most common causes of feline lymphadenopathy, however—all of the infectious diseases and autoimmune diseases—the reasons are less clear. Understanding why lymph nodes swell during infections and autoimmune reactions is essential to understanding animals' responses to and recovery from these syndromes.

LEARNING OBJECTIVES

After reading this chapter, you should be able to

- understand the location, structure, and function of the bone marrow, thymus, lymph nodes, spleen, and MALTs;
- know the origins, characteristics, and physical properties of T lymphocytes, B lymphocytes, macrophages, and DCs;
- understand the organization and function of the lymphatics.

ORGANS AND CELLS OF THE ADAPTIVE IMMUNE SYSTEM

In 1966, Roy Grist—a pathologist working with a mouse colony in Glasgow, Scotland—discovered a very odd-looking mouse in one of his cages. It was puny, hairless, and short-lived. After Dr. Grist made a brief report of his finding, an Edinburgh researcher asked Dr. Grist if his Edinburgh group could try to establish a line of these mice. Grist agreed and shipped a few mice off to the researcher. Because they were hairless, the mice became known as nude mice (see Figure 7.2).

Beyond their lack of hair, closer examination revealed a much more remarkable finding: these nude mice had no thymuses. In the early

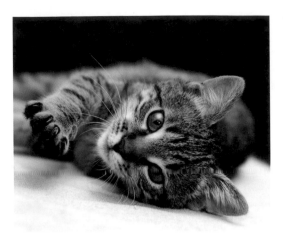

FIGURE 7.1. Domestic cat (© Pashin Georgiy / Shutterstock)

TABLE 7.1. Causes of lymphadenopathy in cats

I. Proliferative and inflammatory lymphadenopathies

  A. INFECTIOUS

   1. Bacterial
     a) Actinomyces app.
     b) Corynebacterium
     c) Mycobacteria
     d) Nocardia app.
     e) Streptococci (contagious streptococcal lymphadenopathy)
     f) Yersinia pestis
     g) Localized bacterial infection

   2. Septicemia

   3. Rickettsial
     a) Feline ehrlichiosis
     b) Hemobartonellosis

   4. Fungal
     a) Blastomycosis
     b) Coccidioidomycosis
     c) Cryptococcosis
     d) Histoplasmosis
     e) Phaeohyphomycosis
     f) Phycomycosis
     g) Sporotrichosis

   5. Parasitic
     a) Cytauxzoonosis
     b) Demodicosis
     c) Toxoplasmosis

   6. Viral
     a) Feline immunodeficiency virus
     b) Feline infectious peritonitis
     c) Feline leukemia virus

  B. NONINFECTIOUS

   1. Dermatopathic lymphadenopathy

   2. Idiopathic
     a) Distinctive peripheral lymph node hyperplasia
     b) Plexiform vascularization of lymph nodes

   3. Immune-mediated disorders
     a) Immune-mediated polyarthritides
     b) Other immune-mediated disorders

   4. Localized inflammation

   5. Postvaccinal

1970s, no one had any idea what thymuses did, and these mice seemed to offer an avenue for greater insight into the role of this organ.

One set of experiments involved transplanting skin from other species onto nude mice. Normally, skin grafts elicit a powerful immune response and do not survive longer than a few days. Nude mice accepted skin grafts from chickens, humans, cats, chameleons, fence lizards, and frogs. Immunologically, nude mice (unlike mice with thymuses) could not distinguish between themselves and chickens, lizards, humans, cats, or frogs (see Figure 7.3A–F).

Clearly, the thymus was critical to developing any immunological sense of self. That discovery added the final piece to the puzzle of the immune system. The thymus, the bone marrow, the lymph nodes, the spleen, and the MALT somehow combine to produce the adaptive immune response.

Primary Lymphoid Organs and Hematopoiesis

BONE MARROW

By the forty-fifth day of gestation, the bone marrow in fetal cats already provides 50 percent of the blood cells. By birth, a cat's bone marrow (as in most mammals) will supply 100 percent of the circulating blood cells. Perinatally, nearly all, if not all, bones contain marrow, the jellylike material where all the cells of the blood originate in a process called *hematopoiesis* (see Figure 7.4).

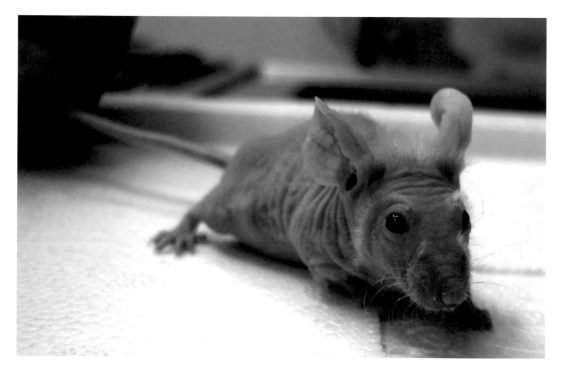

FIGURE 7.2. **Nude mouse (photograph by Armin Kübelbeck)**
This phenotype is the result of a gene mutation involving hair growth and thymus development.

Recall from chapter 2 that all white blood cells, RBCs, and platelets arise from a single pluripotential bone marrow stem cell. Early in hematopoiesis, two distinct cell lineages appear: the lymphoid lineage and the myeloid lineage.

The lymphoid lineage ultimately produces two major types of lymphocytes: T cells and B cells (recall from chapter 2 that the lymphoid lineage also produces NK cells that contribute to innate defense). The T lymphocytes play critical roles in all adaptive immune responses through release of essential cytokines and through direct killing of pathogen-infected cells. The B cells produce antibodies found throughout the body. These antibodies provide a major part of mammalian defense against infections. The B and T lymphocytes are also the only cells with antigen-specific receptors—the BCR (a special form of antibody) and the TCR (see Figure 7.5A–B). Together, T and B cells also produce the remarkable specificity and memory aspects of the adaptive immune response.

The myeloid lineage produces the remaining cells of the blood, many of which participate in innate immune responses, as discussed earlier. After they migrate out of the blood vessels and into the surrounding tissues, monocytes differentiate into macrophages—phagocytic cells found throughout the body—that are of critical importance to innate defense. Other phagocytic cells, the DCs, are specialists in acquiring and presenting antigens. Once a DC has acquired antigen, the cell moves through the lymphatics to the nearest lymph node and presents that antigen to T lymphocytes.

Mast cells begin in the marrow and move into the circulation and from there into the surrounding tissues, where they play major roles in innate responses, especially inflammation. Granulocytes—so named because they contain

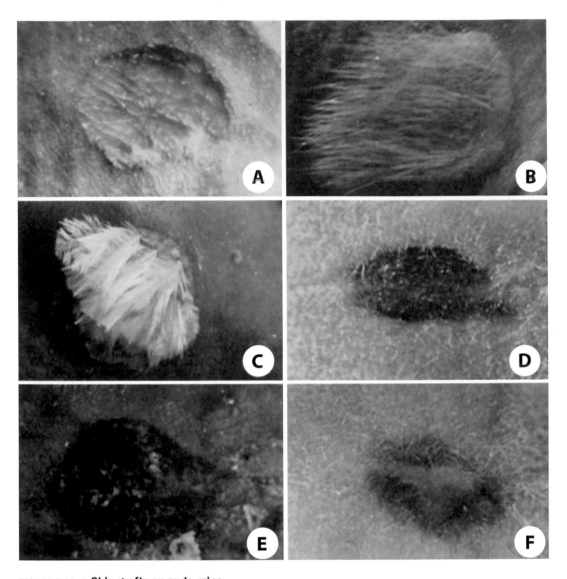

FIGURE 7.3A–F. **Skin grafts on nude mice**

Panel A shows human (mammal) skin after 60 days. Panel B shows cat (mammal) skin at 51 days. Panel C shows chicken (bird) feathers at 32 days; the feathers were already present when the graft was made. Panel D shows chameleon (reptile) skin at 41 days. Panel E shows fence lizard (reptile) skin at 28 days. Panel F shows tree frog (amphibian) skin at 40 days. © 1973 Rockefeller University Press. (Originally published in Manning, Reed, and Shaffer, 1973, *J. Exp. Med.* 138:488–494.)

cytoplasmic granules (active in inflammatory and other pathways)—include neutrophils, basophils, and eosinophils. Neutrophils (also known as polymorphonuclear leukocytes because their nuclei come in many shapes and sizes) are the most numerous of all white blood cells in mammals. Of the three granulocytes, the functions of neutrophils are clearest, but all play important roles in innate defense. (See chapters 2–6.)

THYMUS

Although all lymphocytes originate in the bone marrow, only B lymphocytes mature there

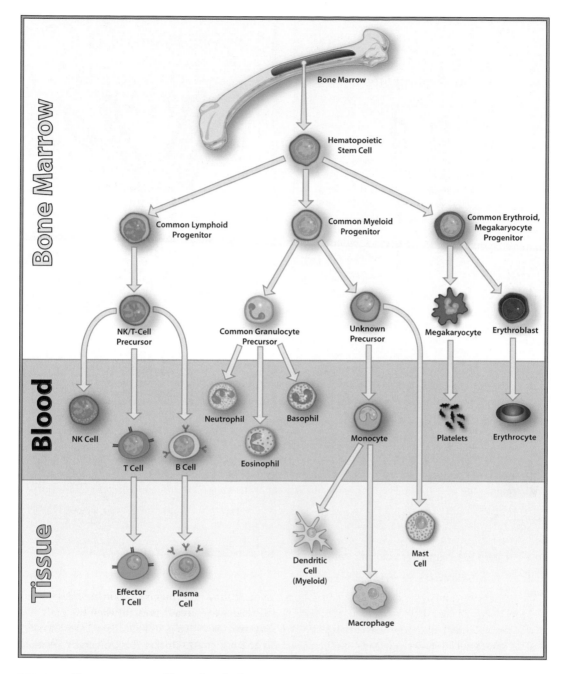

Bone Marrow

Bone Marrow

Hematopoietic Stem Cell

Common Lymphoid Progenitor

Common Myeloid Progenitor

Common Erythroid, Megakaryocyte Progenitor

NK/T-Cell Precursor

Common Granulocyte Precursor

Unknown Precursor

Megakaryocyte

Erythroblast

Blood

NK Cell

T Cell

B Cell

Neutrophil

Eosinophil

Basophil

Monocyte

Platelets

Erythrocyte

Mast Cell

Tissue

Effector T Cell

Plasma Cell

Dendritic Cell (Myeloid)

Macrophage

FIGURE 7.4. **Bone marrow and hematopoiesis**

A single pluripotential bone marrow stem cell gives rise to all of the cells of the blood. Among these are the cells most important to the adaptive immune response, particularly B and T lymphocytes and monocytes, which differentiate into macrophages and DCs.

or in other specialized organs such as the bursa of Fabricius in fowl. In vertebrates, another set of lymphocytes migrates, via the blood, from the bone marrow to the thymus, where these cells become T lymphocytes. This step is essential in developing a functional immune system,

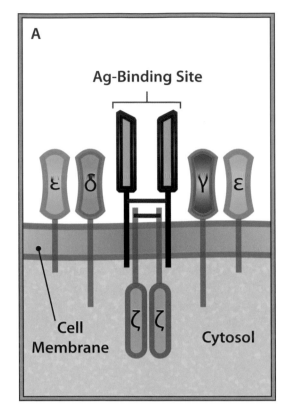

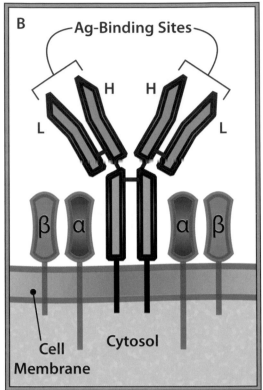

FIGURE 7.5A–B. **Antigen-specific receptors on T and B cells**

T (panel A) and B (panel B) lymphocytes—essential components of immune responses—are the only antigen-specific cells in animals. Distinct antigen-specific receptors on each of these cell types allow for direct interactions with pathogens and their antigens. The left panel shows the TCR embedded in the membrane of a T cell. The right panel depicts the BCR embedded in the membrane of a B cell. Ag = antigen.

and if it does not happen (as in nude mice), animals lack any sense of immunological self or non-self.

The mammalian thymus lies right above the heart and is largest shortly after birth; it then decreases significantly in size and function after sexual maturity. However, the thymus functions in all mammals throughout adult life.

The outer or cortical region of the thymus contains many lymphocytes called thymocytes (while they are in the thymus; see Figure 7.6). The inner or medullary region of the thymus contains mostly epithelial cells. Somehow, inside this organ, T cells acquire the ability to react with non-self.

Secondary Lymphoid Organs

Because the thymus generates T lymphocytes and the bone marrow (and the bursa of Fabricius) generates B lymphocytes, these organs are sometimes referred to as the primary lymphoid organs. The secondary lymphoid organs are the sites where the cells of the immune system and pathogens meet and immune responses occur. In animals' bodies, infections may begin in three major places: the interstitial fluid between the cells, the blood, and mucosal surfaces. Specialized lymphoid tissues or organs have evolved to deal with each. Lymph nodes screen interstitial fluid (lymph) draining from peripheral tissues, the spleen screens the

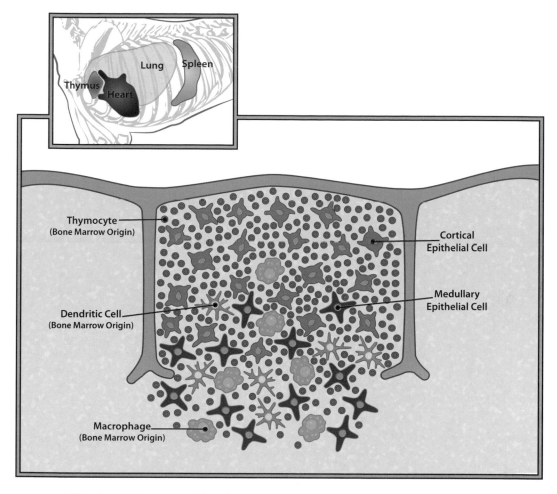

FIGURE 7.6. Structure of the mammalian thymus

The thymus contains several lobules, each of which can be divided into cortical (outer) and medullary (central) regions. The cortex contains immature dividing cells, and the medulla contains more mature cells. Many of these cells (thymocytes) are in the process of becoming T lymphocytes. In addition, thymic epithelial cells populate both cortical and medullary regions. Finally, the medulla also contains both macrophages and DCs that originated in the bone marrow.

blood, and the MALT monitors the mucosal tissues.

LYMPH NODES

All mammals have two circulatory systems: cardiovascular and lymphatic. The cardiovascular system is a closed system of arteries and veins that moves blood through the body to the heart, to the lungs, to the heart, and back to the body. Along the way—especially in the capillary beds—a lot of fluid leaks out into the tissues that surround the blood vessels. This fluid—which is a lot like plasma, minus some of the big proteins—is called lymph. The total volume of lymph that forms every day in most animals is nearly equal to the total plasma volume. Some means for collecting lymph and returning it to the circulation is essential, and that is the function of the lymphatics (see Figure 7.7).

Each of the vessels of the lymphatics terminates in a fingerlike projection with inward-

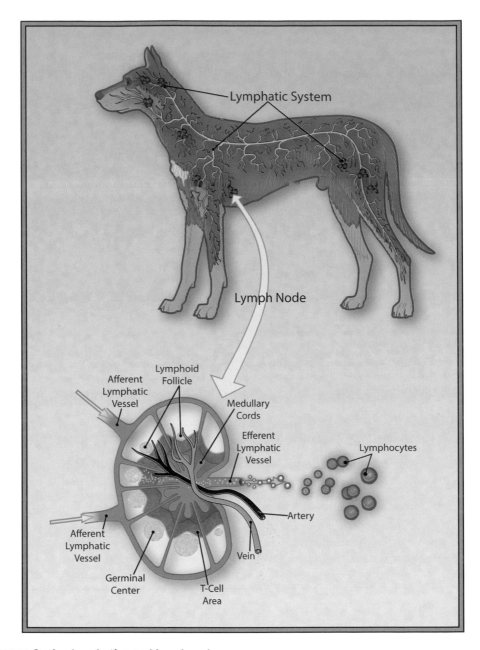

FIGURE 7.7. Canine lymphatics and lymph nodes

Lymphatics (upper portion) are a system of open-ended vessels that return extravascular fluid from the periphery to the heart and blood. Distributed throughout the lymphatics are a series of small filtering stations called lymph nodes. Each node has both cortical and medullary regions where different aspects of immune responses occur. The medullary regions contain B cells, DCs, T cells, and macrophages. The cortical regions contain structures called lymphoid follicles. During an immune response, germinal centers form inside of the lymphoid follicles. Germinal centers contain T cells, FDCs, and other DCs and some resting as well as rapidly dividing B cells. Each lymph node connects to the lymphatics via multiple afferent (inflowing) and one efferent (outflowing) lymphatic vessel as well as to the circulatory system by an arteriole and a venule.

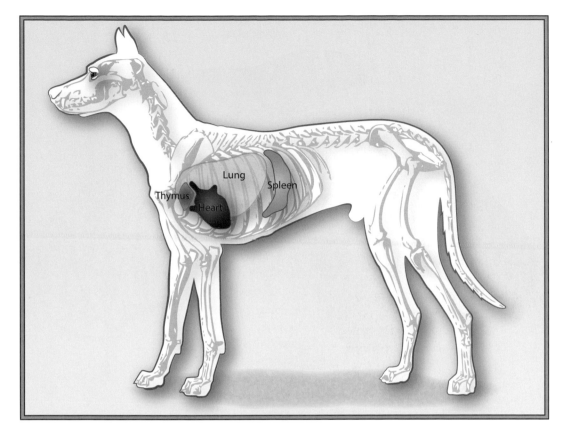

FIGURE 7.8. Canine spleen

The spleen (in green) is the site of most immune responses against blood-borne pathogens.

opening valves. Lymph flows out of the capillaries, into the interstitial tissue spaces, and through the valves into the lymphatics. Once inside the lymphatics, lymph (driven by the contraction of skeletal muscles) moves ultimately to the thoracic duct and to the right subclavian vein and into the heart. Along the way, many small nodes appear; these lymph nodes (see Figure 7.7) are filtering stations. During infections, DCs from the periphery deliver antigens to the lymph nodes. Blood delivers T cells and B cells to lymph nodes.

Inside of lymph nodes, T and B cells as well as macrophages and DCs interact to produce immune responses. The cortical regions of lymph nodes contain lymphoid follicles and germinal centers where B cells proliferate. The paracortical areas (between the cortex and the medulla), however, contain mostly T cells.

SPLEEN

Although spleen size varies considerably among mammals, the basic structures of all spleens are the same. Immunologically, the spleen does for blood-borne antigens what lymph nodes do for lymph-borne antigens (see Figure 7.8). In addition, with the help of resident macrophages, the spleen recycles some senescent RBCs.

Within the spleen, the white pulp contains the lymphoid tissues. Here, T-cell–rich regions surround the splenic arterioles to form a structure called the periarteriolar lymphoid sheath.

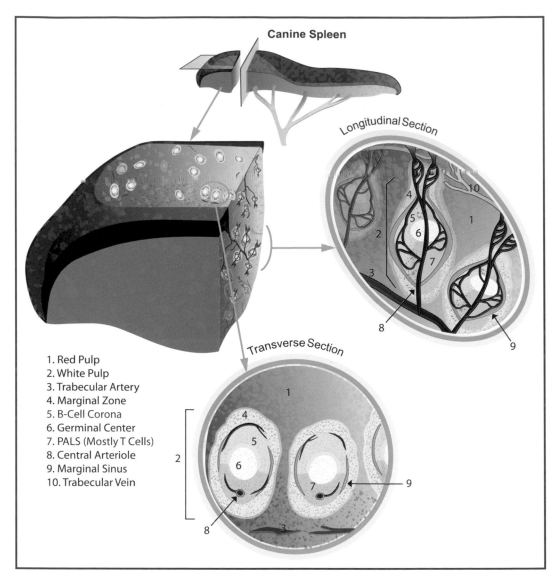

FIGURE 7.9. Structure of lymphoid tissue in the mammalian spleen

PALS = periarteriolar lymphoid sheath

Nearby are B-cell–rich areas that also contain germinal centers (see Figure 7.9).

The red pulp areas are sites of red blood cell destruction; the white pulp areas contain the lymphoid tissues in the periarteriolar lymphoid sheaths. As in lymph nodes, the T and B cells are unevenly distributed between germinal centers and the surrounding tissues. Also as in lymph nodes, germinal centers develop in the spleen when immune responses occur.

Mucosa-associated lymphoid tissues

The epithelial mucosa of all animals are, throughout their lives, constantly exposed to and colonized by potentially infectious agents, especially bacteria. The largest of these surfaces are the lungs and the gut. All mucosal tissues contain specialized lymphoid aggregates called MALT.

Gut-associated lymphoid tissues (GALT)—a part of MALT—include Peyer's patches in the small intestine and the cecal tonsils. The lymphoid tissues of the Peyer's patches are the most organized and possibly most important of these tissues (see Figure 7.10A–B). In the intestine, specialized epithelial cells called M cells transport antigens from the gut lumen into the lymphocyte-rich areas of the Peyer's patches. Approximately thirty to forty groups of Peyer's patches appear in an animal's intestine as elongated areas without villi.

These lymphoid tissues monitor the pathogens in the gut and deal with pathogenic organisms, usually without harming the normal gut flora. Mucosal immunology remains relatively poorly understood, but it is unquestionably one of the keys to understanding animals' immune systems and animal health.

Bronchus-associated lymphoid tissues—another part of MALT—are not as structured as GALT. However, the process by which they deal with inhaled pathogens is very similar to what occurs in GALT. Somewhat similar lymphoid tissues also appear on other mucosal surfaces such as the urethral and vaginal epithelia.

Despite their structural differences, the lymph nodes, spleen, and MALT—with few exceptions—all deal with antigens in very similar ways using the same types of cells.

CLINICAL CORRELATION: FOLLOW-UP

During discussions, the cat's owner shared that about a week before the cat's bout of lethargy and fever, the cat had killed and partially eaten a small feral rabbit. Wild rabbits are known reservoirs for tularemia, a sometimes fatal infectious disease in cats. The examining veterinarian requested a lymph node biopsy and a serum titer for *Francisella tularensis,* the causative agent for tularemia.

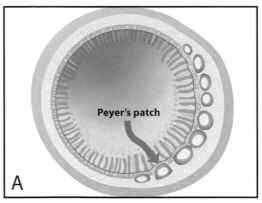

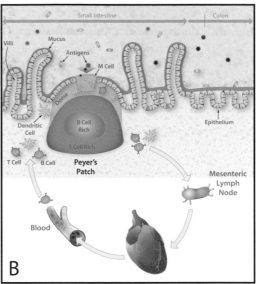

FIGURE 7.10A–B. Lymphoid tissues in the small intestine

Panel A is a diagram of a thin section of small intestine. Within this section, the dark purple–rimmed ovoid areas represent specialized lymphoid tissue called Peyer's patches—sites of immune responses in the intestine. Panel B is a diagrammatic representation of the interaction between the cells of a Peyer's patch and an enteric pathogen. M cells carry antigens from the gut lumen into the Peyer's patch where DCs process and present these antigens to the immune system. As with splenic lymphoid tissues, there are discrete T-cell–rich and B-cell–rich areas where immune responses begin. From these areas, cells enter the lymphatics and eventually the blood. From the blood, immune B and T cells return to mucosal tissues and mediate protection.

The biopsy revealed areas of focal necrosis and lymphoid hyperplasia, whereas the serum exhibited a titer of 1/80 for *F. tularensis*. Apparently, the observed lymphadenopathy was lymphadenitis, a result of the bacterial infection as well as the cat's immune response to the bacterium. After antibiotic treatment, the lymphadenopathy resolved, and the cat recovered.

Student Considerations

After having read this chapter and considered the nature, distribution, and function of lymph nodes, you should be able to offer at least two possible explanations for the symptoms observed in the patient described at the beginning of this chapter.

Possible Explanations

The association of lymphadenopathy with infectious diseases occurs for at least two reasons. First, it is possible for the nodes themselves to become infected, resulting in inflammation (lymphadenitis). This lymphadenopathy results from the inflammation and the movement of cells and fluid out of the blood and into the lymph nodes. Much more commonly, lymphadenopathy is the result of protective immune responses against infectious agents. Once antigens (pathogens or pieces of pathogens), T cells, and B cells arrive inside of lymph nodes, immune responses develop. Each of these immune responses involves massive proliferation of lymphocytes or lymphoid hyperplasia. These expanding cell populations cause lymph nodes to swell well beyond their normal size, as with human mandibular nodes during respiratory infections. This swelling is a reflection of the essential role of the lymph nodes in immunity and defense against infections.

Regardless of the cause, antibiotic therapy would be the appropriate course of action for the attending veterinarian. In this case, the nature of tularemia and the fact that the mandibular and cervical nodes showed areas of focal necrosis suggested that lymphadenitis was the cause of the swollen lymph nodes. The presence of antibody against *F. tularensis* indicates the cat had eaten an infected tick while killing or feeding on the rabbit, and the presence of this bacterium in the lymph nodes was the underlying cause of the lymphadenitis.

Gerald N. Callahan

Antigens and Antigen Processing

Chapter 8

10.5876_9781607322184.c008

CLINICAL CORRELATION: CAPRINE ARTHRITIS ENCEPHALITIS

When caprine arthritis encephalitis virus (CAEV) infects a herd of goats (Figure 8.1), most animals remain healthy even if infected. An unfortunate few, however, develop untreatable, debilitating diseases that manifest as polyarthritis and occasionally in kids as encephalomyelitis. Because CAEV infection is common and causes lifelong infections, several nations will not accept goats from countries where CAEV is enzootic, such as the United States.

Genetic studies of symptomatic and asymptomatic goats have yielded some of the most significant insights into the pathogenesis of CAEV. Genetically, a major difference exists between unaffected and affected goats. That difference maps onto a particular region of the caprine genome known as the major histocompatibility complex, or MHC.

Goats that develop arthritis, encephalitis, or both are more likely to carry one or both of two MHC alleles, Be1 and Be14. This finding suggests that the products of these MHC genes play major roles in the pathogenesis of CAEV. Associations between diseases and MHC alleles are not unique to goats. The first of these associations was identified in humans, and it showed a clear link between expression of a particular MHC class I allele, human leukocyte antigen–Bw27, and ankylosing spondylitis, a debilitating autoimmune disease. Other studies soon uncovered similar associations in most species of mammals. Table 8.1 shows MHC alleles associated with various diseases in cattle. The MHC alleles of cattle are also called bovine leukocyte antigen alleles.

Today, it is clear that MHC genes play a role in a variety of diseases in many mammalian species. But how MHC genes affect disease processes remains murky. A more complete understanding of the relationship between MHC and disease is likely to offer new insights into disease prevention and therapy.

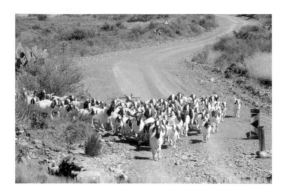

FIGURE 8.1. **South African goat herd (© WOLF AVNI/ Shutterstock)**

LEARNING OBJECTIVES

After reading this chapter, you should be able to

- distinguish among pathogens, antigens, immunogens, and epitopes;
- know the properties that make a molecule antigenic;
- know the general character of the mammalian MHC;
- distinguish between class I and class II MHC genes and molecules;
- understand how MHC molecules bind antigens and the differences between antigens bound by class I or class II molecules;
- know the different classes of APCs and their distributions;
- understand how APCs process and present antigens and the roles of MHC class I and class II molecules in this process;
- explain why certain MHC genes may predispose animals to some diseases.

STIMULATORS OF ADAPTIVE IMMUNITY: PATHOGENS, ANTIGENS, AND EPITOPES

The word *antigen* apparently arose as a condensation of the words *antibody generator,* but that is not exactly what all antigens are. More accurately, antigens are molecules or pieces of molecules that bind to antibodies, MHC molecules, or TCRs. The two antigen subcategories are immunogens—substances capable of stimulating an immune response—and haptens—substances that will not by themselves produce an immune response but can do so when complexed with a larger molecules, such as a host protein.

Despite these different ways of speaking about molecules that interact with immune systems, in practice, most immunologists refer to all immunogens and haptens simply as antigens. In the remainder of this book, we consider antigens to be any molecules that can stimulate adaptive immune responses.

Because of their roles in defense, immune systems are generally thought to focus on non-self—things foreign to hosts. But not all foreign things are antigenic, and sometimes parts of self may be antigenic. How do molecules that are antigenic and those that are not differ?

To be capable of stimulating an adaptive immune response a substance must be

- complex,
- organic,
- degradable,
- large.

These properties are necessary for a molecule to be antigenic, but not all complex, organic, degradable, large molecules are antigenic in any given animal. For example, bovine serum albumin fulfills all of these conditions and is, thus, antigenic in mice, but under normal conditions bovine serum albumin is not antigenic in cattle. So, often (but not always), an antigenic molecule must, in addition to all of the preceding properties, be recognizably foreign.

All living things carry unique chemical signatures, which is what separates one animal or even one bacterium from another. Among those chemical signatures, proteins are the most individually distinct. Among the biological macromolecules, no other group so finely differentiates individual organisms.

TABLE 8.1. Cattle MHC alleles and disease susceptibility

Disease	Breed	Bovine major histo-compatibility system	Effect
ENZOOTIC BOVINE LEUKOSIS			
Seroconversion	Holstein	A14	Late
	Holstein	A15	Rapid
	Guernsey	A21	Late
	Guernsey	DA6.2, A12	Rapid
Peripheral lymphocytes and B-cell numbers	Shorthorn	DA7	Resistance
	Shorthorn	DA12.3	Susceptibility
	I. Shorthorn	A6, EU28R	Susceptibility
	I. Shorthorn	A8	Resistance
	Holstein	A12 and A15	Susceptibility
	Holstein	A14 and A13	Resistance
	Holstein	DRB22A	Resistance
	Holstein	DRB21C	Susceptibility
	Holstein	DRB3(ERmotif)	Resistance
	Holstein	DRB3(ERmotif)	Resistance
MASTITIS			
Clinical mastitis	Norwegian Red	A2	Resistance
	Norwegian Red	A16	Susceptibility
	Swedish Red & White	DQ1A	Susceptibility
	Holstein	A11	Resistance
	Holstein	CA42	Susceptibility
Subclinical mastitis (cell count)	Icelandic	A19	Susceptibility
	Simmental (S) or S × Red Holstein	A15	High
	Danish Black Pied	A11, A30	Low
	Danish Black Pied	A21, A26	High
California Mastitis Test	Holstein	A14	Low
HELMINTHS			
Nematodes	Belmont Red	A7, CA36	Resistance
	Africander × Hereford	A9	Susceptibility
PROTOZOA			
Theileria parva	Bos indicus	Class I	Parasite entry
TICKS			
Boophilus Microplus	Brahman × Shorthorn	A6, CA31	Susceptibility
Posterior spinal paresis	Holstein	A8	Susceptibility
Ketosis	Norwegian Red	A2, A13	Resistance
Retained placenta	Dutch Friesian	Compatibility	Susceptibility

Proteins make all life possible. Proteins are, of course, strings of amino acids linked by peptide bonds. But unlike carbohydrates or nucleic acids, at every position in a protein there are twenty possible amino acids to choose from. That makes proteins unique identifiers—markers that set each animal apart from all the rest. Adaptive immune systems exploit those differences.

Proteins are the most potent of all antigens, and the antigenicity of most pathogens depends on their protein components. Whether a protein stimulates an immune response, however, depends on the properties of that protein.

Artificial proteins constructed from a single amino acid—for example, homoalanine—elicit no immune responses. Complexity appears to be an absolute requirement for antigenicity. Similarly, a protein constructed from D-amino acids will not stimulate an immune response in any animal. All naturally occurring amino acids are L-amino acids. Because of that, all naturally occurring proteases have evolved to focus on L-amino acids and cannot split peptide bonds formed between D-amino acids. To be antigenic, a protein must be complex and degradable by naturally occurring proteolytic enzymes.

Enzymatic degradation of proteins is essential, because T cells—essential components of all immune responses—cannot recognize intact proteins. Before an immune response can begin, antigenic proteins must be chopped into pieces and presented by an MHC molecule, and MHC molecules only bind to peptide bits of protein antigens.

Small proteins ($<2,500$ molecular weight) make poor antigens, and inorganic molecules—unless coupled to proteins—generally do not elicit immune responses. Inorganic molecules are not usually major parts of the pathogenic world. Also, of course, immune systems have evolved to focus on pathogens—transmissible agents of disease: viruses, bacteria, fungi, and parasites.

Almost all pathogens induce a wide range of immune responses. Interestingly, though, not all pathogen parts are equally antigenic, not even all the proteins. Beyond that, not all parts of pathogen-derived antigenic proteins are equally antigenic (see Figure 8.2). Some pieces of the pathogen's proteins stimulate strong responses, whereas others go unrecognized. For example, Figure 8.2 shows antigenic portions of proteins that stimulate immune responses (red or yellow) and other portions that fail to stimulate immune responses (green).

The parts of proteins that stimulate immune responses are called antigenic epitopes (or simply epitopes) and come in at least two forms—continuous and discontinuous. A continuous epitope is the product of the contiguous amino acids in the primary sequence of the protein. A discontinuous epitope involves noncontiguous amino acids and results from the secondary, tertiary, or quaternary structure of the protein, as shown in Figure 8.2. Because of the manner in which they acquire antigens, MHC molecules bind only continuous antigenic epitopes. Only B-cell receptors and antibody molecules (see chapters 11 and 12) recognize and bind to discontinuous antigenic epitopes.

MAJOR HISTOCOMPATIBILITY COMPLEX

History of the Major Histocompatibility Complex

Nearly as long as people have known about the origins of cancers, scientists have been interested in the role of immunity in defense against tumors. As discussed further in chapter 17, in the early 1960s Sir MacFarlane Burnet and Lewis Thomas even went so far as to propose that a primary role of mammalian immune systems was to detect and destroy tumors. This proposal came to be called the theory of immune surveillance.

To investigate this theory, scientists began studying mouse tumors. Initially, those studies focused on transplanting tumors from mouse to mouse. Some transplanted tumors grew well

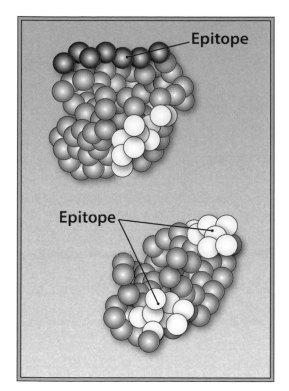

FIGURE 8.2. Antigenic epitopes of an immunogenic protein

Not all portions of a protein activate the host's immune system. Those segments that do stimulate immunity are antigenic epitopes. They can be of two types: continuous epitopes involving adjacent amino acids (shown in red) or discontinuous epitopes formed by the secondary or tertiary structure of the protein (shown in yellow). Here, each ball represents an amino acid.

in some mice, but not in others. For this reason, some investigators thought they had discovered tumor-specific factors that might be manipulated for cancer treatment. But in similar experiments using normal tissues, scientists got the same results. Instead of something unique to tumors, what these scientists had discovered was a group of genes whose products determined the immunological compatibility of tissues (malignant and otherwise) transplanted from one mouse strain to another.

Studies with other mammalian species yielded similar results: the success or failure of al-

lografts depended on the similarity or dissimilarity of only a few genes. Because these genes had a major effect on tissue (or histo-) compatibility, they were called the major histocompatibility complex, or MHC.

Each species has its own set of MHC genes and, within each species, a unique name for the MHC. Because these molecules were originally found on white blood cells, almost every MHC name contains the words *leukocyte antigen*. The MHC in humans is also called the HLA (human leukocyte antigen) complex, in monkeys it is also called the RHA (rhesus leukocyte antigen) complex, in cattle it is BLA (bovine leukocyte antigen) complex, and so on. Only mice and rats depart from this general rule. The MHC of mice is called H-2 and the MHC of rats is called RT1.

Although they were discovered during transplantation experiments, these genes did not evolve simply to frustrate transplant surgeons. Instead, the products of MHC genes bind and present antigens to T cells, and those T cells direct immune responses. Sometimes those immune responses cause graft rejection, but more often they help to protect animals from the pathogenic world.

Major Histocompatibility Complex Genetics

The basic structure of the MHC is similar in all mammals. Figure 8.3A–C shows the MHCs of horses, humans, and mice.

Within each MHC are three distinct gene types: MHC class I, MHC class II, and several other genes called MHC class III. Also, the products of DM, DN, and DO genes in humans and H-2M in mice, although structurally homologous to other MHC class II molecules, are much less variable and function differently than other MHC class II gene products.

From end to end, the MHC in mice and humans spans about 4×10^6 base pairs. Each MHC contains multiple genes encoding class I MHC molecules and multiple genes encoding class

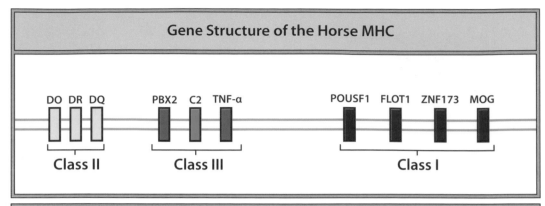

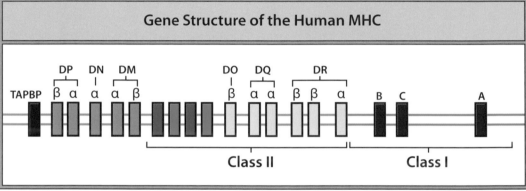

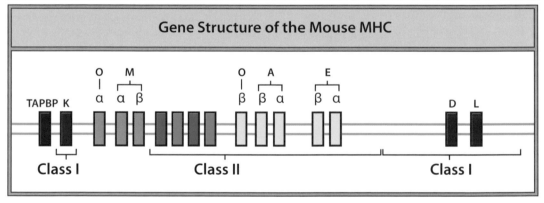

FIGURE 8.3A–C. Diagrammatic representation of the chromosomal organization of MHCs of horses, humans, and mice

MHC class I genes are shown in red, and MHC class II genes are shown in yellow. All mammalian MHCs contain additional genes (sometimes called class III genes) that are involved in some immune and non-immune functions unrelated to the roles of MHC class I and II genes (shown in green and blue).

II MHC molecules. In the mouse MHC, three separate loci code for three different MHC class I molecules, and two distinct regions code for MHC class II molecules. In horses, four sepa-rate loci encode four distinct MHC class I mol-ecules, and five separate regions produce five separate MHC class II molecules. Expression of MHC class I and II genes is codominant, mean-

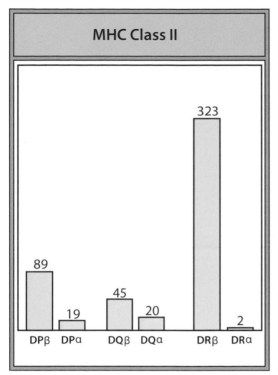

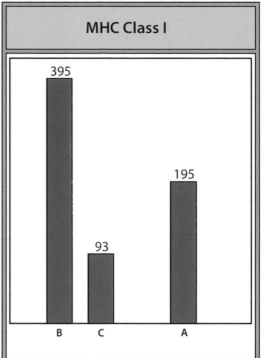

FIGURE 8.4. MHC gene polymorphism

Except for the DRα locus, each MHC class I and MHC class II locus has many possible alleles, which means that among populations of mammals enormous variety is present in the genetic characteristics of the MHC.

ing that each animal expresses the alleles on both parental chromosomes.

MHC proteins, as mentioned earlier, bind bits of protein antigens and present them to T cells. If that does not happen—if some pathogen escapes MHC molecules—the host animal is more likely to succumb to that infection. To deal with this potential problem, each MHC molecule has evolved to bind a variety of antigens, but in spite of that evolutionary pressure, no one MHC molecule can bind all potential antigens. Instead, over time, the MHC of mammals has grown to include multiple loci encoding class I and II MHC molecules. Those additional loci add another level of protection. Multiple loci encoding MHC class I and class II molecules reduce the chance of an animal's encountering a pathogen that can escape the

animal's immune system. Up to a point, the more MHC molecules an animal has, the more pathogens it can effectively present to its immune system. Therefore, multiple loci help to protect each mammal from a diverse and evolving pathogenic world.

Beyond multiple loci, the genes of the MHC are the most polymorphic genes in mammals. Thus, at every locus that encodes an MHC molecule, there are many possible alleles. For example, humans have six loci involved in producing MHC class II molecules—DPα, DPβ, DQα, DQβ, DRα, and DRβ. Every human has all of these loci, but not all humans have the same allele at each locus. The human population has at least 20 different alleles possible at the DQα locus, 89 at the DPβ locus, 45 at the DQβ locus, 20 at the DQα locus, 323 at the

DRβ locus, and 2 at the DRα locus (see Figure 8.4).

As a result, in addition to multiple MHC loci in each individual, there are multiple alleles at each MHC locus in the population at large. So, although every human being has a DRβ locus, it is rare for two unrelated people to have the same allele at that locus, meaning that among humans, as with most other animal populations, finding two human beings with the same set of genes in their MHCs is extremely improbable (except for identical twins). Because the products of these genes also play a role in graft rejection, MHC polymorphism is a major reason for the difficulties in finding compatible kidney, heart, or liver donors for identified recipients. Much more important, MHC polymorphisms offer essential protection for both individuals and species.

Usually, when an infectious disease strikes a population of animals, some individuals will die and others will survive. One significant difference between survivors and fatalities is often the complement of MHC molecules present in each individual. Some animals will have the MHC molecule needed to present the critical antigenic epitope or epitopes to the immune system and neutralize the pathogen, and others will not.

Thus, species-wide MHC polymorphisms dramatically reduce the likelihood that a single infectious agent will destroy an entire population of animals. Some notable exceptions to this include African cheetahs, Florida panthers, and the lions of Ngorongoro crater in Tanzania.

Between 10,000 and 20,000 years ago, the cheetah population dwindled to one or two mating pairs. All of the cheetahs alive today came from those mates. Because of this, cheetahs are now genetically nearly identical. This sort of event is called genetic bottlenecking.

Cheetahs are now so similar, they do not reject skin grafts from one another, their MHCs are nearly identical, and when their hides are stacked atop one another, all of the spots line up perfectly. In a population such as this one, if

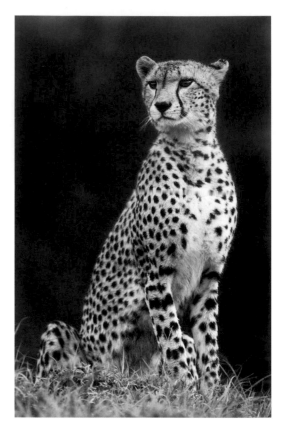

FIGURE 8.5. **African cheetah (© Anna Omelchenko / Shutterstock)**

African cheetahs are genetically very homogeneous and at risk for decimation by infectious pathogens.

an infectious disease kills one animal, it is likely that it will kill every animal.

For the lions of the Ngorongoro crater, geographical isolation led to genetic bottlenecking. The result, however, was the same. In 1962, an infestation of biting flies and their parasites killed all but ten or so of these lions.

Much more recently, genetic bottlenecking happened in the Florida panther. All of the Florida panthers alive in the twentieth century appear to have come from a single female. Disease and human pressures nearly destroyed this population. In 1995, five Texas pumas were introduced into panther habitat, and the resulting hybrids appear to be doing well. However,

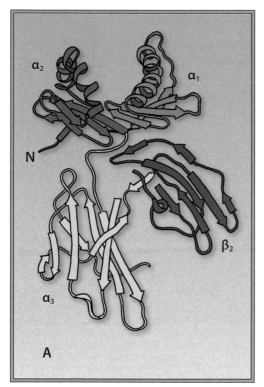

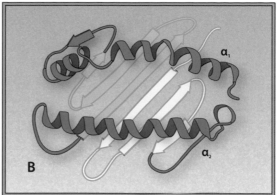

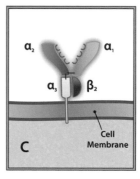

FIGURE 8.6A–C. MHC class I structure

Approximate representations of MHC class I molecules. Panel A shows a ribbon diagram of the MHC class I α chain (MHC derived) and β_2-microglobulin. The tertiary structure of the class I α chain contains three separate structural domains: α_1, α_2, and α_3. The α_1 and α_2 domains form a cuplike groove near the N-terminal region of the molecules and form the peptide–antigen binding site. Flat ribbons ending in arrows indicate regions of β-pleated sheet, and the helical ribbons indicate regions of α-helix. Panel B shows a top view of the MHC class I peptide–antigen binding site. Note how the α-helical regions frame the flat segments of β-pleated sheet to form the binding site. Panel C shows a diagrammatic representation of an MHC class I molecule including the transmembrane domain of the α chain. The purple band across the figure bottom represents the lipid-bilayer outer membrane of a eukaryotic cell. (Panels A and B adapted from C. Janeway, P. Travers, M. Walport, and M. Shlomchik, 2006, *Immunobiology*, 122)

because of the MHC homogeneity in these species, some scientists predict that none of these populations will survive the next few decades.

Structure and Distribution of Major Histocompatibility Complex Class I and Class II Molecules

Both MHC class I and II molecules are cell-surface glycoproteins composed of two polypeptide chains. MHC class I molecules contain an MHC-encoded α chain and a smaller molecule called β_2-microglobulin. Both of the two chains of MHC class II molecules, α and β, come from genes within the MHC (see Figure 8.6A–C).

Although MHC class I and II molecules have similar tertiary and quaternary structures, these MHC molecules are chemically distinct. Those chemical distinctions result in some important structural differences at the antigen-

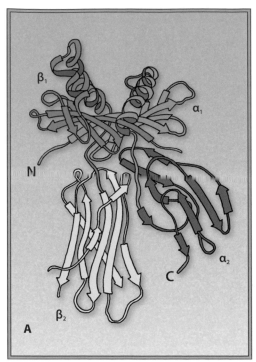

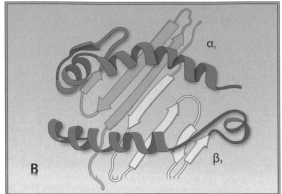

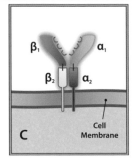

FIGURE 8.7A–C. MHC class II structure

Approximate representations of MHC class II molecules. Panel A shows a ribbon diagram of the MHC class II α chain and β chain. Each chain contains three separate structural domains: α_1, α_2, and α_3, as well as β_1, β_2, and β_3. The α_1 and α_2 domains, along with the β_1 and β_2 domains, form a cuplike groove near the N-terminal region of the molecules and form the peptide–antigen binding site. Panel B shows a top view of the MHC class II peptide–antigen binding site. Panel C shows a diagrammatic representation of an MHC class I molecule including the transmembrane domain of the α and β chains. The purple band across the figure bottom represents the lipid-bilayer outer membrane of a eukaryotic cell. (Panels A and B adapted from C. Janeway, P. Travers, M. Walport, and M. Shlomchik, 2006, *Immunobiology*, 123)

binding site. For this reason, MHC class I and class II molecules bind distinct sets of antigenic peptides. In addition, the biosynthetic pathways of MHC class I and class II molecules differ (discussion follows). Because of that difference, class I and II molecules bind antigenic peptides in different intracellular compartments and present these antigens to distinct subsets of T cells.

In MHC class I molecules, only the α chains are encoded in the MHC. The first and second domains of these α chains—where all of the allelic polymorphisms reside—form the antigen-

binding grooves. Only the α chain spans the lipid bilayer. β_2-microglobulin binds noncovalently to the MHC class I α chain and is monomorphic. Two short stretches of α-helix above a relatively flat plane of β-pleated sheet (all part of the MHC class I α chain) frame the antigen-binding groove of MHC class I proteins (see Figure 8.6A–C).

Both the α and β chains of MHC class II molecules come from the MHC region, both span the cell membrane, and both contribute to the antigen-binding groove of the molecule. Again, two coils of α-helix above a plane of β-pleated sheet create the groove itself. In MHC class II molecules, however, the ends of the α-helices are further apart than in MHC class I molecules, leaving open ends to the groove. Because of this, MHC class II molecules can bind slightly larger peptides than those bound by MHC class I molecules. However, the peptides bound by MHC class I or II molecules are not large enough to have significant secondary or tertiary structure. As a result, only linear, continuous antigenic epitopes bind to MHC molecules. Together, the binding cleft of MHC molecules and their bound peptides create the ligands recognizable to T lymphocytes.

Still, MHC class I and class II molecules play very different roles in developing immune responses, and the tissue distribution of MHC class I and class II molecules reflects their unique roles. MHC class I antigens appear on all or nearly all nucleated cells, whereas MHC class II molecules appear only on APCs. Recall from earlier chapters that macrophages and DCs are APCs, as are B cells and other cells such as astrocytes in the central nervous system and thymic epithelial cells.

Antigen–Major Histocompatibility Complex Interactions

As mentioned, each MHC molecule will bind multiple (but not all) antigenic peptides, which means the interactions between antigens and MHC molecules have some specificity. That specificity comes from noncovalent interactions between certain amino acids in the binding cleft and amino acids in the antigenic peptide (see Figure 8.8).

MHC class I molecules bind eight- to ten-amino-acid-long peptides (see Figure 8.8 and Figure 8.9), but not all of the amino acids in each peptide are equally important to the binding affinity. Instead, MHC class I–peptide interactions depend on as few as two amino acids. The spacing of those two amino acids is critical, because they must line up with corresponding amino acids in the binding cleft of

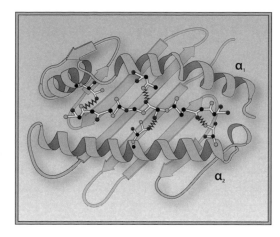

FIGURE 8.8. Antigen binding by MHC class I molecules

This ribbon diagram shows an approximation of an MHC class I molecule–peptide complex from above. Two stretches of α-helix near the N-terminal portion of the α chain form the boundaries of the binding cleft. The antigenic peptide lies in the binding cleft of the MHC class I molecule. The diagram also shows the noncovalent interactions (in red) between amino acid side chains of the MHC α chain and the peptide. (Adapted from C. Janeway, P. Travers, M. Walport, and M. Shlomchik, 2006, *Immunobiology*, 125)

the MHC molecule, but the rest of the peptide is irrelevant to MHC binding. That degenerate specificity allows MHC molecules to bind many different antigenic peptides. As a result—using a relatively small amount of DNA—mammals are capable of defending themselves against most pathogens.

MHC class II molecules bind peptides of varying lengths (typically from twelve to twenty-four amino acids). Because the binding cleft of MHC class II proteins is open at both ends, the absolute length of the peptide is less important than is the position of certain amino acids relative to one another (see Figures 8.10 and 8.11). Again, not all of the amino acids in the peptide bind to the MHC class II molecule, and as few as two amino acids may determine the

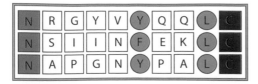

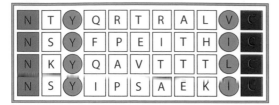

FIGURE 8.9. **Molecular properties of peptides bound by MHC class I molecules**

Upper and lower panels show the amino acid sequence of peptides that bind to two different MHC class I alleles. Although all of the peptides differ, the green amino acids indicate the features they share. In the first set of peptides, the amino acid found at position 5 must be either phenylalanine (F) or tyrosine (Y), and the amino acid found at the C-terminal position must be leucine (L). Similarly, peptides that react with the second MHC class I allele must contain tyrosine at position 2 and a C-terminal valine (V), leucine, or isoleucine (I). In addition, the length of the peptides is critical. For the first MHC class I allele, each peptide must be exactly eight amino acids long, whereas for the second allele, each peptide must be exactly nine amino acids long. The critical points of interaction for the first allele are the amino group at the peptide's N-terminus, amino acids 5 and 8, and the hydroxyl group at the C-terminus. The amino acids at all of the other positions in these peptides are irrelevant to the peptide's MHC class I binding affinity. This specificity is relatively degenerate, meaning that any given MHC class I allele will bind many peptide antigens, but not all. (Adapted from C. Janeway, P. Travers, M. Walport, and M. Shlomchik, 2006, *Immunobiology*, 126)

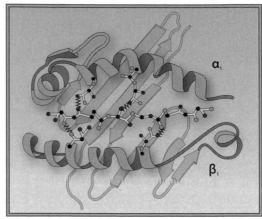

FIGURE 8.10. **Antigen binding by MHC class II molecules**

This ribbon diagram shows an approximate representation of an MHC class II molecule–peptide complex from above. Two stretches of α-helix—one from the N-terminal portion of the α chain and the other from the N-terminal portion of the β chain—form the boundaries of the binding cleft. The antigenic peptide lies in the binding cleft of the MHC class II molecule. In addition, the diagram shows the noncovalent interactions between amino acid side chains of the MHC α and β chains and the peptide in red. (After C. Janeway, P. Travers, M. Walport, and M. Shlomchik, 2006, *Immunobiology*, 127)

MHC class I and II molecules also routinely bind and present self peptides. MHC molecules bind and present almost all intracellular and extracellular proteins—self or non-self. For a variety of reasons (discussed in subsequent chapters), this does not routinely result in autoimmune destruction of self tissues. As you will see, though, in type II hypersensitivities and other disorders, self-presentation and autoimmunity are at the root of many animal diseases.

ANTIGEN ACQUISITION, PROCESSING, AND PRESENTATION

Antigen-Presenting Cells

The function of MHC class I and class II molecules is to present peptide antigens to T lym-

capacity of a peptide to bind to an MHC class II molecule.

It is important to recognize that, although this discussion focuses on the antigens of pathogens,

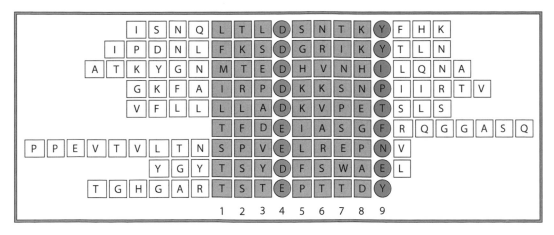

FIGURE 8.11. Antigen-binding motif of MHC class II molecules

Because the ends to the antigen-binding cleft of MHC class II molecules are open, the molecules bind peptides of varying lengths (typically twelve to twenty-four amino acids). The gray regions represent the portion of the peptide containing the anchor residues—the amino acids actually within the binding site of the MHC class II molecule. The peptides that bind to this particular MHC class II molecule range from thirteen to nineteen amino acids long. However, among all of these peptides, only amino acids 4 and 9 appear critical for binding to this MHC class II allele. Amino acid 4 must be aspartic acid (D) or glutamic acid (E). Amino acid 9 must usually be a hydrophobic or uncharged amino acid—tyrosine (Y), isoleucine (I), proline (P), threonine (T), phenylalanine (F), asparagine (N), or glutamic acid. As with MHC class I molecules, this specificity is relatively degenerate (especially compared with the specificities of B- and T-cell receptors). So, each MHC class II molecule can bind many different, but not all, peptides. (Adapted from C. Janeway, P. Travers, M. Walport, and M. Shlomchik, 2001, *Immunobiology*, fig. 3.26)

TABLE 8.2. Distribution and properties of APCs

	Macrophage	*DC*	*B cell*
MHC-II expression	Low levels; induced by PAMPs, DAMPs, and cytokines	Always expressed	Always expressed; inducible on activation
Antigen type and presentation by MHC	Extracellular antigens: presentation via MHC II	Intracellular & extracellular antigens: presentation via MHC I & MHC II	Extracellular antigen binds to specific Ig receptors: presentation via MHC II
Location	Lymphoid tissue Connective tissue Body cavities	Lymphoid tissue Connective tissue Epithelium	Lymphoid tissue Blood

phocytes. The cells that use MHC class I and class II molecules to perform this function are APCs. Outside the primary lymphoid organs and the central nervous system, macrophages, DCs, and B cells are the major APCs (see Figures 8.12–8.14).

All of these cells share certain characteristics, but each excels at acquisition of certain types of antigens (see Table 8.2), and each APC has a unique distribution in peripheral tissues and secondary lymphoid organs. In addition, these cells differ in how they acquire antigen and what they do with it (see Figures 8.12, 8.13, and 8.14).

There are several important DC subsets, including lymphoid, plasmacytoid, myeloid, and

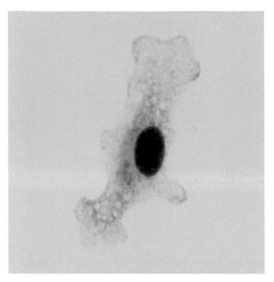
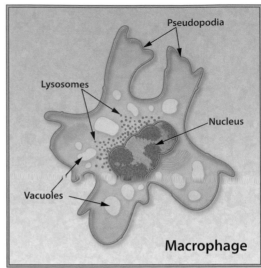

FIGURE 8.12. **Macrophage photo and drawing**

The large cell in the center is a macrophage with pseudopodia. Macrophages acquire antigens by phagocytosis and endocytosis.

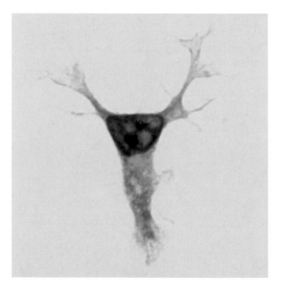
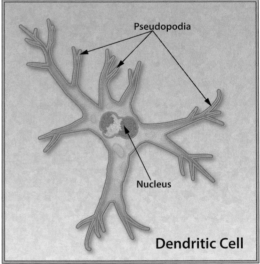

FIGURE 8.13. **DC: photo and drawing**

This cell is called a DC because of the long processes. These cells also acquire antigens through phagocytosis or endocytosis.

follicular. Each differs in location and effectiveness as an APC. In peripheral tissues, myeloid DCs seem to be most common. We focus primarily on myeloid DCs.

Macrophages and DCs acquire antigens in several ways—through fluid-phase macropinocytosis, endocytosis, and phagocytosis of whole pathogens. Endocytosis and phagocytosis can

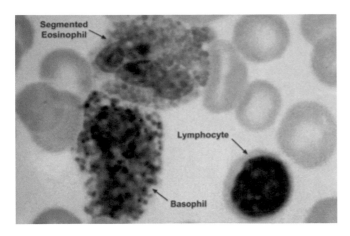

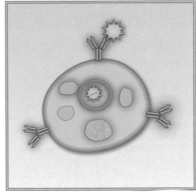

B Cell

FIGURE 8.14. B cells

Graphic representation of mammalian B cell (right panel) and micrograph of a B cell (labeled "lymphocyte" in left panel). This mononuclear cell is one of two types of white blood cells called lymphocytes, a B lymphocyte or B cell. It is the ultimate source of antibody molecules. B cells use BCRs to specifically bind antigen, endocytose it, and process it.

occur via PRRs such as the MR and scavenger receptor (see chapters 3 and 6). Simple high-mannose glycoproteins are present in greatest quantities on prokaryotic organisms, because these organisms do not have Golgi apparati where most complex sugar modifications occur in eukaryotes.

B cells acquire antigens only through receptor-mediated endocytosis. For this purpose, B cells use a unique receptor—the BCR. The antigen-binding part of that receptor is, of course, the same as the antigen-binding region of an antibody molecule. B cells are the only APCs that acquire antigens in an antigen-specific manner.

Major Histocompatibility Complex Class I Antigen Processing and Presentation

Inside animals are two spaces where infectious agents may proliferate—inside of cells (intracellular) and outside of cells in fluid spaces (extracellular). For an immune system to be protective, it must have information about events in both of those two spaces. MHC class I molecules mostly present intracellular antigens, and MHC class II molecules mostly present antigens from outside of the cell (extracellular antigen).

A subset of all proteins produced in the cytosol of eukaryotic cells includes misfolded, mutant, damaged, and excess proteins. To maintain cellular homeostasis, the cell needs to divest itself of these proteins. For this purpose, eukaryotic cells have evolved specialized cellular structures called proteasomes—large barrel-shaped protein complexes in the cytosol of eukaryotic cells. Proteolysis (the breakdown of proteins) occurs within the core of proteasomes. Each proteasome core contains one α ring at each end and two β rings in between (see Figure 8.15).

Beta rings have three enzymatically active sites with three separate specificities. B1 cleaves on the C-terminal side of hydrophobic residues; B2 cleaves on the C-terminal side of basic amino acids; and B3 cleaves on the C-terminal side of acidic residues. As a result, intact proteins enter one end of the proteasome, and peptides of various lengths exit the other end of the proteasome. Although they all perform

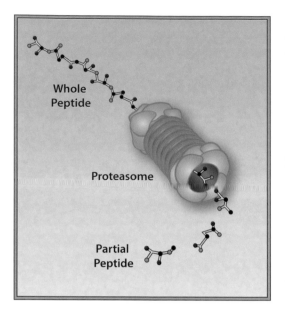

Proteasomes are cellular structures that digest intracellular proteins into short stretches of linear polypeptides and are essential to normal antigen processing.

similar functions, not all proteasomes are alike. At least two proteasome subtypes have been identified—immunoproteasomes and thymoproteasomes. How these subtypes affect immune responses remains unclear. Regardless, one end of cellular proteasomes collects representatives of all intracellular proteins (self or non-self) and digests them into smaller peptides. Mammalian immune systems use those peptides and transporters associated with antigen presentation (TAPs) to deliver those peptides into the endoplasmic reticulum (ER).

In the absence of infection, the proteins entering and the peptides leaving proteasomes are all parts of self. As we discuss later, immune systems—for the most part—ignore self. However, if an intracellular virus or bacterium is actively assembling itself inside of a host cell, the proteasomes will also be delivering peptides derived from that virus or bacterium.

The first phase of MHC class I molecule assembly occurs on the ribosomes of the rough ER. As each MHC protein assembles, the product extrudes into the lumen of the ER. Inside the ER, nascent MHC class I molecules, associated with chaperone proteins, bind $\beta 2$-microglobulin, acquire peptide antigens, and assume their final configurations. Because of TAP transporters, the peptides available to MHC class I molecules include not only those present in the ER but also those created in the cytosol (see Figures 8.16 and 8.17).

As MHC class I α-chain proteins extrude off ribosomes and into the ER, they associate with a series of molecular chaperones. These molecules, along with β_2-microglobulin, force the α-chain–β_2-microglobulin complex into an antigen-binding form. After antigen binding, the MHC α-chain–β_2-microglobulin complexes, along with the bound antigen, move from the ER to the Golgi complex and finally to the cell surface. This process occurs inside most mammalian cells. For this reason, most cells present an exterior image of internal events. As you will see, a particular T-cell subset—CD8$^+$ T cells—takes advantage of this image to find and destroy infected cells.

Major Histocompatibility Complex Class II Antigen Processing and Presentation

What about extracellular infections, microbes that never reside in a cell's cytosol, or organisms such as leishmania that grow inside of intracellular vesicles? Monitoring for extracellular and intravesicular infections is the function of MHC class II molecules. As with MHC class I molecules, class II molecules are also synthesized on and extruded into the lumen of the rough ER (see Figures 8.18 and 8.19).

Unlike class I molecules, as soon as MHC class II α and β chains associate inside the ER, a protein called the invariant chain (Ii) binds to and blocks the antigen-binding cleft. Because of this, no antigenic peptide inside of the ER can bind to an MHC class II molecule. Also, unlike MHC class I molecules, after MHC class II

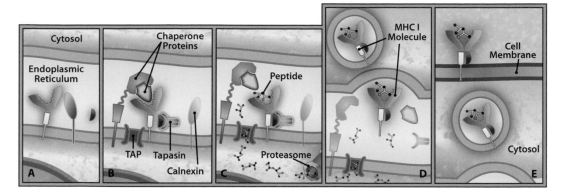

FIGURE 8.16. Antigen processing and presentation by MHC class I molecules

As with all proteins destined for the cell surface, MHC class I molecules, as they are synthesized, insert their N-termini into the ER but remain anchored in the ER membrane (A). Inside the ER, the body of MHC class I α chains interact with a series of chaperone proteins (shown here in gray) that, along with $β_2$-microglobulin (purple), force the α chain into its final configuration (B). A subset of all proteins made in the cytosol collects in proteasomes where enzymes cleave the proteins into small peptide fragments. The TAP moves these peptides into the lumen of the ER (C). Once inside the ER, the peptides encounter MHC class I molecules. Under the right conditions, the peptides bind into the antigen-binding groove of MHC class I molecules. The chaperone proteins detach (D), and the MHC class I–peptide complex continues on to the Golgi complex and then to the cell surface (E).

molecules pass through the Golgi complex, they move—via the trans-Golgi network—into acidic vesicles that fuse with lysosomes.

Pathogens and other antigens acquired by macropinocytosis, phagocytosis, or receptor-mediated endocytosis end up in endosomes or phagosomes that eventually fuse with lysosomes. So in the end, endosomes and lysosomes contain extracellular antigens and MHC class II molecules.

Recall from chapter 6 that lysosomes are acidic compartments filled with proteolytic enzymes. As endosomes or phagosomes carrying exogenously acquired antigens (which may include pathogens) fuse with lysosomes, protein antigens are quickly chopped into peptides. The enzymes in lysosomes also remove most of the Ii from MHC class II molecules. The last piece of Ii—the CLIP—remains bound to the binding groove until the very last, when an MHC class II surrogate molecule (human leukocyte antigen-M in humans) alters the structure of MHC class II molecules in such a way that the

CLIP dissociates. Removal of CLIP leaves the antigen-binding groove empty so that exogenously acquired antigenic peptides can bind to the MHC class II molecule. All of this ensures that most MHC class II molecules bind antigens that came from outside of the APCs.

From the endolysosome–phagolysosome compartment, MHC class II molecules, along with bound antigens, move to the surface of the APCs, where they present an antigenic picture of what is happening in the extracellular space near the APC and within vesicles inside the APC. A T-cell subset—CD4[+] T cells—monitors MHC class II molecules and their contents and, when appropriate, initiates immune responses.

Cross-Presentation

As we have discussed, generally MHC class II molecules present extracellular antigens, and MHC class I molecules present intracellular antigens, which allows for presentation to specific

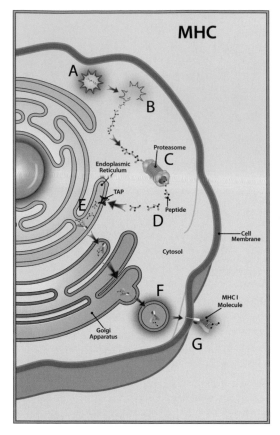

FIGURE 8.17. Overview of antigen processing and presentation by MHC class I molecules

As antigens are synthesized inside of cells (A), a portion of the antigenic proteins (B) enter cellular proteasomes (C). Those organelles digest these antigenic proteins into peptides. TAPs (D) deliver these peptides into the ER.
(E) There, antigenic peptides bind with MHC class I molecules, and endosomes (F) transport them to the cell surface (G), where they present these peptides to T cells.

T-cell subtypes best equipped to respond to antigens, based on whether a given antigen is extracellular or intracellular.

For instance (discussed in later chapters), $CD4^+$ T (Th) cells are most effective against extracellular pathogens. These cells recognize antigens bound by MHC class II molecules. However, $CD8^+$ T cells (Tc cells) are most effective against intracellular pathogens (such as viruses). These cells recognize antigens bound by MHC class I molecules and destroy infected cells.

However, many effective immune responses require antigen presentation to both Th and Tc cells. For example, effective immune responses to virus infections often require both antibody and Tc cells. Antibody production usually involves $CD4^+$ Th cells that require antigen presentation via MHC class II molecules. $CD8^+$ Tc cell activation, however, requires antigen presentation in the context of MHC class I molecules. Thus, the virus would have to both infect the DC cell (entering the cytosol, a traditional pathway for MHC class I presentation) and enter the endosomal pathway through phagocytosis for MHC class II presentation. Phagocytosis of viral particles by DC cells occurs regularly and efficiently. However, virus infection of DC cells is a relatively rare event.

To deal with this, DCs have evolved cross-presentation, a process that allows extracellular antigen to be processed and displayed in MHC class I molecules (in addition to MHC class II molecules). When a DC phagocytoses a dead cell containing viral particles, the DC can shuttle viral antigens into both the MHC class II and the MHC class I processing pathway and present to both $CD4^+$ and $CD8^+$ T cells.

The cellular mechanisms by which DCs cross-present extracellular antigens to MHC class I molecules are still obscure. Some antigens appear to be simply exported from the phagolysosome to the cytoplasm where proteasomes process them. The TAP moves the resulting peptides into the ER lumen for loading onto MHC class I molecules. Other antigens seem to be cross-presented without the involvement of the proteasome and TAP. In this case, it may be that MHC class I molecules interact with antigens in specialized endosomes. Regardless, cross-presentation is an important process by which APCs can monitor antigens within the cytoplasm of other host cells and potentially stimulate T-cell responses that most effectively deal with intracellular infections.

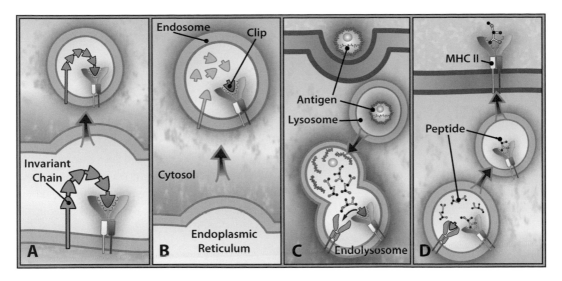

FIGURE 8.18. Antigen presentation by MHC class II molecules

MHC class II molecules are also synthesized on ribosomes and extruded into the lumen of the ER. However, as MHC class II proteins arrive inside the ER, another molecule—the invariant chain, or Ii (shown here in orange)—binds to them (A). The Ii covers the antigen-binding site and prevents MHC class II molecules from presenting the same set of peptides bound by MHC class I molecules. The MHC class II–Ii complex then enters the endolysosomal pathway (B) and eventually ends up inside of endolysosomes. There, a protease removes all but a small piece of Ii from MHC class II molecules. That small remaining piece is called class II–associated Ii peptide (CLIP). As APCs acquire pathogens from their surroundings via phagocytosis and endocytosis, the resultant phagosomes and endosomes containing extracellular antigens eventually fuse with lysosomes to form phagolysosomes and endolysosomes. Inside of these compartments, proteolytic enzymes cleave the pathogen's proteins into peptides (C). At the same time, the CLIP leaves the antigen-binding site of the MHC class II molecules, which allows for binding of antigenic peptides in the endolysosome. Portions of the endolysosome along with MHC–antigen complexes then return to the cell surface via recycling endosomes, which fuse with the cell membrane (D).

The end result of antigen acquisition, processing, and presentation within MHC molecules is a cell-surface representation of everything occurring in and around host cells. Mammalian immune systems rely on this information to detect and respond to infectious nonself and sometimes to mutant self.

CLINICAL CORRELATION: FOLLOW-UP

As we said at the beginning of this chapter, only a few goats infected with CAEV develop disease. Exactly why remains unclear. A major factor seems to be the makeup of the goats' MHCs. Goats that develop arthritis or encephalitis often carry one or both of two MHC genes—Be1 and Be14—and disease-free goats have a higher incidence of Be7.

Among infectious diseases of goats, CAEV is one of the most common. As with other retroviruses, these infections are lifelong, and recrudescence or transmission of the virus may occur at any time. Goats most commonly pass the virus to kids in the colostrum and milk of infected dams. Goats exposed to CAEV often develop persistent infections, slowly developing arthritis of their carpal joints and mastitis. Only rarely do adult goats develop encephalitis.

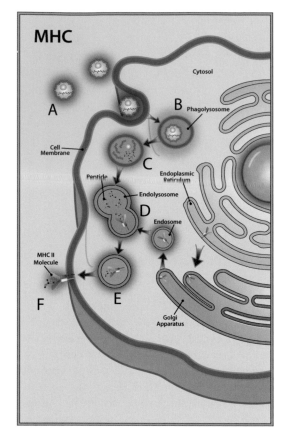

FIGURE 8.19. Overview of antigen processing and presentation by MHC class II molecules

APCs ingest extracellular antigens (A) and enclose them in endosomes or phagosomes. These phagosomes and endosomes eventually fuse with lysosomes (creating hybrid organelles—phagolysosomes and endolysosomes—where proteases digest the antigens into peptides. These phagolysosomes and endolysosomes then fuse with endosomes containing MHC class II molecules (E). At this point the CLIP is removed from the MHC class II molecules and replaced with antigenic peptides. MHC class II–antigen complexes then return to the cell surface, where they present these peptides to T cells.

Genes Be1, Be14, and Be7 all encode MHC class I proteins. Goats carrying either Be1 or Be14 genes are more likely to develop arthritis after CAEV infection, and goats carrying the Be7 gene are less likely to develop disease. This

sort of association is not unique to goats. So far, it appears that MHC–disease associations occur in all mammals.

Student Considerations

Why might a particular MHC allele make an animal more or less susceptible to a certain disease? From what you have just learned about the function of MHC molecules, you should be able to offer one or two explanations for the association between CAEV and MHC genes—explanations that apply to any association between a disease and an MHC allele.

Possible Explanations

The exact reasons for these associations remain unknown, but at least two possibilities seem obvious. Because of the roles of MHC class I and class II molecules in antigen binding and presentation, a disease might arise in an animal that was unable to present a critical antigen and mount a protective immune response. For example, a protective immune response against pathogen X occurs only if the host animal recognizes antigenic epitope Y. If an animal expresses MHC alleles whose protein products do not bind and present antigen Y, then that animal will succumb to the infection.

Alternatively, the disease might result from an overreaction or cross-reaction of the immune system. Let's say pathogen X also carries an antigenic epitope Z that looks a lot like a protein on synovial cells. If an animal infected with pathogen X carries a certain MHC allele and the product of that allele binds to the antigenic epitope Z, then when this animal's immune system reacts to epitope Z on pathogen X, it may inadvertently also strike the synovial cells and cause a progressive arthritis. Although one usually thinks of immune responses as being protective—the ultimate defense against infectious diseases—under certain circumstances, immune responses can harm host animals. Goats might also develop CAEV because their immune re-

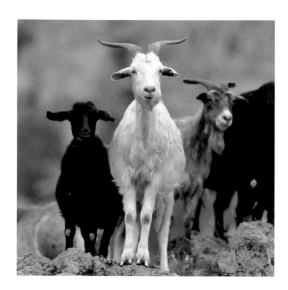

FIGURE 8.20. **Domestic goats (© Mircea Bezergheanu / Shutterstock)**

sponses against CAEV cross-react with and damage host tissues.

MHC class I and class II gene products bind wide varieties of (but not all) antigenic epitopes derived from pathogens. In goats, it could be that among the possible MHC class I alleles at a particular MHC locus, the only ones that fail to bind and present the critical CAEV epitope are Be1 and Be14. If that is true, then goats with either or both of these alleles would mount ineffective immune responses, the infection would go unchecked, and these goats would develop arthritis and sometimes encephalitis.

One more observation about CAEV points, however, toward an alternative explanation for the observed differences in susceptibility. In one study in which goats were intentionally infected with CAEV, researchers found that immunosuppression of goats reduced the likelihood that these goats would develop arthritis. Although the pathogenesis of CAEV remains largely unknown, this finding suggests that, in addition to the virus, an inappropriate immune response plays a role in the pathogenesis of CAEV.

Of the two possibilities discussed, the immunosuppression studies have pointed toward overactive immune responses as the probable cause of CAEV. The association of this disease with MHC class I alleles Be1 and Be14 demonstrates the importance of these genes and their protein products in antigen presentation and protective immunity or destructive autoimmunity.

CLINICAL CORRELATION: SEVERE COMBINED IMMUNODEFICIENCY DISEASE IN ARABIAN FOALS

Every year, about 3 percent of U.S.-born Arabian foals (Figure 9.1) exhibit a devastating and uniformly fatal affliction. This disease—called severe combined immunodeficiency disease (SCID)—manifests as repeated and eventually fatal opportunistic respiratory infections, including adenovirus, *Pneumocystis carinii,* and assorted bacterial infections, especially streptococci. Clinical analyses of these foals indicate dramatically low lymphocyte counts and, at necropsy, severe atrophy of their thymuses and lymph nodes.

The only antibodies found in SCID foals are remnants of those maternally transferred through colostrum. Breeding studies have shown that among Arabian foals, SCID is due to an autosomal recessive mutation, meaning that the sire and the dam have both contributed one defective gene to an afflicted foal. More recently, studies have identified the relevant gene as a DNA-dependent phosphokinase. How does such a mutation make these foals so susceptible to infection?

LEARNING OBJECTIVES

After reading this chapter, you should be able to

- understand the structure and function of the TCR and the CD3 complex;
- describe the unique arrangement of TCR genes;
- understand the process and products of genetic rearrangement of TCR gene families;
- describe the process and outcome of positive and negative selection of T cells in the thymus;
- understand the origins of double-positive and single-positive T cells and the roles of CD4 and CD8 molecules on T cells;
- describe the characteristics of naive T cells that emigrate from the mammalian thymus;
- explain the nature of and evidence for central and peripheral tolerance.

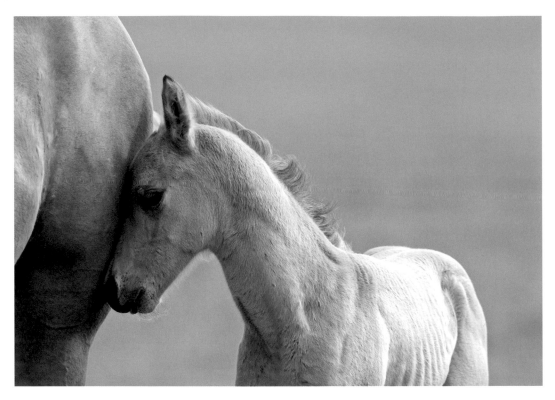

FIGURE 9.1. **Arabian foal (© Pictureguy / Shutterstock)**

T-CELL RECEPTOR GENES

Structure of the T-Cell Receptor

Immunity—the ability to detect and respond to potentially pathogenic microorganisms—depends on an animal's ability to distinguish self from non-self—a critical distinction that keeps us all alive.

Among all the cells of the body, only lymphocytes have antigen-specific receptors. On T cells, these molecules are the TCRs (see Figure 9.2). In their functional state, the N-termini of these molecules project into T cells' surroundings, and the C-termini extend into the cytosol.

These receptors contain two polypeptide chains—either α and β or γ and δ—that together form the antigen-binding site at their membrane-distal N-termini. Both the α and β chains and the γ and δ chains span the plasma membrane with their C-termini extending into the cytosol. Together, α and β or γ and δ de-

termine the antigen specificity of the receptor. Also, both α/β and γ/δ chain pairs associate with CD3—a complex of four different polypeptides (γ, δ, ε, and ζ) that together form the signal-transduction machinery of TCRs. Beyond this, the similarities between α/β and γ/δ TCRs are few.

The α/β TCRs recognize antigens only after processing and presentation inside of MHC class I or II molecules. The γ/δ TCRs recognize intact antigens in the absence of classical MHC class I or II molecules. The structural variability among α/β TCRs is much greater than that among γ/δ TCRs. Also, γ/δ TCRs seem to have evolved to recognize a relatively narrow range of specialized antigens, including the lipids of mycobacteria, some phosphorylated ligands, and heat-shock proteins. Here, we focus primarily on α/β TCRs, the most common form in most mammals, although species variations can be substantial.

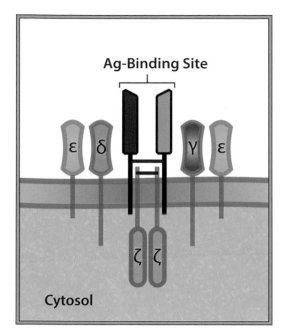

FIGURE 9.2. T-cell α/β antigen-specific receptor
The complete TCR includes an α and a β chain or a γ and a δ chain that together form the antigen-binding complex. In addition, functional TCRs include a series of associated molecules collectively called CD3. These include the γ, δ, ε, and ζ chains that transduce activation signals after antigen binding. Ag = antigen.

The N-terminal (antigen-binding) regions of α and β chains have highly variable amino acid sequences, whereas the C-terminal regions are invariant. These chemical differences reflect the functional differences in these two regions of TCRs—antigen binding versus membrane anchoring and signal transduction.

Amino acid sequence analyses of these receptors have revealed three clusters of variability in the N-termini of α and β chains and γ and δ chains. These regions are called hypervariable regions 1, 2, and 3, or—more commonly— complementarity-determining regions (CDRs) 1, 2, and 3 because these regions determine the complementarity of the fit between TCR and antigen, like a lock and a key.

TCRs are highly specific—nearly one TCR for each antigen. In spite of that, most animal species can respond to essentially every potential pathogen. Considering the enormity of the antigenic universe, that means that every animal must be able to make a nearly unlimited number of TCRs—literally trillions upon trillions of TCRs. How is that possible?

T-Cell Receptor Gene Families

The essentially unlimited diversity among mammalian TCRs is the result of a unique genetic mechanism that operates only inside of T and B lymphocytes: the random rearrangement of germline gene segments. Most of the original insights into gene rearrangement came from studies of genes inside of B cells. However, T cells use the same mechanisms for generation of diversity. T-cell DNA-sequencing studies revealed the remarkable finding that TCR genes are not in contiguous segments of DNA. Rather, the DNA that eventually encodes a TCR is in segments strung out along the DNA strand. Moreover, for each of the final pieces of a TCR, there are multiple possible segments on the chromosome (see Figure 9.3).

Gene Rearrangement in the Thymus

The assembly of a TCR α chain begins with a genetic rearrangement that randomly brings together one V_α segment and one J_α segment. The intervening DNA loops out and is excised. Then ligases join the V and J segments. This VJ segment is then joined to the C_α constant region segment (see Figure 9.4). After transcription, spliceosomes remove all of the excess RNA from the nuclear transcript, and the messenger RNA encodes a single α chain from N- to C-terminus, including the constant region.

The assembly of a β-chain gene is slightly more complicated. This process begins with a genetic rearrangement that loops out intervening DNA and randomly brings together one D_β segment and one J_β segment. The resulting DJ segment then randomly combines with one V_β segment to generate a VDJ segment that

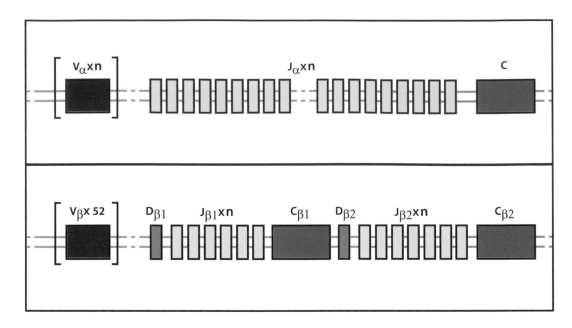

FIGURE 9.3. Arrangement of TCR genes on mammalian chromosomes

The genetic material that encodes TCR α and β chains is not contiguous. Instead, it exists in segments. These segments include variable (V), joining (J), diversity (D), and constant (C) region segments. The numbers above each gene segment indicate the total number of distinct segments found in each region of each animal. This figure shows human α (upper panel) and β (lower panel) gene families. Each species has a unique number of each gene segment.

encodes the variable region of a TCR β chain, which is then joined to a C_β gene segment to form a complete gene. Again, spliceosomes remove intervening RNA and convert the nuclear transcript into messenger RNA that encodes a complete β chain from its variable N-terminus to its constant C-terminus.

As with all molecules destined for the cell surface, the synthesis of TCR chains begins on the surface of the rough ER. As they grow, these polypeptides extrude into the lumen of this organelle. Inside the ER, disulfide bonds join the two chains. Later, inside the Golgi complex, enzymes add sugars to these glycoproteins, which then move to the surface of T cells and join with the CD3 complex to form the TCR.

This random association of V and J or V, D, and J gene segments allows for a variation, similar to shuffling a large deck of cards and selecting two or three cards at a time. Using the mathematical power of random combination, it dramatically increases the number of possible TCRs that a T cell can generate from a fixed amount of DNA. In addition, it appears that any TCR α chain can pair with any TCR β chain, which creates even more diversity.

By themselves, though, genetic rearrangement and random pairing of α and β chains cannot account for the astronomical array of TCRs inside of every mammal. The real secret to TCR diversity lies in the ways in which the gene segments join during genetic rearrangement—a process called junctional diversification.

Physically, rearrangement of TCR gene segments occurs after looping out and excision of intervening DNA to join randomly selected gene segments (as with TCR α chain in Figure 9.5).

The products of two genes—*RAG1* and *RAG2*—drive this process. The protein products

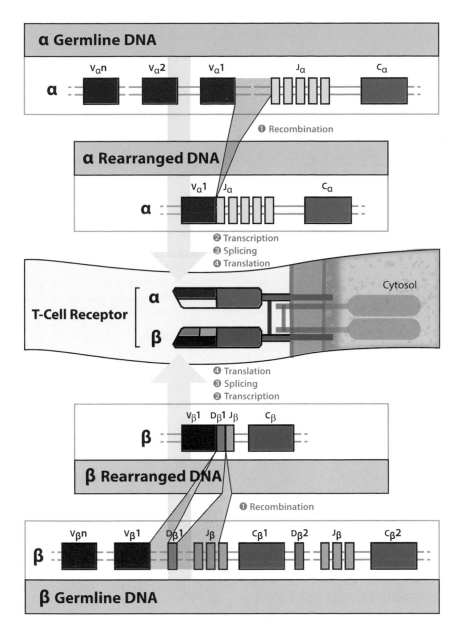

FIGURE 9.4. Assembly of an α/β TCR

Formation of an α/β TCR begins with rearrangement of β-chain genes (lower half of figure) with the random joining of a D_β and a J_β gene segment. The gray areas between the lines indicate the excised segments of DNA. Enzymes then randomly link this new DJ_β segment with a V_β segment to form the variable region of a β chain. Spliceosomes convert this nuclear RNA transcript into messenger RNA encoding a complete β chain. Once a complete β-chain polypeptide appears, rearrangement of α-chain gene segment begins (upper half of figure). First, a randomly selected V_α and a J_α pair of gene segments are joined to form complete α-chain variable region. Then, the VJ segment is joined with a C_α constant region segment. After splicing, a complete α-chain message forms. After translation, the α-chain polypeptide joins the β-chain polypeptide and the α/β TCR appears on the cell surface. (Note: For clarity, only a few gene segments are shown in this drawing.)

TABLE 9.1. TCR diversity (adapted from C. Janeway, P. Travers, M. Walport, and M. Shlomchik, 2006, *Immunobiology*, 151)

Element	Immunoglobulin		α:β receptors	
	H	L	ß	α
Variable segments (V)	65	70	52	~70
Diversity segments (D)	27	0	2	0
D segments read in 3 frames	rarely	—	often	—
Joining segments (J)	6	5(κ) 4(λ)	13	61
Joints with N- and P-nucleotides	2	50% of joints	2	1
Number of V gene pairs	3.4×10^6		5.8×10^6	
Junctional diversity	$\sim 3 \times 10^7$		2×10^{11}	
Total diversity	$\sim 10^{14}$		$\sim 10^{18}$	

of these genes combine to form the lymphoid-specific components of the VDJ recombinase. This enzymatic complex—along with several other enzymes, including essential DNA-dependent protein kinases—accomplishes the rearrangement steps shown in Figure 9.5A–D. First, complexes of *RAG1* and *RAG2* bind near relevant gene segments. The RAG proteins then bind to one another, looping and excising the intervening DNA.

During joint formation, enzymes, including DNA-dependent protein kinases, cut away the hairpin loop and leave single-stranded DNA ends behind. The enzyme, terminal deoxynucleotidyl transferase (TDT), then randomly adds complementary nucleotides to both strands, and DNA polymerases fill the resultant gaps. During the process, at least one-third of the time, TDT creates new codons that code for new amino acids at the VJ and VJD joints (see Figure 9.6A–D). In the final tertiary structure of the TCR, the VJ and VDJ joints form CDR3, one of the most variable regions of the TCR and the region that directly contacts antigenic peptides during antigen presentation to T cells. Thus, as a result of junctional diversification, the diversity of possible TCRs increases exponentially, and the number of TCRs with unique antigenic specificities inside one animal appears to be effectively limitless (see Table 9.1). Because of this, an animal will rarely encounter a pathogen or an antigen that the animal cannot recognize and respond to. However, that incredible diversity comes at a price. Also shown in Figure 9.6, during joint assembly, enzymes add or remove nucleotides randomly. At least two-thirds of the time, this results in a frameshift mutation and no TCR. Only when a full codon appears or disappears will the rearranged gene produce a functional TCR.

As we show later, T cells that do not form functional TCRs die. If instead the cell assembles and expresses a functional TCR, TCR gene rearrangement ceases, which means that all the TCRs on a given T cell have exactly the same antigenic specificity. No T cell ever expresses more than one TCR or more than one antigenic specificity.

Similar to those of the gene families of α/β TCRs, the gene families used to produce γ/δ receptors appear in the genome as a series of fragments (see Figure 9.8). In fact the δ-chain gene family nests within the family of gene segments that encode the α chain of the α/β TCR. All of the processes that operate in the generation of α/β TCRs also operate in the generation of γ/δ TCRs. As mentioned, though, γ/δ T cells are much less diverse and recognize antigens in a distinct manner.

The human TCR γ locus resembles the TCR β locus: it has two C genes, each with its own set of J gene segments. The mouse γ locus (not shown) has a more complex organization and three functional clusters of γ gene segments.

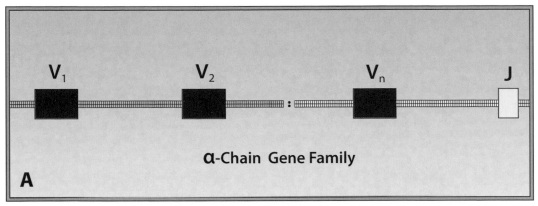

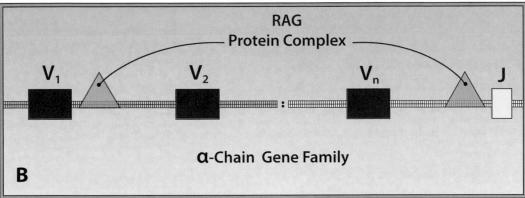

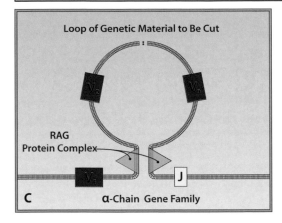

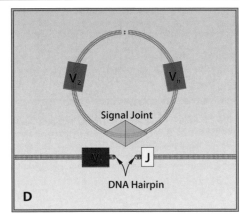

FIGURE 9.5A–D. DNA rearrangement during TCR α-chain formation

Alpha-chain gene family (panel A); attachment of recombination activating gene (RAG) protein enzymatic complexes (panel B); looping out intervening DNA (panel C); and excision of intervening DNA and formation of DNA hairpin loops (panel D).

Panel A shows a representative α-chain gene family with V segments from 1 to n and a J segment. Panel B shows the attachment of RAG complexes—the initiation of rearrangement. Panel C shows how the RAG complexes bind to one another and loop out intervening DNA between randomly selected V and J segments. Panel D shows how enzymes, including DNA-dependent protein kinase, excise the intervening DNA. The space with the two dots indicates an indeterminate amount of DNA.

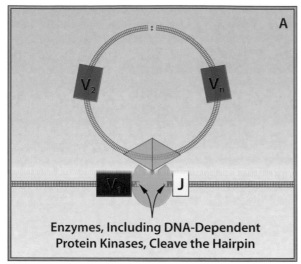

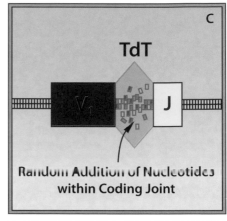

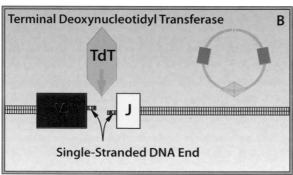

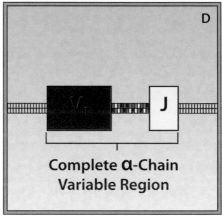

FIGURE 9.6A–D. **Junctional diversification**

Cleavage of DNA hairpins (panel A); random deletion of nucleotides and activation of terminal deoxynucleotidyl transferase (TDT) (panel B); junctional diversification (panel C); and DNA ligation and formation of VJ joint (panel D).

During the final steps of gene rearrangement, a process called junctional diversification introduces additional diversity into the TCR α-chain gene. Panel A shows the final excision of the loop of intervening DNA, the formation of singled-stranded DNA ends with a final hairpin loop, and enzymatic cleavage of the hairpin. In Panel B, the enzyme TDT binds into the remaining gap in the DNA and, in Panel C, begins to randomly add nucleotides, completing the DNA gap between V and J. Finally, as shown in Panel D, DNA ligases join the now double-stranded DNA ends and complete the VJ joint.

Each contains V and J gene segments and a C gene. Rearrangement at the γ and δ loci occurs in the same way as in the other TCR loci, with the exception being that during TCRδ rearrangement, both D segments can be used in the same gene. The use of two D segments greatly increases the variability of the δ chain, mainly because extra N-region nucleotides can be added at the junction between the two D gene segments as well as at the V–D and D–J junctions.

T-CELL SELECTION IN THE THYMUS

Products of T-Cell Receptor Gene Rearrangement

Beyond the potential frameshift inefficiency, random rearrangement and insertion and dele-

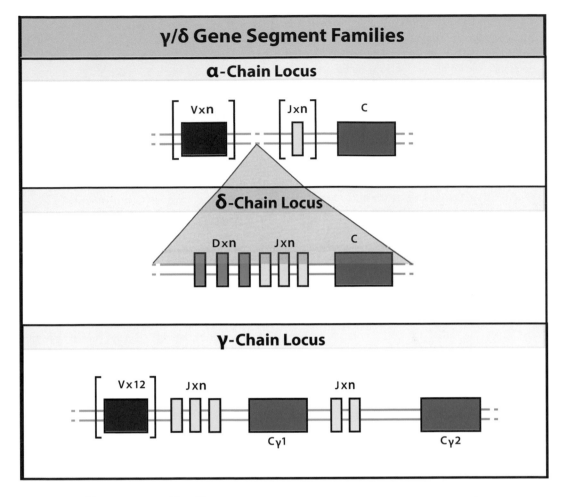

γ/δ Gene Segment Families

α-Chain Locus

Vxn   Jxn   C

δ-Chain Locus

Dxn   Jxn   C

γ-Chain Locus

Vx12   Jxn   Jxn

Cγ1   Cγ2

FIGURE 9.7. γ/δ gene segment families

The TCR γ and TCR δ loci—as with the TCR α and TCR β loci—have discrete V, D, and J gene segments and C genes. In humans, the locus encoding the δ chain is entirely within the α-chain locus.

tion of nucleotides has another downside: the specificity of the resultant TCR is unpredictable. Because these processes are random, they may generate T cells with no functional TCRs, T cells with self-reactive TCRs, or T cells with non-self-reactive TCRs. The first group is useless, the second dangerous, and only the third can be safely expanded and exposed to the tissues of an animal's body.

In most mammals, T-cell development begins well before birth. During the last one-third of gestation, a large population of lymphocytes leaves the bone marrow and migrates to the thymus (see Figure 9.8).

When these lymphocytes arrive in the thymus, the thymic stroma delivers a signal that activates the *Notch 1* gene, and TCR gene rearrangement begins. Because these early-stage thymocytes lack CD4 and CD8, they are double-negative cells. Three TCR gene families begin rearranging simultaneously—the β-chain, the γ-chain, and the δ-chain families. If the cell successfully rearranges and synthesizes a complete β chain first, the cell goes on to

FIGURE 9.8. T-cell development

All lymphocytes originate in the bone marrow. Some of these lymphocytes emigrate from the bone marrow and travel—via the blood—to the thymus. Whether these cells are identifiably different from other lymphocytes in the bone marrow is unclear. Once inside the thymus (probably through activation of the *Notch 1* gene), most of the newly arrived lymphocytes begin to differentiate, which results in the activation of gene rearrangement among the β, γ, and δ gene families. Depending on the outcomes of these rearrangements, the cells begin to express α/β and CD4 and CD8 cell-surface proteins or γ/δ TCRs. After positive selection, α/β T cells no longer express either CD4 or CD8 and differentiate along two independent lines as either CD4$^+$ Th cells or CD8$^+$ Tc cells.

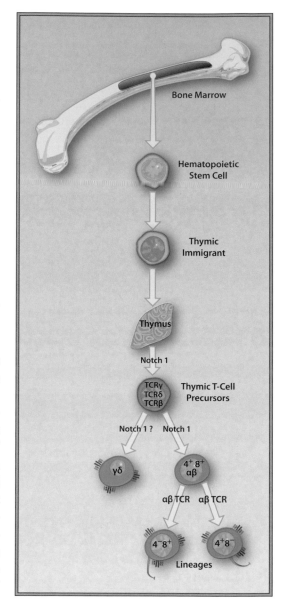

become an α/β T cell. If γ- and δ-chain genes successfully rearrange first, the cell goes on to become a γ/δ T cell.

Inside the thymus, gene rearrangement proceeds one allele at a time; that is, it begins on only one of the two parental chromosomes. If rearrangement at the first allele fails, only then does gene rearrangement begin at the second allele. Because of this, TCRs always represent the products of only one parental allele. However, the opportunity to rearrange gene segments on both parental chromosomes means that each lymphocyte has two opportunities to produce a functional gene rearrangement of each of the chains of the TCR.

Obviously, the success of this whole process is essential to an animal's survival—useless T cells have to be disposed of, self-reactive T cells have to be destroyed, and somehow non-self-reactive T cells have to be identified and preserved. To meet these needs, mammals have evolved a means to monitor TCR gene rearrangement. Ultimately, the thymic stroma is responsible for this monitoring.

For monitoring to be successful throughout T-cell development, each successive rearrange-

ment event has to be detectable at the surface of the T cell. With α/β T cells, rearrangement begins with the β-chain gene family. Even if the T cell manages to successfully rearrange a β chain, TCR β chains by themselves cannot insert into the cell's membrane. Only α/β pairs arrive at the cell surface, but α-chain gene rearrangement cannot begin until it is clear that a functional β chain exists. Somehow, the developing T cell has to signal the thymic stroma that it has successfully rearranged a β-chain gene.

To provide that signal, T cells use an α-chain surrogate called pre-Tα. When pre-Tα joins with an assembled β chain, the complex inserts into the developing cell's membrane and, along with the CD3 complex, forms the pre-TCR. The appearance of the pre-TCR signals the thymic stroma that the cell has created a functional β-chain molecule. In turn, the thymic stroma delivers a signal that ends β-chain gene rearrangement and initiates α-chain gene rearrangement. Once the cell has assembled a functional α chain, the full TCR appears on the cell surface along with two other molecules—CD4 and CD8. CD4 and CD8 are cell-surface proteins that interact with constant regions of MHC class II and class I molecules during antigen presentation (see Figure 9.9).

Positive Selection of Functional T Cells

At this point in thymocyte development, the thymocyte has on its surface an α/β TCR (or not, because many rearrangements go wrong), the CD3 complex, and CD4 as well as CD8. Because these thymocytes now express both of the markers of mature T cells (CD4 and CD8) they are called double-positive cells.

Ultimately, this complex of molecules is destined to interact with the MHC–antigen complex on the surface of APCs. To be useful, this newly formed TCR must show signs that it is capable of detecting those complexes. Because the processes of gene rearrangement and nucleotide deletion and insertion all occur randomly, this newly formed TCR might be useless, dangerous, or potentially protective. It is the job of the thymus and its components to sort out the useless and dangerous T cells and destroy them. This sorting or selection process occurs in two steps—positive selection and negative selection.

To be of use, the T cell must express a functional TCR: a TCR that can recognize and react

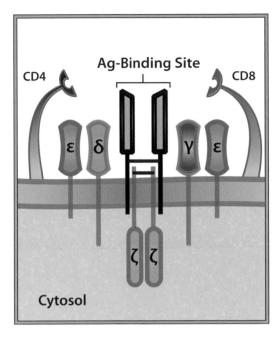

FIGURE 9.9. The fully assembled α/β TCR

C-termini of the α and β chains both span the cell membrane while the membrane-distal N-termini form the MHC–antigen (Ag) binding site. In addition, all α/β T cells express CD4 and CD8 before positive selection. These cell-surface molecules bind to constant regions of MHC molecules: CD4 binds MHC class II, and CD8 binds MHC class I. In the T-cell membrane, the α/β heterodimer associates with another group of molecules collectively called CD3. These include the γ, δ, ε, and ζ molecules, either alone or in pairs.

with the MHC–antigen complex on the surface of an APC (see Figure 9.10).

Positive selection tests whether a newly created TCR can bind to the MHC class I or MHC class II molecules on thymic cortical epithelial cells (these cells are also APCs). This binding is likely a low-affinity interaction between MHC and TCR. Most (maybe as much as 96 percent of) thymocytes fail positive selection and undergo apoptosis. Remember, genetic rearrangement and reassembly are not only random but perhaps as much as two times more likely to generate no or nonfunctional TCRs.

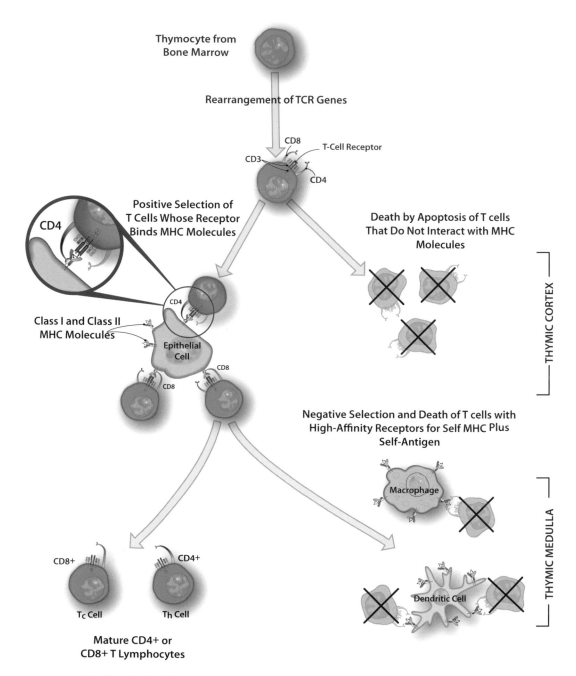

Thymocyte from
Bone Marrow

Rearrangement of TCR Genes

CD8

T-Cell Receptor

CD3

CD4

Positive Selection of
T Cells Whose Receptor
Binds MHC Molecules

Death by Apoptosis of T cells
That Do Not Interact with MHC
Molecules

CD4

CD4

Class I and Class II
MHC Molecules

Epithelial
Cell

CD8

CD8

CD8

Negative Selection and Death of T cells with
High-Affinity Receptors for Self MHC Plus
Self-Antigen

Macrophage

THYMIC CORTEX

CD8+

CD4+

Dendritic Cell

THYMIC MEDULLA

Tc Cell

Th Cell

Mature CD4+ or
CD8+ T Lymphocytes

FIGURE 9.10. T-cell selection in the thymus

Once formed, the α/β TCR must react with MHC molecules present on APCs (including thymic epithelial cells) in the thymic stroma. The first of these tests, positive selection, determines whether the new TCR can bind with low affinity to the MHC portion of an MHC–antigen complex on thymic epithelial cells. If a T cell fails positive selection, it dies by apoptosis. If it survives positive selection, the T cell must pass a second test—negative selection—a test for self-reactivity. If the new TCR strongly binds to an MHC–antigen complex presented on bone marrow–derived macrophages or DCs in the thymus, those T cells also undergo apoptosis. Only non-self-reactive cells emigrate from the thymus.

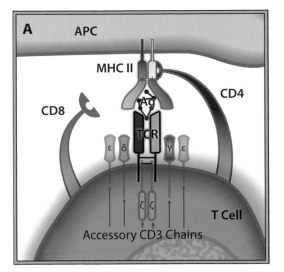 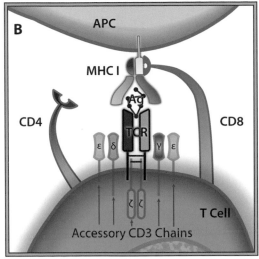

FIGURE 9.11. The roles of CD4 and CD8 molecules

By binding to a constant region found on all MHC class II proteins, CD4 molecules on Th cells increase the TCR's avidity for the MHC class II–antigen complex on the APC (A). By binding to a constant region found on all MHC class I proteins, CD8 molecules on Tc cells increase the TCR's avidity for the MHC class I–antigen complex on the APC (B). Once a TCR has bound to an MHC class I molecule, that T cell ceases to express CD4. Likewise, once a TCR has bound to an MHC class II molecule, that T cell ceases to express CD8. Neither CD4 nor CD8 contributes to the antigenic specificity of the TCR, but the combination of TCR and CD4 or CD8 binding leads to activation of the T cell via signals transduced through the CD3 complex of molecules.

CD4, CD8, and Major Histocompatibility Complex Recognition

Also during positive selection, thymocytes transform from double-positive cells to single-positive cells. This transformation occurs during the interaction of the newly formed TCR with an APC. If the TCR has an affinity for an MHC class I molecule, the thymocyte turns off the CD4 gene and begins to express solely CD8. That cell then commits for life to MHC class I molecules and their antigens. CD8 is a cell-surface protein dimer that binds to constant regions of MHC class I molecules (see Figure 9.11). For reasons that will become apparent later, CD8+ T cells are also called Tc cells.

Conversely, if the newly formed TCR has affinity for MHC class II molecules, that lymphocyte switches off the CD8 gene and expresses only CD4. CD4+ T cells recognize antigens only in the context of MHC class II molecules. CD4 is a cell-surface protein that binds to the constant region of MHC class II molecules (see Figure 9.11). CD4+ T cells are also known as Th cells, because they assist several other cell types during immune responses.

Negative Selection of Self-Reactive T Cells

Through the preceding process, positive selection eliminates thymocytes that either have failed to assemble a TCR or have assembled a useless TCR and seals a T cell's fate, committing it to a CD4+ or a CD8+ lineage. However, even after positive selection, the remaining thymocytes are as likely to have self-reactive TCRs as they are to have non-self-reactive TCRs.

Because of their potential danger, the process of negative selection has evolved to eliminate these self-reactive T cells.

Inside the thymus, if a T cell's TCR binds with high affinity to an MHC-antigen complex present on an APC, the T cell usually dies through apoptosis (see Figure 9.11). Because a blood–thymus barrier keeps non-self out of the thymus, any reactive T cell in the thymus is a self-reactive T cell. The process of negative selection eliminates most thymocytes that react with self as represented in the thymus.

On the surface, although this process seems to be an effective means for eliminating useless and dangerous T cells, it also seems as though it might eliminate only those cells reactive with self presented in the thymus, which might represent only a small portion of the total variety of self molecules.

To deal with this, the thymus has evolved a genetic mechanism that allows for a much broader representation of self on APCs in the thymus. A gene known as the autoimmune regulator, or *AIRE,* gene allows thymic epithelial cells to express many of the proteins usually found on other tissues of the body (see Figure 9.12). The result is that most cells leaving the thymus are tolerant of (will not react to) self antigens. This form of tolerance is called central tolerance, and it results from the process of negative selection in the thymus.

Although negative selection on APCs expressing the *AIRE* gene eliminates most self-reactive T cells, a subset of these cells (T-regulatory [Treg] cells) survives and differentiates into a group of cells expressing FoxP3 molecules. Ultimately these cells, and probably at least a few other cell types, help maintain some aspects of self-tolerance beyond the thymus. Tolerance maintained outside the thymus is called *peripheral tolerance.*

Despite central and peripheral tolerance, it is obvious—because of autoimmune disease—that some self-reactive cells do escape and, under the right circumstance, can attack self and create diseases such as autoimmune hemolytic anemia in dogs and cats. The reasons for this are not clear.

T-Helper, Cytotoxic T, and T-Regulatory Cells

Those T cells that survive positive and negative selection leave the thymus via the blood. Along with NKT-lymphocyte cells (an innate subgroup of T cells), these T cells include at least three populations of cells: α/β Tc, α/β Th, and α/β Treg cells, as well as γ/δ T cells.

Tc cells express CD8 molecules on their surfaces and react with antigens in the context of MHC class I. These cells are largely responsible for the destruction of pathogen-infected cells.

After leaving the thymus, and reaction with their specific antigens, CD4$^+$ Th cells differentiate into several distinct subsets, including Th1, Th2, Th17, and probably some types of regulatory cells (see chapter 10). Th cells are active in almost all aspects of every immune response. Th1 cells activate macrophages, sometimes assist Tc cells, and activate some NK cells and B cells. Th2 cells drive the proliferation and differentiation of B cells into antibody-secreting plasma cells. Th17 cells promote inflammation, and Th3 cells probably help suppress autoimmunity. Some T-regulatory cells differentiate in the thymus but operate outside the thymus to help suppress self-reactive T cells that leave the thymus.

γ/δ T Cells

The γ/δ T cells make up only a small fraction of the T-cell population in mice and humans. In ruminants and chickens, however, the majority of T cells are γ/δ T cells. In some species, γ/δ T cells line the epithelia of the gut and the reproductive system, whereas in other species, most γ/δ T cells are at the same sites as α/β T cells. The majority of γ/δ T cells express neither CD4 nor CD8 molecules. In addition, most γ/δ T cells use very few V gene segments during assemblies of TCRs and may, therefore,

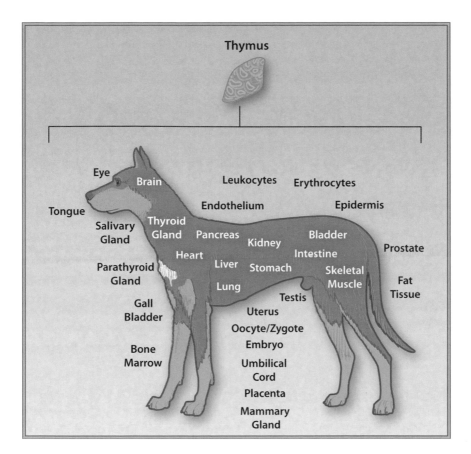

FIGURE 9.12. Expression of self in the mammalian thymus and the role of the _AIRE_ gene

Because of the _AIRE_ gene, APCs in the thymus express and present many peptides derived from non-thymic tissues.

have a significantly narrower diversity than that seen in α/β T cells. However, because of frequent and substantial nucleotide deletion and addition during gene rearrangement, the CDR3 region of the δ chain is the most diverse of all the antigen-specific receptors in mammals.

The γ/δ T cells recognize unprocessed antigens, including intact pathogens, and classical MHC class I and II molecules are not involved in presentation of antigens to γ/δ T cells. Only a few of the antigens that γ/δ T cells recognize have been identified, and the role of these antigens in disease processes is not always clear. For example, one subset of γ/δ T cells recognizes a group of molecules called MHC class Ib molecules. These molecules resemble classical MHC class I molecules but are monomorphic in animal populations, are not encoded by genes within the MHC, and do not seem to be involved in classical antigen presentation. These MHC class Ib proteins present some unprocessed antigens, such as certain phosphoproteins present on cell surfaces. After interaction with their target antigens, γ/δ T cells respond in the same ways as CD8⁺ α/β cells. That is, both cell types secrete cytokines and induce apoptosis in the cells bearing their target antigens. Because γ/δ T cells are widespread in the animal kingdom, and because—in some species—these T cells make up a significant part of the T-cell population, γ/δ T cells must be important to immune-mediated protection,

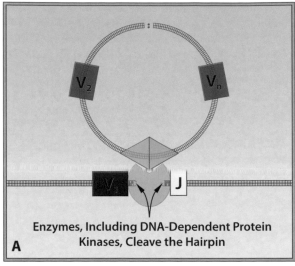

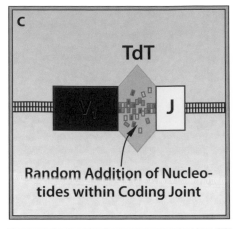

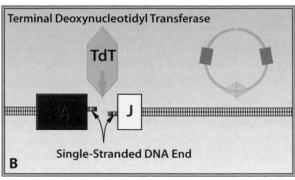

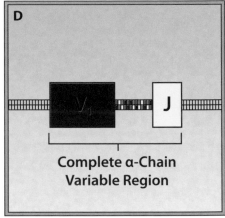

FIGURE 9.13A–D. **The role of DNA-dependent kinases in gene rearrangement**

Cleavage of DNA hairpins (panel A); random deletion of nucleotides and activation of TDT (panel B); junctional diversification (panel C); and DNA ligation and formation of VJ joint (panel D). Note the essential role the DNA-dependent protein kinase plays in excision of intervening DNA and formation of the new DJ joint. (For a complete description of these events, see Figure 9.6.)

but the exact nature of that importance is only beginning to appear.

CLINICAL CORRELATION: FOLLOW-UP

Student Considerations

SCID in Arabian foals manifests as severe repeated infections, often respiratory infections. These foals invariably die from these infections by age five months. SCID results from an autosomal recessive mutation in a gene encoding a DNA-dependent phosphokinase. Knowing this, and the material covered in this chapter, you should be able to offer a complete explanation for the clinical laboratory and necropsy findings with SCID foals and the reason they all die so young.

Possible Explanations

During genetic rearrangement of TCR V, D, and J segments, a DNA-dependent phosphokinase aids in cleaving the intervening DNA and ligating the new joint between the rearranged segments (see Figure 9.13A–B). Without that enzymatic event, rearrangement is impossible, and functional TCRs cannot be assembled (see Figure 9.13A–D).

During maturation in the thymus, thymocytes without functional TCRs die during positive selection, which means that in affected Arabian foals, no functional T cells ever emigrate from the thymus. Also (as you will see in chapter 11), the same enzymes drive the rearrangement of BCRs. In the absence of functional receptors, B cells die. The inability to produce either B or T cells explains the marked lympho-penia and atrophy of both thymus and lymph nodes.

The reason that some of these foals survive for as long as five months is that antibody-containing colostrum—transferred from mare to foal shortly after birth—provides temporary protection against infection. Because these antibodies have a limited half-life in the foals' blood, protection wanes by five months. Left defenseless, these foals rapidly succumb to infections.

T-Cell Activation

10.5876_9781607322184.c010

CLINICAL CORRELATION: CANINE X-LINKED SEVERE COMBINED IMMUNODEFICIENCY

In 1978, a local breeder brought a litter of basset hound pups (Figure 10.1) to the Genetics-Pediatrics Clinic of the University of Pennsylvania Veterinary Teaching Hospital. The litter included five males and five females. At about age three weeks, two of the male pups developed superficial pyoderma—a bacterial infection of the skin common in dogs—over their hindquarters. The attending veterinarians began antibiotic therapy, but over time the infections

worsened. About three weeks later, one of these pups developed signs of a systemic infection, and the owner took the dog to the hospital. The animal was small and underweight and exhibited a large papular–pustular dermatitis, and the examining veterinarian could find no peripheral lymph nodes. More antibiotics were prescribed as well as adjunctive therapy, but at eight weeks old, the pup died, apparently from pneumonia. At about the same time, the other pup that had early symptoms of an infection worsened and began to show the same symptoms as the first pup. Antibiotic therapy had no effect, and a suppurative otitis developed. After vaccination with a canine distemper–hepatitis live-virus vaccine, this pup developed symptoms of hepatitis, became hypothermic and icteric, eventually slipped into a coma, and was euthanized.

Later, the same breeding pair of hounds produced a second litter of eight pups—seven males and one female. All appeared normal at birth. By age two weeks, one male pup exhibited skin lesions, and two more male pups developed similar symptoms at age three weeks. All the lesions resolved after antibiotic treatment. None of these pups had palpable lymph nodes or a detectable thymus gland. Between twelve and sixteen weeks, all three of the affected pups developed canine distemper and were euthanized. Even though all were unvaccinated, none of these pups' littermates developed canine distemper.

At necropsy, all the affected pups showed signs of extensive infections, including canine

TABLE 10.1. B and T cells in dogs with X-linked SCID (adapted from Felsberg, Somber, Harnett, Henthorn, and Carding, 1988, *Immunologic Research*, 17: 63)

Cells	<4 Week		>8 Week	
	Normal	*XLSCID*	*Normal*	*XLSCID*
B Cells	14.3 ± 15.9[a]	66.3 ± 4.6	12.9 ± 2.5	49.7 ± 15.1
T Cells	58.2 ± 4.6	1.4 ± 1.9	68.1 ± 5.8	23.7 ± 21.4
CD45RA*+ T cells[b]	92.5 ± 2.6	88.1 ± 4.6	90.6 ± 3.2	8.0 ± 0.6

Notes:

a Percentage ± SD.

b Percentage of T cells that are CD45RA+.

* CD45RA+ represents naive T cells.

distemper, hepatitis, and pneumonia. The thymuses of all affected animals were severely atrophied and mostly acellular. (See thymocyte cell counts from affected animals in Table 10.1.)

Overall, T-cell counts were dramatically lower in affected littermates. An interesting finding was that affected animals had higher-than-normal B-cell counts. On the basis of these and other data, it appeared that the affected pups' thymocytes had some sort of defect that prevented their normal proliferation during thymic development.

Further investigations have confirmed that this, in fact, is the case. Because the relevant gene is on the X chromosome of these dogs, and the mutation results in a broad-spectrum immunodeficiency, this disease—which has counterparts in other species—is known as X-linked severe combined immunodeficiency (XLSCID).

More recent studies have shown that the affected gene encodes a protein known as the cytokine receptor common γ chain, or simply γc. Receptors for several distinct IL receptors, including IL-2R, IL-4R, IL-7R, IL-9R, IL-15R, and IL-2R, contain γc (or CD132). Furthermore, γ_c is also among the family of molecules called type I cytokine receptors and is expressed on most lymphocytes. The gene for γc is on the X chromosome of mammals. Somehow, the effects of the XLSCID mutation in dogs result in a profound immunodeficiency as well as dramatic atrophy of the thymus and near to complete absence of lymph nodes.

LEARNING OBJECTIVES

After reading this chapter, you should be able to

- describe the nature of the first, second, and third signals necessary for T-cell activation;

- explain the consequences of each of these signals on the process and direction of T-cell differentiation;

- describe the role of the CDR1, CDR2, and CDR3 regions of the α/β TCR in binding to MHC–antigen complexes;

- list differences and similarities in the activation signals for activation of Th and Tc cells;

- describe the differences in the requirements for naive T-cell and effector and memory T-cell activation;

- explain the origins and functions of the major classes of effector Th cells, including Th1, Th2, Th17, Tfh, and Treg cells;

- explain the actions of Tc cells on infected target cells.

ANTIGEN RECOGNITION BY T CELLS

First Signal: T-Cell Receptors and Major Histocompatibility Complex–Antigen Interactions

Inside of the thymus, T cells acquire a TCR, a CD4 or CD8 molecule, and the CD3 complex (see Figure 10.2). The TCR contains an α and β chain or a γ and δ chain that together form the antigen-binding site. Once the TCR has bound

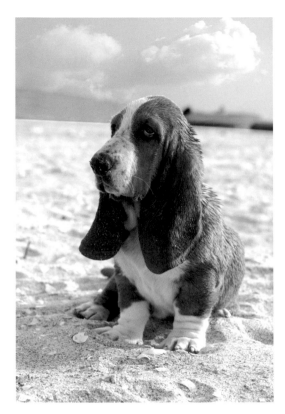

FIGURE 10.1. **Basset hound (© caimacanul / Shutterstock)**

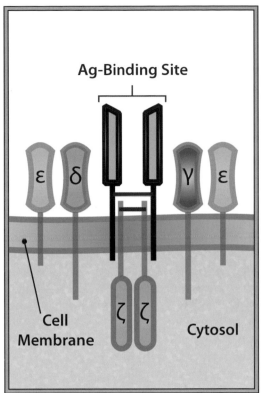

FIGURE 10.2. **T-cell antigen-specific receptor**

antigen, signal transduction occurs via the CD3 complex, which includes γ, δ, ε, and ζ chains. Mature T cells also express either CD4 or CD8 (not shown here), molecules that are not part of the TCR but do help determine whether a T cell will react with antigen in the context of MHC I or II molecules.

Each of these molecules has an important function, but only the α and β chains (or γ and δ chains) directly interact with both antigen and MHC molecules in MHC–antigen complexes. Thus, the α and β chains (or γ and δ chains) determine all of the antigenic specificity of a TCR.

After differentiation in the thymus, two populations of mature, naive T cells emigrate to the thymus—CD4$^+$ Th cells and CD8$^+$ Tc cells. Naive T cells are those T cells that have left the thymus but have not yet encountered their spe-

cific antigen–MHC target. It now appears that both of these populations of naive T cells can only be activated by antigen–MHC complexes on DC APCs (most commonly in secondary lymphoid tissues). Once activated, however, both Th and Tc cells respond to other types of APCs, including B cells, macrophages, and infected self cells. Also, activated T cells, including effector and memory T cells, react more rapidly during antigen presentation, require fewer antigen–MHC complexes, and require less or no costimulation. For now, we focus on activation of mature naive T cells.

As mentioned in chapter 9, the N-terminal (membrane-distal) regions of the TCR α and β chains contain most of the chemical variation seen between TCRs of differing antigenic specificity. Within those N-terminal regions, the greatest variation lies in the so-called CDRs. Each TCR chain has three CDRs, designated

CDR1α, CDR2α, and CDR3α for the α chain and CDR1β, CDR2β, and CDR3β for the β chain. Together, these CDRs form the antigen–MHC contact face of the TCR (see Figure 10.3).

Crystallographic studies of TCR and MHC–antigen complexes revealed first that the TCR interacts simultaneously with both the MHC molecule and the antigenic peptide. Furthermore, during this interaction each of the CDRs of the α and β chains plays a different role. During binding, CDR1α, CDR2α, CDR1β, and CDR2β bind to the α-helical portions of the antigen-binding cleft of either MHC class I or II molecules. Remember that positive selection of T cells inside the thymus relies on the TCRs' ability to bind to MHC molecules. Different T cells have affinities for different MHC molecules. These affinities result from the interactions of CDR1α, CDR2α, CDR1β, and CDR2β with either MHC class I or II molecules.

However, CDR3α and CDR3β bind directly to the antigenic peptides in MHC molecules' binding clefts. As described in chapter 9, CDR3α and CDR3β are the most variable portions of TCR α and β chains. An animal must generate TCRs reactive with relatively few MHC molecules. Those MHC molecules, though, may hold a nearly infinite number of antigenic peptides. So it makes sense that the most variable parts of TCRs would be those that bind directly to antigens.

The binding of TCRs to antigen–MHC complexes is as specific as antigen–antibody interactions but of lower affinity, which means that nearly one TCR exists for every possible antigen. The lower affinity means that TCRs by themselves are not enough to anchor a T cell to its target.

Second Signal and Major Histocompatibility Complex–CD4/8 Interactions

Interactions between a TCR and an antigen–MHC complex are essential but not sufficient (by themselves) to activate a naive T cell. At

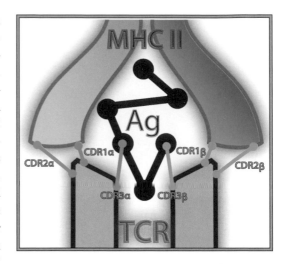

FIGURE 10.3. Interaction of TCR and antigen–MHC complex

The N-terminal (membrane-distal) regions of both the α and β chains of the TCR directly interact with the antigen–MHC complex. From crystallographic studies, it is apparent that CDR1α and CDR2α as well as CDR1β and CDR2β interact most directly with the MHC molecule, whereas the CDR3 regions of both chains interact most directly with the antigenic peptide in the MHC binding cleft.

least two other interactions must occur between T-cell and APC cell-surface molecules. The first of these involves two molecules discussed in chapter 9: CD4 and CD8.

As T cells undergo positive selection in the thymus, they switch from being double positive (expressing both CD4 and CD8) cells to expressing only CD4 (MHC class II–specific) or CD8 (MHC class I–specific) molecules. CD4 and CD8 molecules strengthen the bond between TCRs and MHC molecules by binding to a constant region (the same regardless of encoding allele) of an MHC molecule. Overall, this bond with the constant region of the MHC molecule increases the avidity of the TCR for the APC but has no effect on the antigenic specificity of the TCR (see Figure 10.4A–B). All Th cells express CD4 molecules that bind to antigen–MHC class II complexes. All Tc cells express

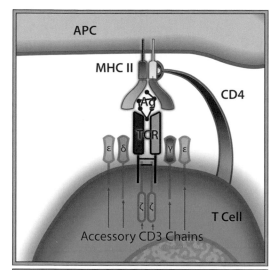

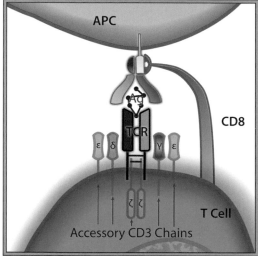

FIGURE 10.4A–B. Interactions between CD4 and CD8 molecules with APCs

The CD4 molecule on the surface of Th cells binds MHC class II molecules and strengthens the interaction between Th cells and DC APCs (upper panel). The CD8 molecule on the surface of Tc cells binds MHC class I molecules and strengthens the interaction between DC APCs or target cells and Tc cells (lower panel).

CD8 molecules that bind to antigen–MHC class I complexes.

Beyond CD4 and CD8, T-cell activation requires one more interaction between molecules on T cells and APCs. This interaction involves

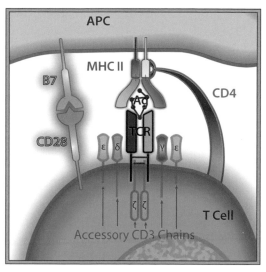

FIGURE 10.5. T-cell costimulation

The initial phase of T-cell activation requires two signals; a primary signal CD3 delivers after the TCR has bound to the MHC–antigen complex on an APC and a secondary signal CD28 delivers after it has bound to B7 on the APC.

CD28 on the T-cell surface and B7 molecules on the APC surface. Although we focus only on T-cell activation, it is also possible for APCs to deliver negative or inhibitory signals to T cells, which may be important in both downregulation of immune responses and self-tolerance.

Complete activation of T cells is a two-step process. In the first step, after TCR binding of antigen–MHC complex, CD3 delivers a primary signal to the T-cell nucleus. In the second step, B7 (CD80 and 86) on the APC delivers a secondary signal through CD28 on the T cell (see Figure 10.5). Only after both interactions occur successfully will a T cell respond.

Because inappropriate activation of T cells may pose a threat to self, as with MHC class II molecules, B7 molecules appear only on APCs. Moreover, until pathogens, cytokines, or T cells activate them, most APCs express fairly low levels of B7.

If a T cell receives only signal 2, nothing happens. But when a T cell receives signal 1 alone, that T cell becomes anergic (unreactive) to further antigenic stimulation (see Figure 10.6A–B). This requirement further guards against T-cell activation by non-APCs or APCs that have not been previously activated by danger signals (PAMPs, DAMPS, or both), because these cells are likely presenting only self antigen.

Signal Transduction and T-Cell Activation

The first lymphocytes activated during most adaptive immune responses are Th cells. Once a Th cell receives both signals from an APC, a series of events follows.

Through a series of phosphorylations and dephosphorylations inside the T cell, as well as the activation of enzymes and nuclear factors such as NFAT and NF-κB, nuclear gene expression changes. The pivotal role of these steps is most apparent after treatment with corticosteroids, which inhibit the activation of NF-κB and result in marked immunosuppression.

Under normal circumstances, though, T-cell activation induces several Th-cell genes to cease or begin producing proteins. One particularly important change is induction of expression of the high-affinity IL-2 receptor and the cytokine IL-2 (see Figure 10.7A–D).

Naive T cells express an IL-2 receptor (IL-2R) composed of only β and γ chains (a γ chain is common to many IL receptors). This form of the IL-2R has only moderate affinity for IL-2, and the resultant interaction between receptor and ligand is too weak to push the naive T cells into cell division. After a specific interaction with its cognate antigen (the antigen–MHC complex that specifically reacts with the cell's TCR) and costimulation, a T cell begins to express the third (or α) chain of the IL-2R. Once the α chain joins with the β and γ chains, the complete IL-2R develops high affinity for IL-2. At the same time, the newly activated T cell begins to express IL-2. The interaction of IL-2 with the high-affinity IL-2R causes the T cell to begin dividing rapidly, which results in a process called clonal expansion (the rapid expansion of

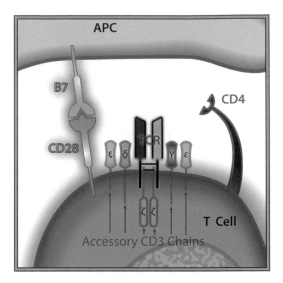

Costimulatory Signal Alone

No Effect on T Cell

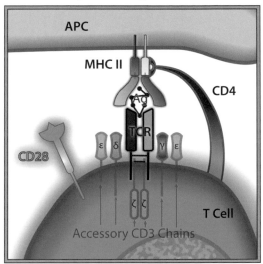

Specific Signal Alone

Inactivates T Cell (Anergy)

FIGURE 10.6A–B. T-cell responses to only primary or only secondary signal

By itself, interaction of B7 and CD28 (second signal) elicits no T-cell response (upper panel). Interaction of TCR with antigen–MHC complex (primary signal) without the second signal, however, renders the T cell unresponsive to this antigen (lower panel).

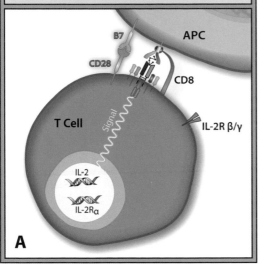

Resting T Cells Express Only a Moderate-Affinity IL-2 Receptor (IL-2Rβ and γ Chains Only)

A

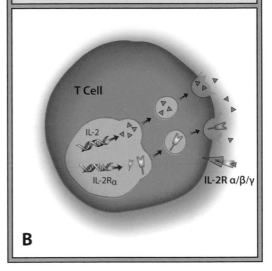

Activated T Cells Express a High-Affinity IL-2 Receptor (IL-2Rα, β, and γ Chains) and Secrete IL-2

B

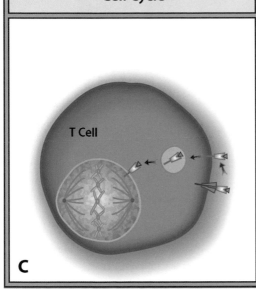

Binding of IL-2 to Its Receptor Signals the T Cell to Enter the Cell Cycle

C

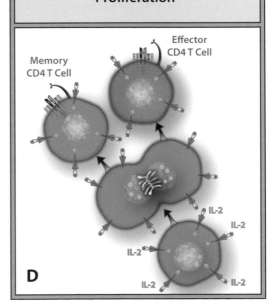

Induces T-Cell Proliferation

D

FIGURE 10.7A–D. T-cell activation and the appearance of the high-affinity IL-2 receptor

After antigen presentation and costimulation (A), T cells begin to express both the α chain of the IL-2 receptor and IL-2 (B). When the completed receptor binds IL-2, a signal is transmitted to the nucleus (C) and the activated T cells begin to proliferate and eventually differentiate into either effector or memory T cells (D).

a single antigen-specific T cell into a clone of millions of identical T cells, all specific for the same antigen). This process is ultimately responsible for the exquisite specificity of adaptive immune responses.

Third Signal and T-Helper Cell Differentiation

After activation, Th cells may follow any one of several paths of differentiation. Understanding this process is essential to understanding animals' immune responses and how to manipulate those responses for maximum benefit—either through vaccination or immune regulation.

Ultimately, DC APCs determine the final directions of naive Th-cell differentiation through selective cytokine secretion (third signal). During interactions with Th cells, APCs secrete specific cytokines that react with specific receptors on Th cells, altering gene expression inside the Th cells and pushing the Th cells down one differentiation pathway or another.

When, during antigen presentation, DCs secrete IL-12, Th0 cells become Th1 cells. When APCs induce Notch-receptor signaling, Th0 cells develop into Th2 cells. When APCs produce IL-6 and TGF-β, Th0 cells become Th17 cells. Some regulatory T cells (in particular, Treg cells) develop in the thymus and become active in the periphery, but other Treg cells develop from Th0 cells outside the thymus, including Th3 and TR1 cells. The formation of these cells requires DC-derived IL-10, TGF-β, or both. No one knows exactly what induces the APC or the Th cell to produce a particular set of cytokines, but it depends, at least in part, on the nature of the innate response that precedes T-cell activation. Different innate responses can alter APCs in several ways, and they direct the Th-cell response down different pathways.

The pathways to Tc-cell activation differ from those leading to Th-cell activation. First, interactions between APCs and CD8+ T cells involve antigens bound by MHC class I (not

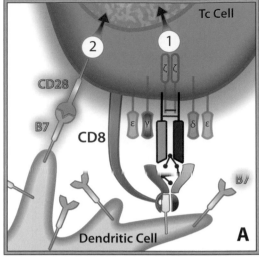

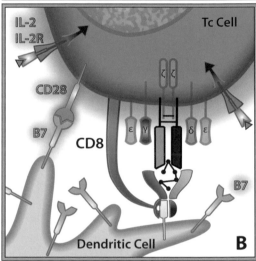

FIGURE 10.8A–B. Direct activation of Tc cells by highly effective APCs

APCs (like DCs) that constitutively express high levels of B7 can provide both first (MHC–antigen) and second (B7) signals to Tc cells (panel A). In response, the T cells begin to express the high-affinity IL-2R and to produce IL-2 (panel B), which leads to activation.

II) molecules. Second, APCs can activate CD8+ cells in more than one way. Highly effective APCs, in particular DCs, that express abundant MHC–antigen complexes and B7 molecules can deliver first and second signals and directly activate Tc cells (see Figure 10.8A–B).

Activation of naive CD8$^+$ cells by other APCs (e.g., macrophages) expressing lower amounts of B7, however, often requires the participation of a Th cell. Constitutively, macrophages express lower levels of B7. After antigen-specific interactions between macrophages and Th cells, macrophage APCs express much higher levels of B7, allowing for effective delivery of the second signal and activation of Tc cells (see Figure 10.9A–B). Regardless of the activation pathway, in the end, the activated Tc cells begin to express the high-affinity IL 2R and IL-2, resulting in rapid expansion of antigen-reactive clones of Tc cells.

The third signal for Tc-cell activation comes from the APC in the form of IL-12. This cytokine strongly directs immune responses toward CD8$^+$–Tc-cell responses, also known as adaptive cellular immune responses.

As you may have noticed, throughout this description—from antigen processing and presentation to final activation of T cells—none of the processes distinguish between self and non-self. APCs are, in fact, just as effective at presenting self antigens as they are at presenting non-self antigens. Clearly, two factors that help to reduce the likelihood of self-reactivity are central and peripheral tolerance. But even beyond that, antigen presentation—self or non-self—fails to activate T cells in the absence of danger signals. Such signals arise when host cells bind to PAMPs and DAMPs from pathogens and the ensuing inflammation. In the absence of danger signals and the resulting expression of costimulatory ligands on the APCs, antigen presentation not only may fail to activate T cells but may even render them tolerant of the presented antigen.

EFFECTOR T CELLS

Effector T-Helper Cells: Th1, Th2, Tfh, and Th17 Cells

After activation, naive T cells become effector T cells capable of mediating their effects in immune responses and other host defenses. As

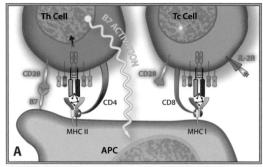

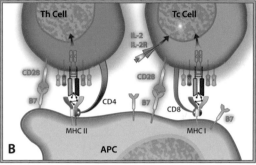

FIGURE 10.9A–B. Th cell–assisted activation of Tc cells

APCs expressing lower levels of B7 may first have to interact with Th cells. That interaction induces activation of the APC and higher levels of expression of B7 and MHC (panel A), which increases the efficiency of the APCs, provides additional IL-2, and leads to activation of the Tc cell (panel B).

mentioned earlier, effector T cells have significantly different minimal requirements for activation, including lower or no requirement for costimulation via B7.

All Th cells begin their lives as naive Th cells (sometimes called Thn cells); after activation, they become Th0 cells. These Th0 cells have the potential to become many other types of Th cells (see Figure 10.10).

As shown in the first set of arrows in Figure 10.10, APC- and Th-cell–derived cytokines direct Th0 differentiation toward one of many possible subsets of Th cells. Despite all the possible outcomes of Th-cell differentiation, all Th cells continue to express CD4 and α/β TCRs and recognize only antigen in the context of

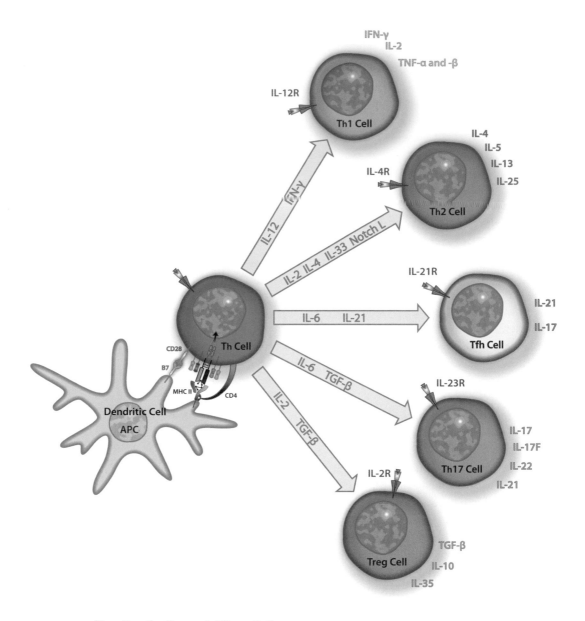

FIGURE 10.10. Th-cell activation and differentiation

After interaction with a DC APC, Th cells may differentiate into several different cell types, including Th1, Th2, Tfh, Th17, Treg, Th3, and Tr1 cells. The pathway of Th-cell differentiation depends on the cytokines produced during antigen presentation (arrows). Each Th-cell type secretes a characteristic set of cytokines (far right) and participates in a unique way in the immune response.

MHC class II molecules. But the similarities end there.

Most immunological studies generally recognize four products of Th0-cell differentiation: Th1, Th2, Th17, and Treg cells. Of these, the most is known about Th1, Th2, and Th17 cells. The Th1 cells participate in inflammatory responses and in the production of certain types of antibodies, and the Th2 cells mostly direct B-cell differentiation and antibody responses.

Th17 cells play their largest roles in inflammatory responses. Differences in the cytokines the cell types produce make this possible.

The largest numbers of Th1 cells develop after infections with intracellular bacteria and viruses. Activated Th1 cells produce a series of proinflammatory cytokines, including γ-IFN, IL-2, TNF-α, TNF-β, Fas ligand (FasL), and others (see Figures 10.11A–D and 10.12). These cytokines affect many different aspects of protective responses, especially innate effector responses. Together, Th1 cytokines (particularly IFN-γ and IL-2) activate macrophages, increase inflammation, stimulate B-cell proliferation and differentiation, and accelerate T-cell proliferation. The Th1-cell–activated macrophages express higher levels of B7 and MHC class II molecules, more effectively destroy ingested bacteria (particularly through upregulation of oxidative radical-generating machinery), more efficiently activate additional T cells (especially Tc cells), and secrete additional TNF-α—a powerful stimulator of inflammation. The Th1-cell–activated macrophages and inflammation are major players in protective responses against bacteria. After secretion, IL-3 induces increased production of macrophages in the bone marrow. TNF-β further contributes to inflammation and emigration of monocytes from the blood and, along with FasL, helps to destroy chronically infected cells and release their contents to fresh macrophages. In addition, Th1 cells secrete macrophage chemotactic protein 1. This cytokine brings more macrophages to sites of inflammation. Th1 cells and their cytokines also favor production of specific antibody types and suppress activation of Th2 cells and some B cells.

In addition, Th1 cells are effective activators of B cells and induce isotype switches to particular Ig isotypes (especially those isotype types that are the best opsonins; see chapter 11) and suppress activation of Th2 cells.

Activated Th2 cells participate most directly in antibody-mediated adaptive immune responses. These cells secrete IL-4, IL-5, IL-13, and IL-25. IL-4 and IL-5 stimulate Th2-cell division, as well as B-cell activation and division, and direct B cells toward the production of specific antibody types, including IgGs and IgE. IL-4 and IL-5 also activate eosinophils (along with IgE, also important in some parasitic infections) and mast cells (see Figure 10.12). Also, IL-4 and IL-13 activate an alternative set of macrophages important for immune response to parasites and tissue repair.

IL-5 stimulates production of granulocytes in the bone marrow, and IL-13 stimulates production of TGF-β—a cytokine that stimulates cellular proliferation and differentiation—whereas IL-25 is another proinflammatory cytokine. At sites of inflammation, IL-5 also serves to activate eosinophils, allowing them to more effectively degranulate and mount antihelminthic responses.

Beyond Th1 and Th2 cells, several additional types of CD4+ T cells play various roles in stimulating or inhibiting immune responses. Other products of Th0 cells, Th17 cells, produce several cytokines (including IL-17, the source of the designation Th17) that favor inflammation. The cytokine IL-17 has multiple effects on events related to inflammation (see Figure 10.13).

In immune reactions to several types of pathogens, this inflammatory enhancement is essential for control and elimination of the pathogen. The cytokines IL-6 and IL-23, from APCs, favor development of Th17 from Th0 cells (see Figure 10.10).

Effector Regulatory T Cells: Treg, Th3, and Tr1 Cells

The last generally recognized group of CD4+ T cells is the regulatory T cells. Some regulatory T cells, specifically Treg cells, arise in the thymus from populations of self-reactive CD4+ T cells that survive negative selection and emigrate to the periphery (see chapter 9). Other regulatory T cells appear to arise after induction outside of the thymus; these cells may be descendants of Th0 cells. The Treg cells play a

FIGURE 10.11A–D. Actions of effector Th1 cells

Activated Th1 cells secrete unique sets of cytokines. Panel A depicts the original activation that leads to the production of IFN-γ, and the other cytokines represented in panels B, C, and D activate macrophages, enhance the killing of bacteria, and induce B-cell differentiation (panel A), kill chronically infected cells (panel B), induce T-cell proliferation (panel C), and activate vascular endothelium to enhance exit of monocytes from blood into inflamed and infected tissues (panel D).

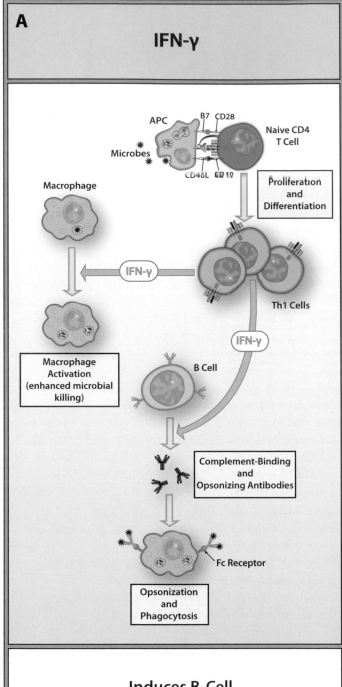

A

IFN-γ

APC   B7 CD28   Naive CD4 T Cell

Microbes

CD40L CD10

Proliferation and Differentiation

Macrophage

IFN-γ   Th1 Cells

IFN-γ

Macrophage Activation (enhanced microbial killing)

B Cell

Complement-Binding and Opsonizing Antibodies

Fc Receptor

Opsonization and Phagocytosis

Induces B-Cell Proliferation and Differentiation, Complement Binding, and Opsonizing Antibodies

B Fas Ligand or TNF-β	C IL-2	D TNF-α + TNF-β
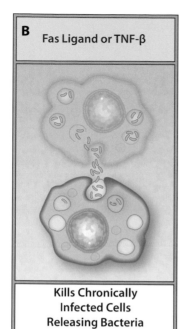	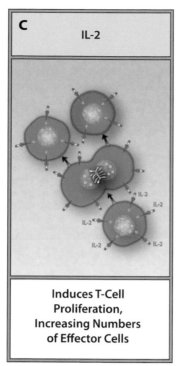	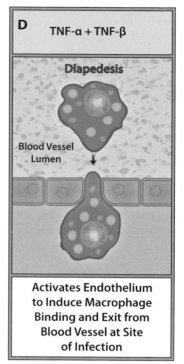
Kills Chronically Infected Cells Releasing Bacteria to Be Destroyed by Fresh Macrophages	**Induces T-Cell Proliferation, Increasing Numbers of Effector Cells**	**Activates Endothelium to Induce Macrophage Binding and Exit from Blood Vessel at Site of Infection**

major role in the suppression of autoimmunity through peripheral tolerance.

To maintain self-tolerance, Treg cells interfere with the normal activation of effector cells or destroy them, but exactly how Treg cells do this is unclear. It now appears that many autoimmune diseases result from dysregulation of, or imbalances among, Treg-cell populations.

Beyond the four generally recognized Th-cell subtypes, other CD4⁺ T cells seemingly participate in certain types of immune responses or immune suppression. The relationships of these cells to commonly recognized Th cells are unclear. Among them are T-follicular helper cells (Tfh). These T cells reside in the follicles inside of lymph nodes and appear to play a role in directing Th-cell differentiation. Because much of Th-cell differentiation occurs after antigen presentation in the lymph nodes, Tfh cells probably play important roles in the lives of Th cells. Whether Tfh cells represent a T-cell lineage distinct from Th1 and Th2 cells, however, is not clear.

Three additional regulatory T-cell categories (Th3, Tr1, and Th9) may also be important in prevention of autoimmunity. But recent evidence has indicated that all three cell types may arise from one of the four major types of Th cells, depending on which cytokines are present.

In summary, Th cells act at many points while innate and adaptive responses are developing. In addition, Th cells help prevent some destructive autoimmune and inflammatory responses. But despite their importance in immunity, the exact number of T-cell lineages and their mechanisms of action are not known. It is clear that Th cells come in many forms and participate in essential ways in all aspects of adaptive immune responses.

Effector Cytotoxic T Cells

In the final steps of CD8⁺-cell activation, APCs provide first signal in the form of antigen presentation in the context of MHC class I molecules and second signal through the inter-

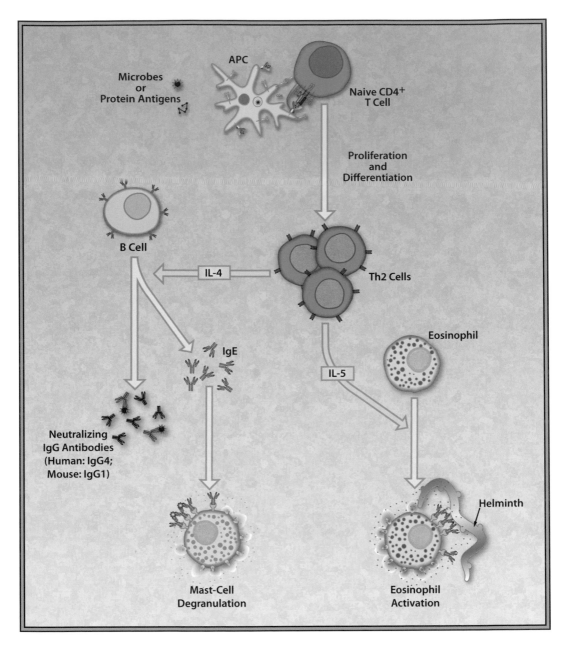

FIGURE 10.12. Actions of activated Th2 cells

Th2 cells secrete several cytokines, including IL-4 and IL-5. These cytokines stimulate proliferation and differentiation, activate mast cells and eosinophils, and stimulate proliferation and differentiation of B cells.

action of B7 and CD28. Once activated, Tc cells no longer require costimulation for further activation. Activated Tc cells migrate from the lymph nodes and circulate in blood and lymph. They can extravasate at sites of inflammation and look for infected cells exhibiting the same MHC class I–antigen complex the APCs first presented to these Tc cells.

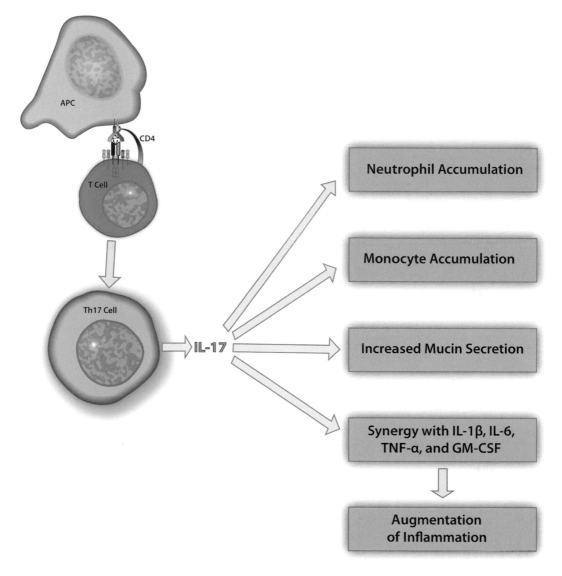

FIGURE 10.13. Effects of Th17-derived IL-17

During responses against bacteria, fungi, and parasites, IL-17 attracts neutrophils and macrophages (derived from monocytes) to sites of inflammation. Once there, this cytokine stimulates mucin secretion and interacts with several other proinflammatory cytokines to enhance and maintain the inflammatory state.

The interaction between effector Tc cells and potential target cells does not begin with MHC–antigen and TCR. Instead, effector Tc cells browse through potential target cells using intracellular adhesion molecules (I-CAMs or simply CAMs) such as leukocyte function-associated antigen-1 (LFA-1) and I-CAM-1. Only after these adhesion molecules anchor a Tc cell is there an opportunity for TCR interactions with specific MHC–antigen complexes. If no TCR binding occurs, Tc cells detach from this potential target and resume their searches for infected cells.

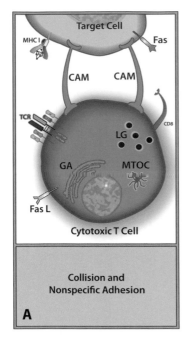 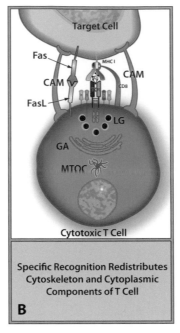 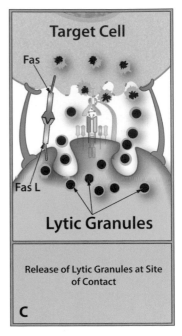

FIGURE 10.14A–C. **Effector Tc cell function**

Tc cells first attach to target cells using CAM (panel A). Then TCR interacts with antigen–MHC complexes, and a shift occurs in the cellular architecture. The Golgi apparatus (GA) aligns between Tc and target cells, the microtubule organizing center (MTOC) realigns the cellular architecture, and lytic granules (LG) appear between effector and target cells (panel B). The release of the lytic granules as well as the interaction between FasL on the Tc cell and Fas on the target cell induce apoptosis in the target cell (panel C).

When a specific interaction occurs between the T cell's TCR and MHC–antigen complexes on the target cell, though, several changes occur inside of the Tc cell (see Figure 10.14A–C). The Tc cell's Golgi apparatus aligns at the point of cellular contact, and lytic granules accumulate in the Tc cell near contact points with the target cell. The cellular architecture shifts as the Tc cell focuses its weapons on the target cell. At this point, the Tc cell releases both perforins and granzymes (a series of serine proteases) and expresses FasL. Perforins open small pores in the target cells' surfaces. When entering through those pores, the granzymes initiate apoptosis in the target cells. When FasL reacts with Fas on the target cell, it also induces apoptosis, and infected cells die without releasing all of their infectious contents. Macrophages then safely clean up the remains of the apoptotic cells, and no inflammatory response follows.

By these means, Tc cells effectively rid an animal's body of infected cells and bring infectious diseases to a healthy conclusion. In summary (see Figure 10.15), APCs activate Tc cells in secondary lymphoid tissues. Activated Tc cells may become effector Tc cells or memory Tc cells. Effector T cells migrate to areas of inflammation and kill infected cells. Memory Tc cells are long-lived and are the first to respond in secondary and subsequent immune responses. After infection, T cells develop into a formidable array of weaponry (see Figure 10.16). Each of these T cells plays a vital role in the developing immune response as well as in the prevention of autoimmunity.

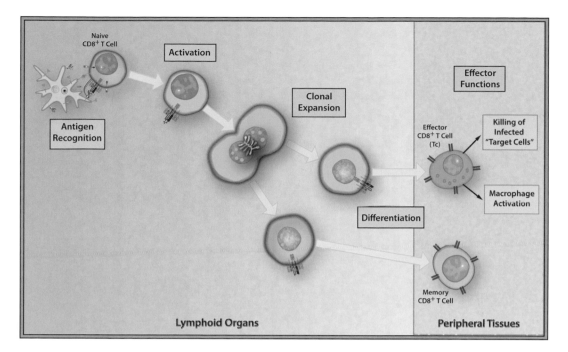

FIGURE 10.15. Life cycle of a Tc cell

APCs activate Tc cells in lymphoid tissues. Activated cells differentiate into memory or effector Tc cells.

CLINICAL CORRELATION FOLLOW-UP

As we said at the beginning of this chapter, XLSCID in basset hounds (Figure 10.17) results in severe atrophy of the thymus and the lymph nodes as well as SCID. Affected animals have dramatically fewer T cells but a normal to above-normal number of B cells. The mutation responsible for XLSCID occurs in the gene that encodes the common γ-chain receptor—a molecule that forms a requisite part of many different IL receptors, including IL-2R, IL-4R, and IL-7R. How could alterations in the γc gene account for the XLSCID?

Student Considerations

On the basis of the material presented in this chapter, you should be able to propose a reason why the absence of IL-2 and IL-4 receptors would result in severely atrophied lymph nodes. Also, on the basis of information from this and previous chapters you should know why the absence of IL-2 receptors might result in thymic atrophy. In addition, you should be able to offer a plausible explanation for the dramatically reduced numbers of T cells.

Possible Explanations

There is no simple explanation for all of the symptoms of XLSCID in basset hounds, but some of the contributing factors seem obvious. The γc chain is an essential component of receptors for IL-2, IL-4, IL-7, IL-9, IL-15, and IL-21.

IL-2 and IL-4 play essential roles in lymphocyte proliferation. Both inside and outside of the thymus, T-cell division depends absolutely on IL-2. Outside the thymus, naive Th cells require IL-2 for proliferation and differentiation. In addition, IL-4 stimulates proliferation and differentiation of Th2 cells and B cells.

A complete lack of IL-2R and IL-4R would result in no lymphocyte proliferation in either

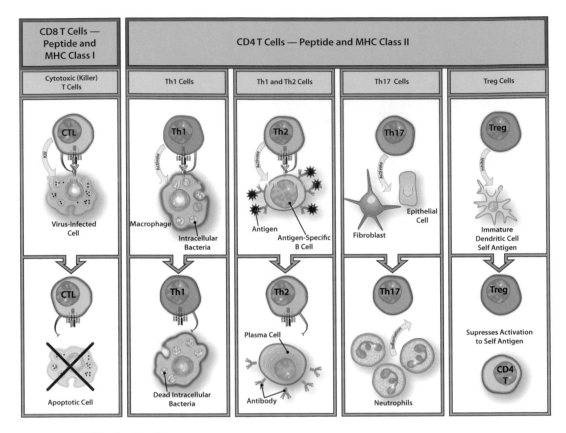

FIGURE 10.16. Effector T cells

After activation by MHC–antigen complexes on APCs, T cells differentiate into a variety of effector cells that drive the progression of a variety of types of immune responses.

the thymus or the lymph nodes and a complete absence of mature B cells. These factors would result in severe atrophy of both primary and secondary lymphoid organs, as seen in these dogs. However, these factors would not explain the continued presence of roughly 30 percent of normal T-cell numbers by age eight weeks old.

In addition, there is the problem of the above-normal B-cell numbers in dogs with XLSCID. Interestingly, all of the B cells in dogs with XLSCID are immature B cells (they only express IgM). Maturation of B cells (see chapter 11) requires interaction with Th cells and cytokines produced by Th cells, such as IL-4. The absence of functional receptors for IL-4, along with the limited number of T cells, explains the absence of mature B cells.

Beyond IL-2 and IL-4, another factor is at play here: IL-7. This cytokine plays a major role in the development of lymphoid progenitor cells in the bone marrow. When pluripotent lymphoid stem cells lack receptors for IL-7, few or no lymphocytes develop in the bone marrow. As a consequence, none go to the thymus, and none leave the thymus to populate the secondary lymphoid tissues. This, too, could explain the absence of palpable lymph nodes and the thymic atrophy in dogs with XLSCID. However, a complete lack of receptors for IL-7 seems inconsistent with the numbers of lymphocytes remaining in basset hounds with

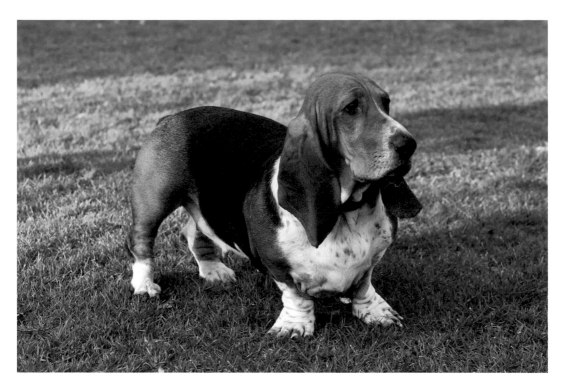

FIGURE 10.17. Tan and white basset hound (© Ewa Studio / Shutterstock)

XLSCID—especially B cells. A complete explanation for this disorder will probably involve reduced numbers of IL-2R, IL-4R, and IL-7R molecules; reduced affinity of these molecules; or both, but it seems likely that other factors contribute as well.

CLINICAL CORRELATION: EQUINE AGAMMAGLOBULINEMIA

Antibody deficiencies, which may be selective or complete, are among the most frequently diagnosed immune deficiencies in mammals. One of these, equine X-linked agammaglobulinemia, provides a useful insight into the nature of B-cell development in horses and probably all other mammals. Among thoroughbred, standard bred, and quarter horses, some afflicted males begin to develop severe bacterial infections at about two to six months of age. These infections include pneumonia, enteritis, and dermatitis. Antibiotics and, interestingly, plasma transfusions provide temporary relief from symptoms and further infections. Hema-

tology testing of these animals shows normal numbers of lymphocytes, but no B cells, no IgM or IgA antibodies, very low concentrations of IgG and Ig(T) (an isotype peculiar to horses) antibodies, and normal T-cell responses in vitro and in vivo. Because shortly after birth most foals receive large amounts of Ig in their dams' colostrum, the immunodeficiencies of the foals become apparent only as maternal Ig disappears from their blood. At this point, these foals often succumb to persistent bacterial infections and die.

Because of the similarities of this disease to X-linked agammaglobulinemia in humans, the underlying cause is likely a defect in a molecule called Bruton's tyrosine kinase (BTK), an enzyme essentially involved in the function of the BCR and other surface receptors. These foals' illness is apparent, but what is less apparent is how a protein-kinase defect could lead to a severe immunodeficiency.

LEARNING OBJECTIVES

After reading this chapter, you should be able to

- describe the structure of the BCR;
- explain the genetic mechanisms responsible for the essentially unlimited diversity of BCRs, including genetic rearrangement and junctional diversification;
- describe the mechanisms and the order of B-cell development, including B-cell selection;
- explain the differences between Ig isotypes and their importance in defense;

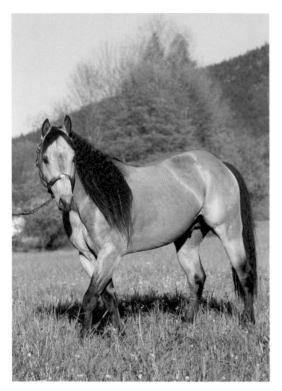

**FIGURE 11.1. American quarter horse (©
Lenkadan / Shutterstock)**

- describe the nature of B-1 and marginal-zone (MZ) B cells and discuss the relevance of these cells to defense against infections.

B CELLS AND THE STRUCTURE OF THE B-CELL RECEPTOR

In mammals, B cells—like all lymphocytes—originate in the bone marrow. Unlike T cells, though, all of the maturation of naive mammalian B cells occurs in the bone marrow; no other organ contributes to the first phases of B-cell development. In birds, however, B-cell development (along with some hematopoiesis) occurs in the bursa of Fabricius, an organ on the dorsal wall of the cloaca. In the teleost fish, the kidneys are the major sites of B-cell development, and in amphibians B cells develop at several sites, including spleen, bone marrow, and kidney.

B cells are the ultimate source of antibodies, the end products of adaptive humoral immune responses—humoral because physicians, such as Galen in the second century BC, once believed that all maladies arose as a result of an imbalance in the humors (black bile, yellow bile, phlegm, and blood) of the circulating fluids. Because of that, factors that appeared in blood were called humoral factors. Because scientists first discovered antibodies in serum, this type of response came to be known as the humoral immune response. B cells come in two forms, B-1 and B-2. In mammals, B-2 B cells are the most numerous and produce the largest variety of antibodies.

Like TCRs, antibodies come in almost limitless forms, each with a unique antigenic specificity, but BCRs contain four polypeptide chains and react with native antigen—that is, with unprocessed antigens and no involvement with MHC molecules (Figure 11.2)

The most common form of mammalian BCRs contains four Ig chains—two H chains and two L chains—all held together by disulfide bonds. This part of the BCR is essentially an antibody molecule with an added membrane anchor. Each of the four chains contains a C-terminal constant region and an N-terminal variable region. Within these variable regions of both H and L chains (just as with TCR α and β chains) are three regions of hypervariability called CDR1, CDR2, and CDR3. Together these regions of one H chain and one L chain form an antigen-binding site—two per BCR.

Unlike TCRs, antibodies exist in two forms, as the cell membrane–bound BCR and as secreted antibodies (see the Order and Regulation of B-Cell Development section) that circulate in blood, extravascular fluids, and lymph. These secreted forms were discovered first and named immunoglobulins or antibodies.

In addition, BCRs associate with two other membrane-bound proteins—Igα and Igβ. Together, these extra two molecules function in signal transduction much as the CD3 complex on T cells. Also like CD3, Igα and Igβ have

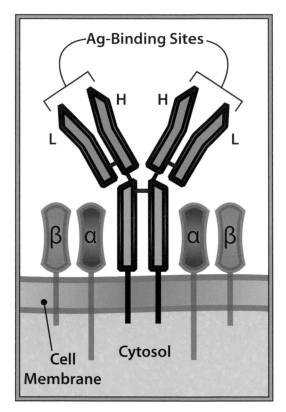

FIGURE 11.2. The common mammalian BCR

The BCR contains four polypeptide chains—two identical H chains and two identical L chains. The L chains are bound to the H chains by disulfide bonds, as the H chains are bound to one another. The C-terminal (membrane-proximal) portions of the H chains span the cell membrane and are identical for each Ig isotype, and the N-terminal (membrane-distal) portions of the H chains are highly variable. Similarly, the C-terminal regions of the L chains are constant within a given type of L chains, and the N-terminal portions are highly variable. Together, the N-termini of the H and L chains make up the two membrane-distal antigen-binding sites. Igα and Igβ molecules associate with the antigen-binding portion of the receptor and are involved with signal transduction. Ag = antigen.

nothing to do with the antigenic specificity of the BCR. That specificity resides completely within the N-termini of the H and L chains.

Unlike TCRs, during its lifetime a B cell may express several different forms of the BCR, all with the same antigenic specificity. Different forms of BCRs and secreted antibodies are called Ig isotypes (see Immunoglobulin Isotypes section). The differences between isotypes are all found in the constant regions of the H chains. The first BCR expressed by developing mammalian B cells is always IgM.

B-CELL GENETICS, DEVELOPMENT, AND CIRCULATION

B-Cell Receptor Gene Families, Genetic Rearrangement, and Junctional Diversity

Once Igs were discovered, it was soon obvious that the chemical diversity among Igs outstripped that of any other animal protein. But only after many years of study was the genetic basis of this structural diversity unraveled. These discoveries actually predated understanding of the genetics of TCRs by a few decades.

The essentially unlimited diversity among the common mammalian BCRs within one animal arises much as does the diversity of mammalian TCRs. Inside the genome of mammals, sequences that encode BCR H and L chains appear in segments or families of genes. H chains have one gene family, and L chains have one or more. As with the TCR gene families, one BCR gene family (H chain) contains variable (V), diversity (D), and joining (J) segments, and the other gene family (L chain) contains only V and J segments (Figure 11.3). Camelids (camels and llamas) are the one known exception to this. Camelid antibodies (not shown) have no L chains. The H chains by themselves form the antigen-binding sites of these antibodies. The Ig gene families of camels and llamas, therefore, do not include L-chain gene segments.

In mammals, bony fish, and amphibians, BCR gene rearrangement begins when the bone marrow stroma signals a developing B cell to start rearranging H-chain genes, which results

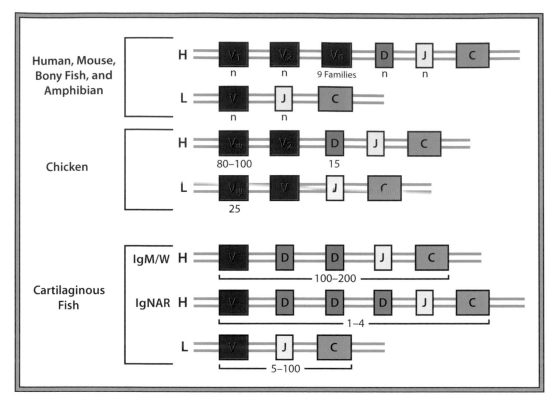

FIGURE 11.3. BCR gene families

The BCR H-chain gene family resides on a single chromosome and contains multiple variable (V_H), diversity (D_H), and joining (J_H) segments. The number of these segments and their arrangements varies between species. The lowercase *n* indicates varying numbers. The Greek letter ψ indicates pseudogenes (incomplete genes), and the numbers under brackets indicate the total number of germline V, D, J, and C complexes. IgW and Ig new antigen receptor (IGNAR) are Ig isotypes unique to cartilaginous fish. BCR L-chain gene families are on separate chromosomes and contain only V, J, and C segments.

in looping out of intervening DNA and juxtaposition of randomly selected D_H and J_H segments. Just as with TCR gene rearrangements, enzymes excise the looped-out DNA and, as the D_H and J_H segments join, additional diversity arises from the process of junctional diversification—the random addition and subtraction of nucleotides as the D_H–J_H joint forms (see Figure 9.6). Next, this DJ segment, through a similar, random process, joins with a V_H segment to create an H-chain variable-region gene complex (Figure 11.4).

After a successful H-chain gene family rearrangement and production of a functional H chain, L-chain rearrangement begins when a randomly selected V_L gene segment associates with a randomly selected J_L segment. Then, following the processes of excision of intervening DNA and junctional diversification, an L-chain variable gene complex appears. Enzymes then transcribe these L-chain and H-chain genes, along with their C segments, into nuclear, or primary, RNA. Then spliceosomes convert these transcripts into messenger RNA (mRNA), which are translated into proteins that join to form a BCR (Figure 11.4).

A final L chain requires one V_L, one J_L, and one C_L segment. The gene rearrangement process

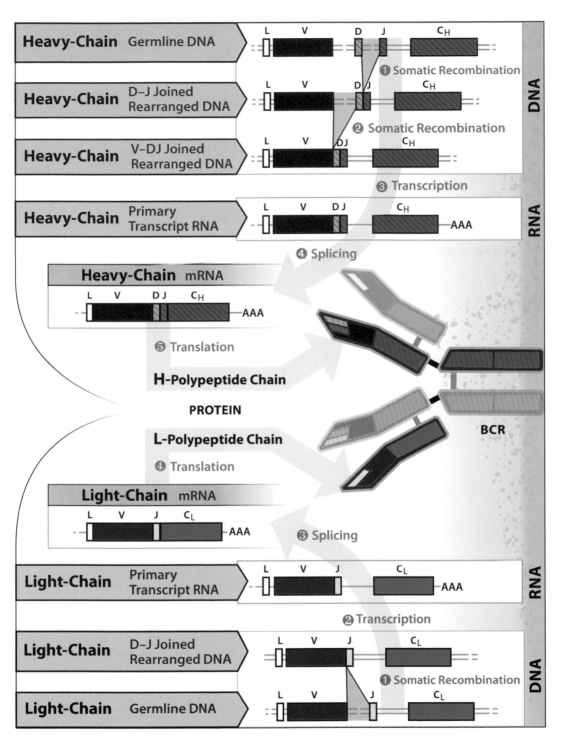

FIGURE 11.4. **Assembly of L chains and H chains**

first randomly couples one V_L and one J_L. The newly formed VJ segment, along with intervening DNA and a C_L segment, are transcribed into a nuclear RNA transcript. Spliceosomes convert this nuclear transcript in mRNA, and ribosomes create the final protein. Similarly, a single H-chain gene begins when rearrangement randomly couples a single D_H segment with a J_H segment. This complex then randomly rearranges to join a V_H segment. The newly created VDJ complex, along with intervening DNA and a C_H segment, produce a nuclear RNA transcript that is converted to mRNA and translated into an H chain. Two identical H and two identical L chains join to form a BCR.

The final products are mammalian BCRs, each with a unique antigen-binding specificity. The nearly unlimited diversity and antigenic specificity of these BCRs is the result of random gene rearrangement and junctional diversification.

Other species use very different mechanisms to generate BCR diversity. For example, in chickens, BCR diversity arises from an entirely different process called *gene conversion* (Figure 11.5).

Chickens have only one V_H, D_H, and C_μ (constant region for the H chain) gene segment. Inside the bursa of Fabricius, genetic rearrangement results in the appearance of the same BCR on all B cells. In addition to the functional gene segments in chicken Ig gene families, however, are multiple pseudogenes—inactive partial genes. During further development in chicken B cells, additional rearrangement randomly inserts pieces of these pseudogenes into the V segments of both H- and L-chain genes, which dramatically increases the variety of BCRs and the capacity for antigen recognition in chickens.

Cartilaginous fish have their H and L genes already connected in the germline genetic configuration (Figure 11.3) and use still another means for diversification. Although structurally unique (no L chains), camelid Ig genes diversify via genetic recombination just as do Ig genes in most other mammals. On the other hand, in sheep and cattle, antibody diversity arises as a

result of somatic hypermutation driven by foreign antigen. But regardless of the underlying mechanisms, the end result is enormous diversity among BCRs and the ability to react with a nearly unlimited variety of antigens.

Order and Regulation of B-Cell Development

Just as with T cells, the development of BCRs is a complex and random process with an equal or greater potential for generating useless or self-reactive molecules over protective BCRs. So the question remains, how is all of this regulated and controlled during B-cell development?

In most mammals, bony fish, and amphibians, B-cell development begins in the fetal liver, spleen, and bone marrow. In chickens, rabbits, and sheep, it begins in the GALT. However, the steps in the developmental processes are similar. First, the bone marrow or other stroma delivers a signal that initiates genetic rearrangement in the pre–B cells. These cells begin rearranging H-chain genes, which starts (as mentioned earlier and shown in Figure 11.4) with random association of D_H and a J_H segment. This DJ complex then randomly associates with a V_H segment, enzymes transcribe the VDJ complex along with a C_H segment—in most cases, a C_υ segment—into nuclear RNA, spliceosomes reform this transcript into mRNA, and ribosomes make H chains from the message.

Pre–B cells that fail to successfully rearrange H-chain genes and express a functional H chain are of no further use, so animals have evolved a means to test for a functional H-chain polypeptide. Just as with T cells, B cells have evolved a special gene to deal with this, a gene called $V_{\lambda 5}$ that produces a surrogate L chain. If the newly formed H chain is functional, it will bind to $V_{\lambda 5}$, and the complex will move to the cell surface where stromal receptors test for the pre-BCR (pBCR). On one hand, if the receptor does not appear, then further rearrangement on that particular chromosome is shut down, and H-chain gene rearrangement begins on the

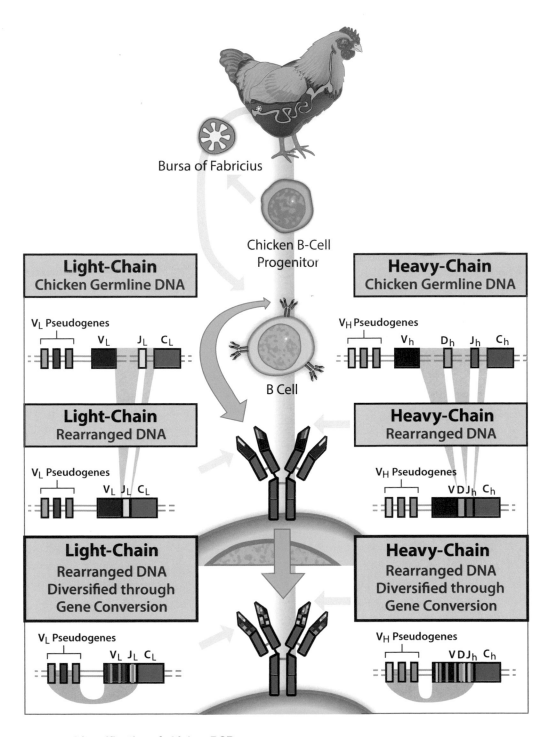

FIGURE 11.5. Diversification of chicken BCRs

Initially, all chicken B cells express the same BCR—the product of only one V_H, one D_H, and one J_H as well as one V_L and one J_L segment. After these cells enter the bursa of Fabricius, they begin to proliferate, and during cell division, pieces of adjacent pseudogenes (normally inactive genes) are inserted into the active H-chain and L-chain genes, adding to the diversity of expressed BCRs.

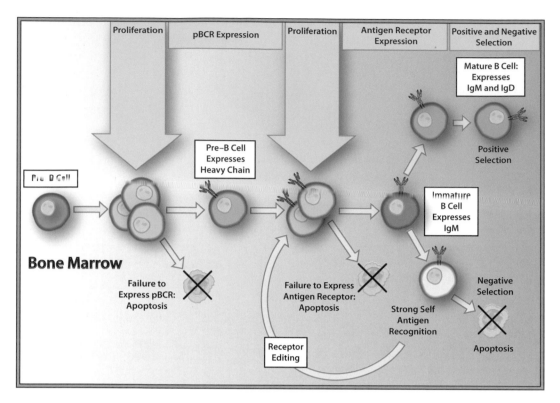

FIGURE 11.6. B-cell development

Gene rearrangement begins as B cells divide in the bone marrow. Cells that fail to produce a functional H chain along with a surrogate L chain die. B cells that produce self-reactive BCRs undergo further rearrangement, called receptor editing. If, after a second gene rearrangement, these B cells still react with self, these cells die.

other chromosome of the parental pair. At the end of that process, the stroma again tests the pre–B cell for the appearance of a pBCR. If at this point the cell expresses no pBCR, the cell dies (see Figure 11.6).

On the other hand, if the receptor appears, the stroma stimulates the initiation of L-chain gene rearrangement. V_L and J_L segments randomly recombine, and a nuclear transcript of this VJ segment, along with a C_L segment, appears. Spliceosomes convert this transcript into mRNA, and ribosomes begin to make L chains. If this rearrangement is successful and a functional L chain appears, it associates with the H chain and moves to the cell surface as a fully formed antigen receptor (BCR). The stroma monitors this process as well. If no BCR ap-

pears, rearrangement of L-chain genes begins on the other parental chromosome. If again no BCR appears, the cell dies. But if a functional BCR does appear, the cell is immediately tested for self-reactivity. Once identified, self-reactive B cells are stimulated to undergo further rearrangement, a process called receptor editing. If these B cells either fail further productive rearrangement or again produce self-reactive BCRs, these cells also die.

Beyond this level of selection, one other process helps to ensure that self-reactive B cells do not attack self outside of the bone marrow. For a B cell to become activated, more than one BCR must bind to an antigen at the same time, and these BCRs must become cross-linked to one another to generate the appropriate intracellular signals. That process requires particulate antigen with a repetitive antigenic epitope, so that two or more BCRs can bind to the same antigen at the same time and induce cross-linking. So, all B cells that react with soluble proteins (which lack repetitive antigenic epitopes), such as serum albumin, become anergic, or unreactive to any further stimulation.

As a result, in a process somewhat similar to T-cell selection, most self-reactive B cells die or are switched off before they can do any damage. B cells with functional BCRs are called naive or immature B cells—naive until they encounter their particular antigens. These B cells exit the bone marrow or bursa of Fabricius and enter the blood. B-cell differentiation does not, however, end in the bone marrow. For all B cells, many steps remain on the way to becoming antibody-secreting plasma cells. After entering the blood, most B cells will eventually make their way into secondary lymphoid tissues, and it is here, especially within the lymphoid follicles, that much of the remainder of B-cell development occurs (see chapter 12).

Immunoglobulin Isotypes

As mentioned earlier, antibodies come in two physical forms—a membrane-bound form as part of the BCR and a soluble form known as antibodies. In addition, both membrane-bound forms and soluble forms of antibodies come in chemically distinct forms known as isotypes (Figure 11.7).

The numbers and characters of Ig isotypes vary markedly between species. Placental mammals express IgM, IgD, IgG, IgA, and IgE. Also, most species that express IgG express multiple forms, or subtypes, of IgG. The same is often true for IgA subtypes. In addition, both IgM and IgA appear in multiple structurally distinct forms (Figure 11.8). As BCRs, both IgM and IgA appear in their monomeric forms (shown in Figure 11.7). When secreted, however, IgM appears as pentamer with ten H chains and ten L chains creating five antibody monomers and

ten antigen-binding sites (Figure 11.9). Secreted IgA antibodies may appear as monomers or as dimers (Figure 11.8). The dimeric form of IgA appears predominantly on mucosal epithelia, so it is sometimes also called secretory IgA.

The feature that distinguishes one Ig isotype from another is the amino acid sequence of the constant region of the H chain. Because of that, different Ig isotypes expressed by single B cells will all have the same antigenic specificity.

How is it possible for one B cell to produce several different isotypes with the same antigenic specificity? The answer is through a combination of selective RNA splicing and genetic rearrangement. In addition to V, D, and J segments, every H-chain gene family has multiple C segments—C_μ, C_δ, C_γ (one or more), C_ε, and C_α (one or more)—corresponding to the H chains for IgM, IgD, IgG, IgE, and IgA (Figure 11.9).

Two distinct genetic mechanisms result in expression of distinct Ig isotypes by developing B cells. All B cells first express IgM, which results from a simple read-through from the VDJ complex to the first two C gene segments, C_μ and C_δ. During production of mRNA, spliceosomes remove the RNA encoding the IgD H-chain C region. Thus, the newly developed B cells express only IgM.

At a later stage in their development, most B cells briefly express both IgD and IgM. This expression results from an alternative mRNA splice (one splice removes C_μ and the other removes C_δ), resulting in the simultaneous production of both isotypes and both types of BCRs. As you will see in chapter 12, at a still later stage in B-cell development, B cells will often switch from expressing IgM and IgD to expressing another isotype—IgG, IgE, or IgA. This process is called isotype switching. It is important to note that isotype switching to IgG, IgE, and IgA occurs only after B-cell activation and expansion, which occurs only if the BCR recognizes an antigen and, usually, receives further signals from Th cells. Exactly how a cell chooses one isotype over another is not clear, but Th cells and their products appear to direct

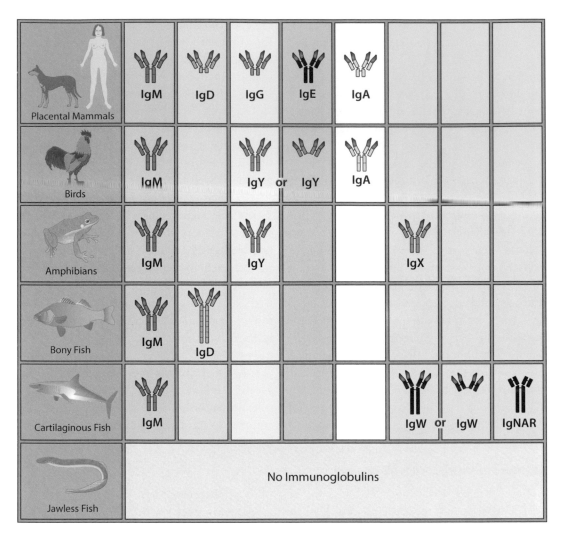

FIGURE 11.7. Ig isotypes

Variations in the constant regions of Ig H chains result in multiple forms of antibodies called Ig isotypes. The number of isotypes, their form, and their designations vary among animal species.

the process. The process of Ig–isotype switch beyond IgM and IgD results not from alternative RNA splicing, but from further genetic rearrangement. For example, inside a cell destined to express IgG, the DNA that encodes C_μ and C_δ loops out, and enzymes excise it. From this DNA, these B cells then begin to make IgG. Because this rearrangement results in changes to the H-chain constant region only, no change occurs in the antigenic specificity of the BCR. The same holds for switches to IgA or IgE.

Occasionally, B cells will make more than one class switch, but these secondary and later switches must involve downstream constant region genes because all of those upstream of the first switch were excised.

The advantage of multiple Ig isotypes is that each antibody isotype appears at varying concentration and distributes differently inside animals' bodies, and each can perform distinct functions after binding to antigen (Figure 11.10 and 11.11).

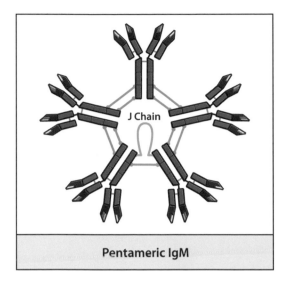

Pentameric IgM

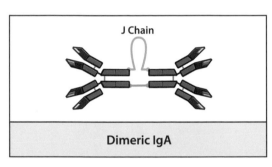

Dimeric IgA

FIGURE 11.8. Polymeric forms of IgM and IgA

As a soluble antibody, IgM always appears as a pentamer with ten H and ten L chains and ten antigen-binding sites. This process may or may not require the participation of another polypeptide called the J chain (unrelated to J_H segments). Also, as a soluble antibody, IgA appears in two forms, monomeric and dimeric, also with a coupling J chain.

Each Ig isotype appears at different concentrations in the serum, with IgG at the highest concentrations. The exact plasma concentrations of each isotype vary among species. For example, numbers for horse Ig isotypes are approximately 1.96 mg/ml for IgA, 27 mg/ml for IgG, 4.19 mg/ml for Ig(T), and 0.7 mg/ml for IgM.

Only IgM and IgG activate complement, an essential element in innate defense against bac-terial and other infections (see chapter 4). Only IgE binds to mast cells, a critical aspect of allergies and defense against parasites. In addition, each isotype has a unique distribution inside an animal's body (Figure 11.11).

OTHER POPULATIONS OF B CELLS

B-1 B Cells

In all mammals so far investigated, there exists a distinct population of B cells called B-1 B cells. The origins and function of these cells are distinct from the B cells discussed so far (sometimes called B 2 B cells or follicular B cells because they are most commonly found in lymphoid follicles). These novel B-1 B cells arise early during fetal development (which is the reason for the B-1 designation) in fetal liver, whereas B-2 B cells arise later, mostly in fetal bone marrow.

Often, but not always, B-1 B cells also express a novel cell-surface molecule called CD5, so B-1 B cells are also called CD5+ B cells. The percentage of the total B-cell population accounted for by B-1 B cells varies among species, from about 5 percent in primates and rodents to the majority of B cells in rabbits and ruminants.

B-1 B-cell Ig gene segments do rearrange during development, but because these cells lack TDT, there is no junctional diversification. In addition, B-1 B cells use only a few DJ and VDJ combinations. Together, these two factors result in a much lower BCR diversity among B-1 B cells than among regular, or B-2, B cells. Also, after maturation in fetal liver, most B-1 B cells migrate to the peritoneal and pleural cavities, not to lymphoid follicles. In the peritoneal and pleural cavities, it appears that further development of B-1 B cells is driven by encounter with a narrow range of specific antigens. The exact nature of these antigens is not always clear, but the most common appear to be bacterial poly-saccharides and lipids, as well as some auto-antigens (self molecules).

After activation, B-1 B cells establish self-renewing populations of active B cells, and

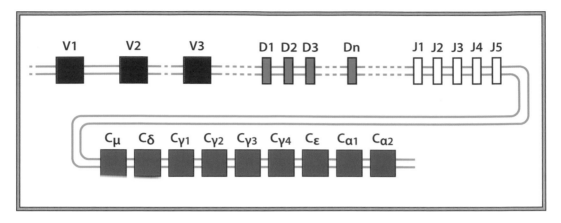

FIGURE 11.9. Ig H-chain constant genes

H-chain gene families contain V, D, and J gene segments that encode the variable region of the H chain. In addition, each H-chain gene family contains multiple C-region gene segments corresponding to multiple Ig isotypes.

	Immunoglobulins								
	IgG1	IgG2	IgG3	IgG4	IgM	IgA1	IgA2	IgD	IgE
Classical Pathway of Complement Activation	++	+	+++	−	+++	−	−	−	−
Lectin Pathways of Complement Activation	−	−	−	−	−	+	−	−	−
Placental Transfer	+++	+	++	−/+	−	−	−	−	−
Binding to Macrophages and Other Phagocytes	+	−	+	−/+	−	+	+	−	+
High-Affinity Binding to Mast Cells and Basophils	−	−	−	−	−	−	−	−	+++

FIGURE 11.10. Properties of primate Ig isotypes

Each mammalian Ig isotype has slightly different properties. These structural differences allow for differences in distribution and function. The data shown in the upper half of this chart were derived from humans and vary among species. IgG crosses the placenta in significant amounts only in mammals with hemochorial (e.g., primates and rodents) or endotheliochorial placentation (e.g., dogs and cats).

they constitute the majority, if not all, of the B-1 B cells present in adult animals. That is, early during fetal development, most mammals generate B-1 B cells in fetal liver. These B cells then migrate to the peritoneal and pleural cavities, where they establish self-renewing

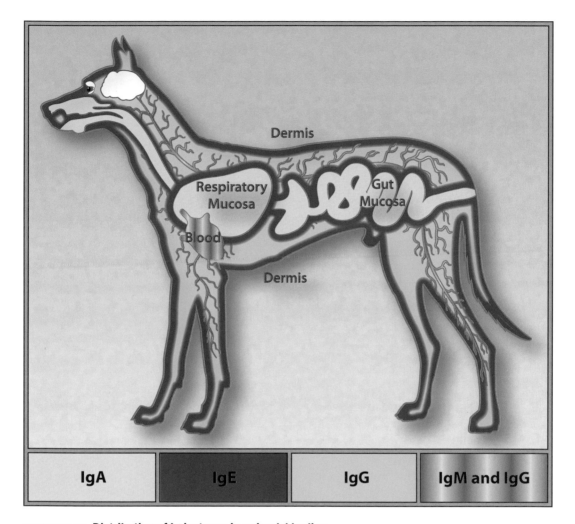

FIGURE 11.11. Distribution of Ig isotypes in animals' bodies

Both IgG and IgM appear in the blood, but extracellular fluid contains mostly IgG and monomeric IgA. Dimeric or secretory IgA is the major isotype on mucosal secretions of epithelia and appears in breast milk. IgE is mostly found bound to mast cells, and mast cells appear in greatest numbers beneath the epithelial surfaces of the respiratory tract, the gut, and the skin. The blood–brain barrier normally partitions Ig from the brain.

populations of B-1 B cells that persist throughout adult life; these are the only B-1 B cells in adults.

B-1 B cells do not require interactions with Th cells to become fully active and differentiate into antibody-producing plasma cells (as do B-2 B cells; see chapter 12). So the antigens that activate B-1 B cells are called thymus-independent antigens (see Figure 11.12). It also appears

that some B-1 B cells can, even in the absence of antigen, differentiate into antibody-secreting plasma cells and are responsible for so-called natural antibodies that appear even in germ-free animals. Most B-1 B cells express only IgM and never switch to another isotype, nor do they further diversify their BCRs in spleen or lymph nodes through the process of somatic hypermutation (as do B-2 B cells; chapter 12).

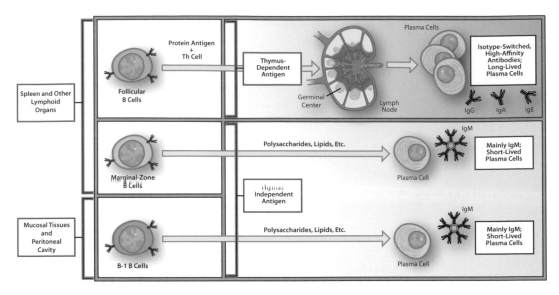

FIGURE 11.12. B-1 B cells and thymus-independent antigens

In comparison with traditional or B-2 B cells, B-1 B cells and MZ B cells recognize distinct sets of antigens called thymus-independent antigens because no T cells are involved in activation of B cells in response to these antigens.

From all of this, it appears that B-1 B cells have evolved to recognize and respond to commonly encountered antigens, such as the components of bacteria. Because bacteria are among the most numerous of all pathogens, it seems reasonable that a rapid response element—such as B-1 B cells—would provide a considerable evolutionary advantage to animals that at birth must unavoidably and immediately deal with a host of bacterial pathogens. The role of B-1 B cells in autoimmunity is also evident, but the mechanisms and evolutionary significance of this aspect of B-1 B cell function are much less clear.

Marginal-Zone B Cells

Inside the marginal sinus of the white pulp of the spleen is yet another population of B cells, the MZ B cells. These cells are physically and functionally distinct from either B-1 or B-2 B cells. The marginal sinus is the site where blood exits the circulation, then traverses a region called the MZ before entering the venous

sinuses and returning to the circulation. Obviously, then, the MZ B cells are well positioned to deal with antigens circulating in the blood and, as it turns out, especially well suited to deal with circulating encapsulated bacteria.

MZ B cells have a greater BCR diversity than B-1 B cells, but not as great as that of B-2 B cells. MZ B cells produce mostly IgM, are longer-lived than B-2 B cells, do not require T-cell help, and appear to have evolved to most effectively deal with circulating pathogens, especially bacteria (see Figure 11.12). From a defense perspective, this is another relatively rapid response mechanism targeted toward bacteria, particularly bacteria in the blood.

To summarize, three distinct populations of B cells have evolved in most mammals to deal with particular infectious threats. B-1 and MZ B cells have relatively limited antigenic repertoires and appear to have arisen to protect animals from commonly encountered pathogens, especially bacteria. B-2 B cells, however, have an almost limitless capacity for BCR diversity and take somewhat longer to respond. But B-2

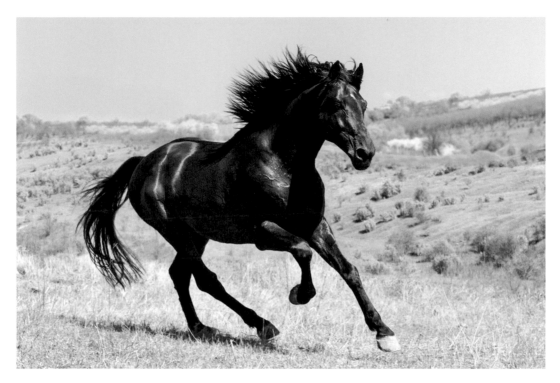

FIGURE 11.13. Thoroughbred horse (© pirita / Shutterstock)

B cells can do something that B-1 B and MZ B cells cannot, and that is, deal effectively with constantly evolving pathogens of all sorts.

CLINICAL CORRELATION FOLLOW-UP

Tyrosine kinases are important components of many signal transduction pathways, and BTK happens to play an especially important role in signal transduction in B cells (see Figure 11.14).

All B cells arise from a common hematopoietic stem cell. Early on, the B-cell lineage diverges from the T- and NK-cell lineages. The first recognizable B-cell precursor is the pre–B cell. Gene rearrangement begins inside of this cell. The first outward sign of successful gene rearrangement is the appearance of the new H chain along with $V_{\lambda 5}$ in the form of the pBCR—the pre–B-cell. For further rearrangement to occur, the bone marrow stroma must deliver a signal through the pBCR to the nucleus of the pre–B-cell to initiate L-chain gene rearrange-ment. The transduction of that signal depends on active functional BTK.

As mentioned, the bone marrow stroma initiates and directs rearrangement of BCR genes.

Student Considerations

On the basis of the material presented in this chapter, you should be able to offer an explanation for the observation that horses with defective BTK enzymes might exhibit a pronounced agammaglobulinemia, have severely atrophied lymph nodes, and, by age six months, uniformly succumb to bacterial infections.

Possible Explanations

As mentioned earlier, B cells (even B-1 B cells) that express the pBCR must receive and deliver another message before L-chain gene rearrange-ment can begin. That signal depends on BTK. In the absence of a second rearrangement signal,

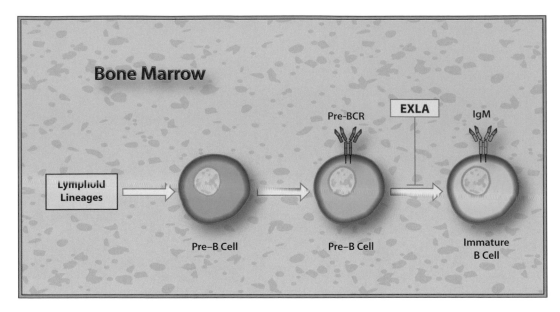

FIGURE 11.14. The role of BTK in equine X-linked agammaglobulinemia (EXLA)

To ensure that each step proceeds normally, B cells have evolved means for signaling the stroma at each major step of development. Rearrangement and production of H-chain genes occurs first, but H chains by themselves cannot assume proper configurations and insert themselves into the cell membrane. Because the cell membrane is the only surface accessible to the bone marrow stroma, B cells have evolved a means to express isolated H chains using a surrogate L chain called $V_{\lambda 5}$. Together, H chain and $V_{\lambda 5}$ form the pBCR at the surface of developing B cells. Normally, the pBCR interacts with stromal receptors and, in return, the stroma delivers a signal through the BCR to pre–B cells' nuclei. The delivery of this signal depends on a complex set of second-messenger molecules. One of these is BTK. In the absence of BTK, further Ig gene rearrangement ceases. These B cells never produce L chains and eventually die via apoptosis.

B cells fail to initiate L-chain gene rearrangement. As a result, these cells never express a functional BCR that will deliver a second signal to the bone marrow stroma and allow the pre–B cells to survive a second round of selection. As a result, animals without functional BTK produce no B cells and no antibodies. Without B cells, lymph nodes atrophy, and no lymphoid follicles or germinal centers appear. As a result, as soon as the maternally transferred antibodies disappear from the foal's blood, massive infections ensue and the animal dies.

CLINICAL CORRELATION: SELECTIVE IMMUNOGLOBULIN A DEFICIENCIES IN DOGS

As many as 80 percent of Chinese shar peis (see Figure 12.1) develop recurrent dermatitises (staphylococcal), demodectic mange (see Figure 12.2), thyroid disease, otitis externa, flea allergies, cystitis, food intolerance, bronchitis, and atopy. Similar disorders also appear in (among others) German shepherds, beagles, Irish wolfhounds, and cocker spaniels.

Most of the symptoms apparent in Chinese shar peis share two features: they involve body surfaces and appear to result from some sort of inherited immune deficiency. Clinical laboratory analyses of serum from affected dogs reveal normal levels of IgG and IgM but depressed levels of IgA. The degree of the suppression varies from no IgA to a less-than-normal level of IgA.

LEARNING OBJECTIVES

After reading this chapter, you should be able to

- describe the manner in which B cells interact with antigens and pathogens;
- understand the role of B cells in antigen presentation to Th cells;
- describe the signals necessary for B-cell activation and their consequences;
- describe the driving forces for Ig isotype switch and the roles of the various Ig isotypes;
- understand the mechanisms, consequences, and importance of somatic hypermutation;
- explain the final differentiation of B cells into plasma cells and the secretion of antibodies;
- explain the process of affinity maturation;
- describe the differences between primary and secondary humoral immune response and the reasons for these differences;
- explain the effector actions of antibodies and their importance in defense;
- explain the various roles of Fc receptors in immune responses and protection.

Two of the most striking features of the immune system and immune responses are antigen specificity and immunologic memory (see Figure 12.3).

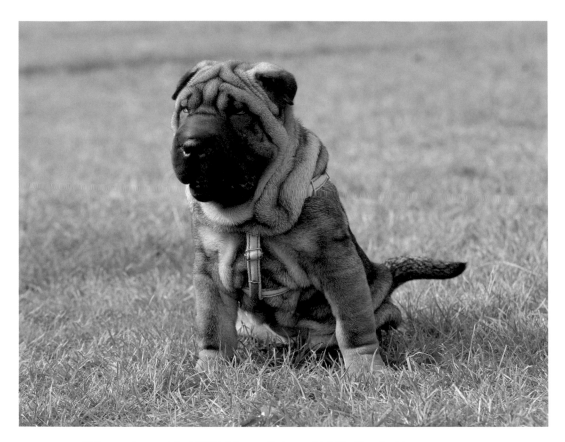

FIGURE 12.1. **Chinese shar pei dog (© Waldemar Dabrowski / Shutterstock)**

After a primary immunization of an animal, no detectable change occurs in blood levels of antibodies for the first seven to ten days. This phase is called the lag phase, and it occurs because it takes time to develop an adaptive immune response. After the lag phase, IgM antibodies begin to appear in the animal's serum. The amount of antigen-specific serum IgM continues to rise for about another seven days and then gradually falls off over the next two weeks to near 0 by day 28. After a secondary immunization with antigen A and antigen B, the lag phase drops to about three days for antibodies to antigen A, followed by a dramatic rise of antibodies to a much higher level than seen in the primary response. In most immune responses, nearly all of these antibodies are IgG (although they could also include IgE and IgA). Also, after secondary immunization, high levels of antibodies persist for very long periods of time—often years or even decades. The immune response to antigen B, injected at the same time as antigen A, exhibits features characteristic of a primary immune response.

Clearly, at day 28 some aspect of the immune system has changed, and it now carries a memory of the previously seen antigen A. Because of this memory, the animal's immune system now does something very different: it produces more antibody, it produces a different type of antibody, it produces it faster, and the antibody persists in the serum for a much longer time. Also, the antibodies produced during secondary immune responses have a much higher affinity for antigen and that affinity continues to increase as the secondary response continues. This progressive increase in affinity is known as affinity maturation, and it occurs in

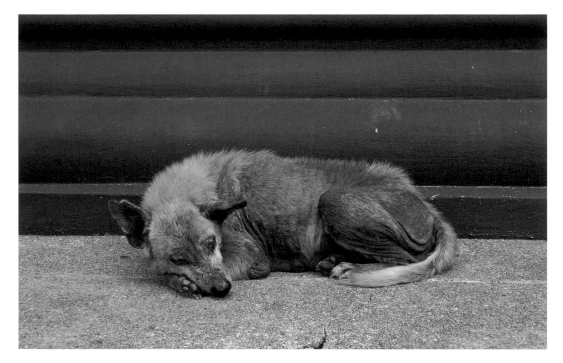

FIGURE 12.2. Dog with severe demodectic mange (© Robert Adrian Hillman / Shutterstock)

Demodectic mange is also known as demodicosis or red mange. A persistent infestation with *Demodex canis*, a mite, causes this mange. It comes in two varieties: localized and generalized. Localized manifests at four or fewer spots of mange. Most normal dogs are not susceptible to demodectic mange.

most immune responses and generates highly antigen-specific antibody. Memory and specificity are the hallmarks of adaptive immunity and result from the characteristics of T and B lymphocytes.

T-DEPENDENT B (B-2) CELLS

Interaction of B Cells with Antigens

The BCR contains not only two H and two L chains, but signal-transduction molecules as well. Igα and Igβ are the same in all BCRs and do not contribute to an antibody's antigen-binding properties. The only parts of the BCR that interact directly with antigens are the variable regions of the L and H chains (see Figure 12.4).

As discussed in chapter 11, within the N-terminus, variable regions of H and L chains are three hypervariable regions, CDR1, CDR2, and CDR3. Essentially, all of the amino acid sequence variability among BCRs lies within the CDRs of the H and L chains (Figure 12.5), the part of the antibody molecule in direct contact with antigen.

As the H and L chains fold into their final conformations, CDR1, CDR2, and CDR3 of both chains come to reside in the antigen-binding site—that is, the portion of the BCR that interacts most directly with antigen.

Unlike T cells, B cells do not require antigen processing before antigen binding, nor is there any involvement of MHC class I or II molecules in antigen binding by BCRs. BCRs bind intact antigens, whether that antigen is a whole bacterium or virus or clumps of denatured proteins, such as the toxoid in tetanus vaccines.

Also, because the regions between the membrane-distal and membrane-proximal regions of the H chains (sometimes called the hinge regions) are very flexible, antibody and BCR

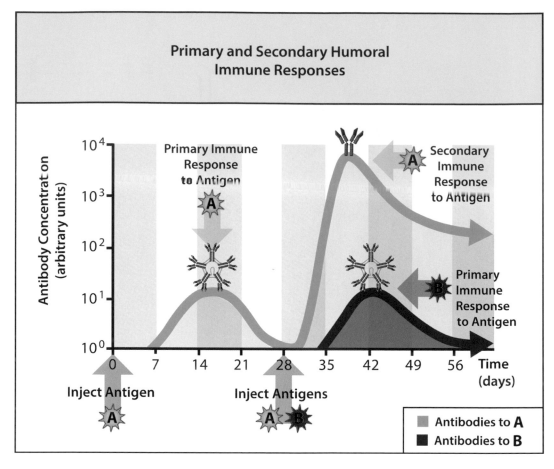

FIGURE 12.3. Primary and secondary humoral immune responses

At day 0, an animal received an injection of antigen A. On day 28, the same animal received an injection of both antigen A and antigen B. From day 0 on, the serum levels of antibodies to antigens A and B were monitored and appear in arbitrary units on the *y*-axis.

molecules can open wide to reach and bind identical antigenic epitopes. That is, antibodies can go from being Y shaped to being T shaped to accommodate the span between epitopes.

The chemistry of antigen–antibody interactions is complex and involves multiple types of bonds, including hydrogen bonds, electrostatic interactions, Van der Wahl's forces, and hydrophobic interactions. Two things all of these types of bonds share is that they are noncovalent and individually weak interactions.

The most important of these chemical interactions varies between antibodies and their antigens, but all antigen–antibody binding involves multiple bonds. The advantage to multiple interactions between antigens and antibodies is that it makes the interaction highly specific. Hydrogen bonds, electrostatic interactions, Van der Wahl's forces, and hydrophobic interactions act over only very short distances, which means that the fit between an antibody and an antigen must be exact or these bonds simply will not form. When the fit is right, though, despite low affinity of individual interactions, the sum of these bonds results in very high overall affinities between antibodies and their antigens. When the fit is imperfect, the affinity decreases (see Figure 12.6)

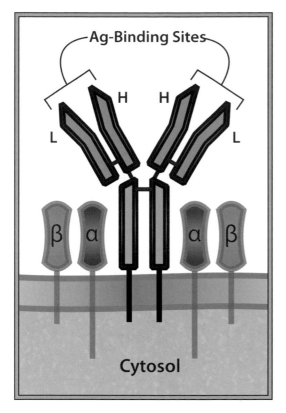

FIGURE 12.4. The common mammalian BCR

This form of the BCR contains four signal-transduction molecules—two Igα chains and two Igβ chains. However, all of the interactions between BCR and antigen (Ag) occur at the N-termini (membrane-distal) portions of the H and L chains.

As a result, a given antibody may bind (with varying affinities) to more than one antigen. For example, a rabbit immunized with bovine serum albumin may produce antibodies with high affinity for bovine serum albumin, but these same antibodies may also bind (with a much lower affinity) to equine serum albumin—an antibody cross-reaction. In spite of their remarkable specificity, essentially all antibodies have some potential for cross-reactivity. This consideration is especially important when using antibodies for immunotherapy or in clinical analyses (see chapter 17).

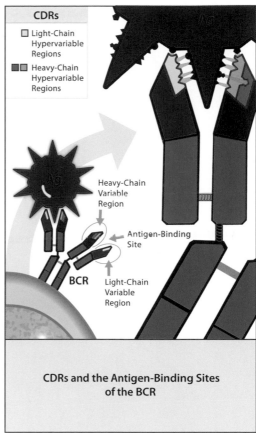

CDRs and the Antigen-Binding Sites of the BCR

FIGURE 12.5. The role of the CDRs in antigen (Ag) binding by the BCR

The N-terminus regions (membrane-distal portions) of H and L chains contain all of the variability found among BCRs of different specificity. Within these variable regions of the H and L chains, the greatest variability lies in three discrete regions called CDR1, CDR2, and CDR3. In the final quaternary confirmation of the BCR, CDR1, CDR2, and CDR3 regions of the H and L chains make up the bulk of the antigen-binding sites and make direct contact with antigens.

Regardless of affinity—high or low—all antigen–antibody interactions are noncovalent and reversible, meaning that antigens are always moving on and off antibody-binding sites at a given rate—simple equlibria determined by

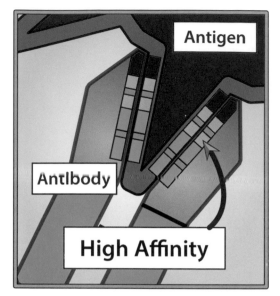

Antigen

Antibody

High Affinity

Antigen

Antibody

Low Affinity

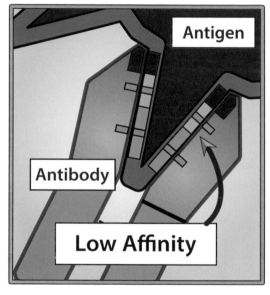

FIGURE 12.6. **The affinity of antibodies for antigens results from the complementarity of fit**

When antigens fit properly within an antibody-binding site, the maximum number of interactions can occur between the two, generating the highest affinity possible (upper panel). If the fit is less good, fewer specific bonds form (indicated in different colors), and the interaction is of lower affinity (lower panel).

the K_{eq} of the reaction. This fact is important to remember in the later discussion of affinity maturation.

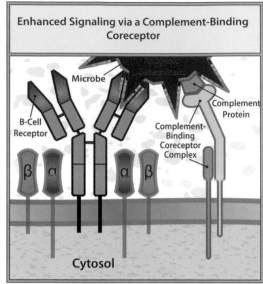

Enhanced Signaling via a Complement-Binding Coreceptor

Microbe

B-Cell Receptor

Complement Protein

Complement-Binding Coreceptor Complex

β α   α β

Cytosol

FIGURE 12.7. **The B-cell coreceptor**

Besides BCRs, B cells express another complex of molecules called the B-cell coreceptor. Together, these molecules bind to fragments of complement proteins and deliver an additional signal to the B-cell nucleus.

As with CD4 and CD8 on T cells, B cells express another group of molecules besides the BCR that are important to B-cell activation—the B-cell coreceptor (see Figure 12.7). The B-cell coreceptor is a complex of molecules that bind a complement protein fragment and transduce a second singal from the B-cell surface to the nucleus to initiate the process of B-cell activation.

As discussed in chapter 4, several pathogens activate complement directly, which results in opsonization of pathogens with complement-derived proteins, especially C3b. IgG or IgM opsonization of pathogens also activates complement and leads to deposition of complement fragments on the pathogen. Binding of the coreceptor to these complement fragments on the antigen, along with the binding of the BCR to antigen, significantly enhances the strength of the binding between B cell and pathogen, leading to more efficient B-cell activation. After

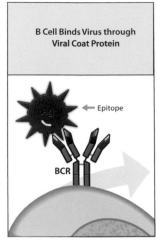
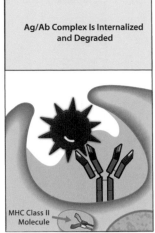
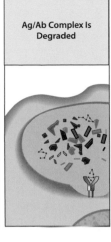
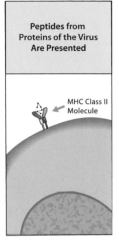

| B Cell Binds Virus through Viral Coat Protein | Ag/Ab Complex Is Internalized and Degraded | Ag/Ab Complex Is Degraded | Peptides from Proteins of the Virus Are Presented |

FIGURE 12.8. B cells as APCs

B cells acquire antigen through the Ig portion of their BCRs. After binding antigen and BCR cross-linking (not shown), B cells internalize the antigen–antibody (Ag–Ab) complexes, and process both antigen and antibody into peptides. MHC class II molecules bind these peptides and present them on B-cell surfaces.

binding of the BCR to antigen and of the B-cell coreceptor to complement fragments, B cells begin to express high levels of MHC class II molecules and B7, making them much more efficient APCs.

So, BCRs can directly bind to native antigen, sometimes with very high affinities, but antigen binding alone (not even antigen binding by the B-cell coreceptor along with BCR binding to antigen) is not enough to activate a B cell and push it into proliferation and differentiation. All B cells, except for B-1 B cells and possibly some MZ B cells, require other signals beyond BCR and coreceptor binding to antigen before activation to proliferation and differentiation. Most of those signals come from Th cells activated by B cells acting as APCs.

B Cells as Antigen-Presenting Cells

After a B cell's BCRs bind to antigen and cross-link to one another, some of the antigens, along with some of the BCRs themselves, are taken into the B cells in a process known as receptor-mediated endocytosis. During this process, the antigen–antibody complexes enter the endosomal pathway, are chopped into pieces, and are bound by MHC class II molecules as described in chapter 8. After this processing step, the MHC class II–antigen complexes move to the surface of B cells, where the complexes become accessible to the TCRs of Th cells (see Figure 12.8).

The same processing and presentation clearly occur with BCR fragments. Because most self-reactive T cells die in the thymus, though, there are usually no Th cells in the periphery that react with self Ig. In fish and amphibians, B cells (as do macrophages and DCs) also directly phagocytose antigens for presentation to Th cells.

After antigen and coreceptor binding, B cells begin to express higher levels of B7 and MHC class II molecules. As a consequence, these B cells transform into highly effective APCs. After antigen-induced activation, B cells also begin to express another molecule called CD40. Ultimately, this molecule will also make B cells better APCs through interaction with CD40 ligand (CD40L) on Th cells. CD40 molecules, in fact, appear on all APCs, but CD40 plays an especially important role in B-cell activation. During interactions between macrophages or DCs, CD40 binding to CD40L causes these APCs to secrete cytokines. In the interaction between B-cell APCs and Th cells, CD40 binding to CD40L provides a costimulatory signal for the B cells and promotes growth, differentiation, and isotype switching (further described in the Isotype Switching section).

B cells may encounter antigen in the periphery or in secondary lymphoid tissues. But regardless of where the antigen-induced activation begins, B-cell development finishes in secondary lymphoid tissues. In our discussion, we focus on lymph nodes.

Activation of B Cells by T-Helper Cells

The final stage of differentiation for most B cells requires the participation of a Th cell that has undergone clonal expansion and further differentiation after activation by an APC other than a B cell, usually a DC. Although the BCR on the B cell binds an antigenic epitope distinct from the one bound by the TCR on the Th cell, the antigen–MHC complex on the B cell must bind to the Th cell's TCR. For all of this to occur properly, T cells, B cells, antigens, and other APCs must all somehow come together inside of lymph nodes.

After antigen binding or ingestion, DCs and some macrophages arrive, along with antigen, in lymph nodes via the lymphatics. Th cells leave the thymus, and B cells leave the bone marrow via the blood. The arterial circulation and the lymphatics have no direct connection, but inside of lymph nodes (and other secondary lymphoid tissues), the endothelia of some of the venules have a unique high-columnar structure and are called high endothelial venules (HEVs). Because of specific interactions between lymphocytes and HEVs, lymphocytes can move through HEVs from blood into lymph nodes, allowing for the direct interaction among B cells, T cells, and antigen (see Figure

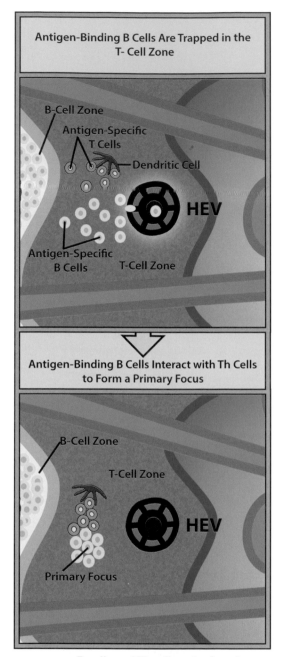

FIGURE 12.9. B cells and Th cells enter lymph nodes through HEVs and interact to effect B-cell activation

Specialized venules inside of lymph nodes and Peyer's patches called HEVs have receptors for cell-surface proteins on T and B cells. This interaction allows the T and B cells to exit the blood and enter lymph nodes. Inside, Th cells encounter antigen-presenting DCs.

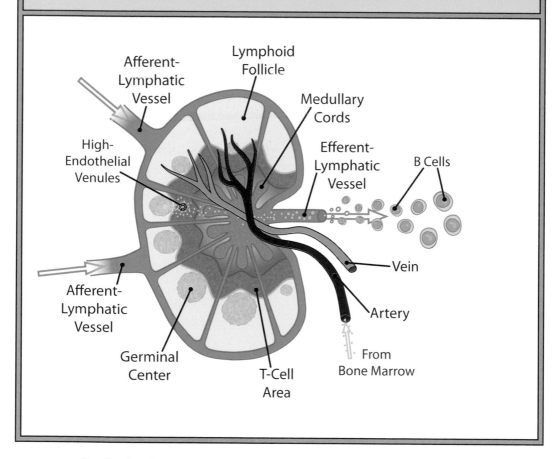

Mature B Cells Travel to the Lymph Node via the Bloodstream and Leave via the Efferent Lymph

Afferent-Lymphatic Vessel

Lymphoid Follicle

Medullary Cords

High-Endothelial Venules

Efferent-Lymphatic Vessel

B Cells

Afferent-Lymphatic Vessel

Vein

Artery

From Bone Marrow

Germinal Center

T-Cell Area

FIGURE 12.10. B-cell migration

Naïve B cells leave the bone marrow via the blood. From there, these B cells may encounter antigen in the blood, lymph, or lymph node. If the B cells fail to bind antigen or fail to find the appropriate Th cell inside a lymph node, they leave nodes via the efferent lymphatics and move on to the next node.

12.9). If, after the antigen-activated B cell enters the lymph node, it does not encounter a T cell with the appropriate TCR, the B cell leaves the node via the efferent lymphatic and moves on to the next node (see Figure 12.10). If, instead, a B cell binds antigen and encounters a Th cell reactive with that same antigen, the Th cell pro-vides the next signal needed to stimulate B-cell division and differentiation (see Figure 12.11).

After interactions with specific antigens pre-sented on APCs, T cells divide, differentiate, and provide necessary, additional signals to B cells that ultimately trigger B-cell division and differentiation. These additional signals come

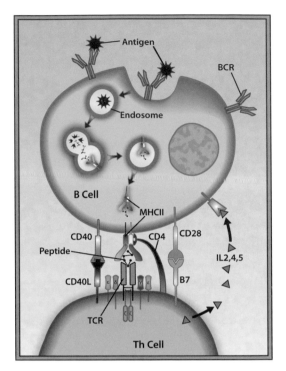

FIGURE 12.11. Antigen processing and presentation by B cells inside of a lymph node

Mammalian B-cell BCRs bind to antigen and then, via receptor-mediated endocytosis, internalize the antigen–antibody complexes (upper portion of figure). The newly formed endosomes fuse with lysosomes that contain both proteolytic enzymes and MHC class II molecules. The antigenic peptides bind to the MHC molecules and the MHC–antigen complexes return to the surface for presentation to Th cells.

in the form of cytokines secreted by Th2 or Th1 cells (see Figure 12.11).

Perhaps most important among the Th2-derived cytokines is IL-4, which (among other things) stimulates B-cell division and induces clonal expansion of B cells. As a result, in a relatively short period of time after exposure, the number of pathogen-specific B cells increases to protective levels. IL-4 also plays a role in Ig class switch (see Isotype Switching section).

In addition, Th2-derived IL-5 stimulates B-cell division, antibody production, and the growth of eosinophils. Similarly, IL-13 stimulates B-cell division and affects Ig class switch, and IL-25 induces production of more IL-4, IL-5, and IL-13 and appears to help protect against certain parasitic worms.

Th1 cells produce IFN-γ, TNF, IL-2, and IL-10. In some species, at least, IFN-γ stimulates B-cell growth and Ig class switching. TNF stimulates inflammation and B-cell differentiation. IL-2 stimulates further T-cell division and also affects class switching. IL-10 has multiple effects on both inflammation and B-cell differentiation.

During primary immune responses, almost all of the available B cells express IgM (as do all naive B cells). After interaction with Th cells, antigen-activated B cells move to the medullary cords of the lymph nodes, differentiate in plasma cells, and begin to secrete IgM—the predominant antibody of primary immune responses (see Figure 12.12). As B cells differentiate into plasma cells, the switch from the membrane-bound form of Ig (the BCR) to the secretion of soluble Ig is the result of an alternative RNA splice that removes the membrane anchor from the Ig H chains and creates a soluble form of the Ig molecule.

Late in the primary response to a persistent antigen and in all secondary immune responses, most B cells will switch to another antibody isotype.

Isotype Switching, Somatic Hypermutation, and Terminal Differentiation of B Cells into Plasma Cells

Some Th cell–activated B cells do not go to the medullary cords. Instead, this population of B cells moves into the lymphoid follicles. There, these B cells interact with additional Th cells and begin to divide, forming germinal centers (see Figure 12.13A–C). As the B cells divide in the germinal centers, Th-cell–derived cytokines induce isotype switching from IgM to IgG or IgA or, occasionally, IgE (see Figure 12.14).

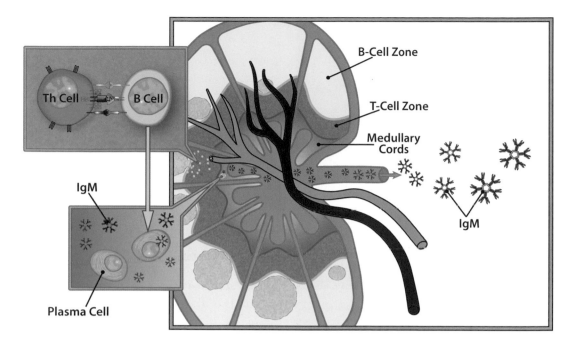

FIGURE 12.12. **The primary immune response**

After the initial interaction between antigen-activated B cells and Th cells, the B cells begin to divide, migrate to the medullary cords, and differentiate into IgM-secreting plasma cells.

After switching isotype, B cells must continue to interact with Th cells that stimulate further divisions, or the B cells will die. During these divisions, mutations begin to accumulate in the B cells' Ig genes at a very high rate—hypermutation. Because hypermutation occurs beyond the B cells developing in the bone marrow, it is called somatic hypermutation. Protein-sequencing studies have shown that these mutations do not occur randomly throughout the sequence of the Ig molecule. Instead, they are concentrated into the CDR1, CDR2, and CDR3 regions of the L and H chains (Figure 12.15).

CDR1, CDR2, and CDR3 regions of the L and H chains are, of course, the segments that make up the antigen-binding sites and directly contact antigen. So mutations that arise as a result of somatic hypermutation have dramatic effects on the antigen-binding affinity of a B cell's BCR. Because somatic hypermutation is a random process, the antigen-binding affinity of the mutated BCR may be the same, better, or worse than that of the original BCR.

To deal with this, animals have evolved a process of selection to eliminate those B cells with unchanged or lower antigen affinity to ensure that the end result of somatic hypermutation is antibody with greater affinity for the immunizing antigen. Overall, somatic hypermutation and selection result in the affinity maturation seen during secondary and subsequent immune responses.

As mentioned earlier, germinal centers also contain cells called FDCs. These cells play a crucial role in affinity maturation. On the surface of FDCs are receptors that bind to antigen–antibody complexes. As antigen–antibody complexes begin to accumulate during the primary immune responses, some are trapped on the surface of FDCs in the germinal centers. The antigens in these complexes serve as a reservoir for B-cell selection.

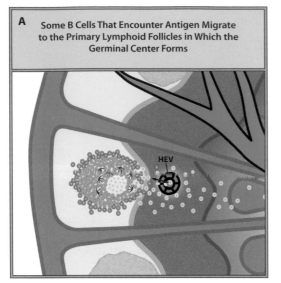

A Some B Cells That Encounter Antigen Migrate to the Primary Lymphoid Follicles in Which the Germinal Center Forms

HEV

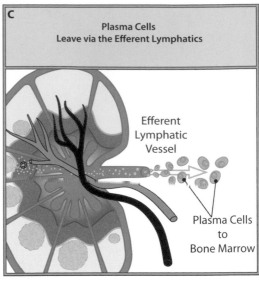

C Plasma Cells Leave via the Efferent Lymphatics

Efferent Lymphatic Vessel

Plasma Cells to Bone Marrow

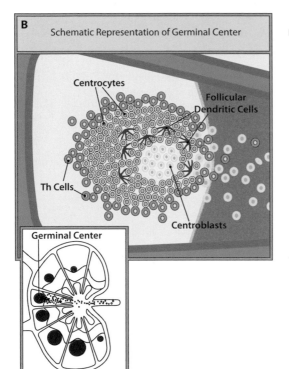

B Schematic Representation of Germinal Center

Centrocytes

Follicular Dendritic Cells

Th Cells

Centroblasts

Germinal Center

FIGURE 12.13A–C. B cells proliferate in lymph node germinal centers

After activation in the medulla, a significant population of B cells moves to the lymphoid follicles (panel A), proliferates, and forms germinal centers (panel B). Dividing B cells are called centroblasts, and resting B cells are called centrocytes. Germinal centers also contain Th cells and FDCs (cells distinct from the antigen-presenting DCs). In the germinal centers, B cells undergo isotype switching and somatic hypermutation, then emigrate the lymph node and differentiate into plasma cells that migrate to the bone marrow (panel C).

Each time a B cell interacts with a Th cell, the B cell is induced to divide. As that B cell comes out of the division cycle—goes from being a centroblast to being a centrocyte—it must again acquire antigen for presentation to another Th cell and enter another round of cell division. If it fails to reacquire antigen, the B cell will die by apoptosis.

The only significant source of antigen in the germinal center is the antigen–antibody complexes on the FDCs. As we have mentioned, all bonds between antigen and antibody are non-

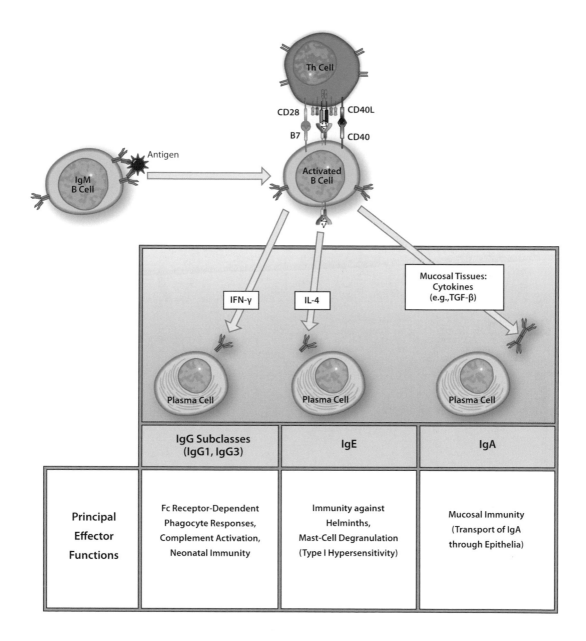

FIGURE 12.14. Cytokine control of isotype switching in germinal centers

In the upper left corner, a B cell first encounters antigen. Inside of a germinal center in secondary lymphoid tissue, this B cell interacts with a Th cell (upper right). Depending on the cytokines produced by the Th cell, the B cell switches from expressing IgM to expressing IgG, IgE, or IgA.

covalent and reversible. If, as the B cell comes out of cycle, its BCR has a higher affinity for antigen than the antibody on the FDC, the new hypermutated BCR can acquire antigen from the complexes on the FDCs and process and, once again, present that antigen to a Th cell and enter a new round of division. If, however, the affinity of new, hypermutated BCR is no better or worse than the affinity of the antibody in the antigen–antibody complexes on the FDCs, the

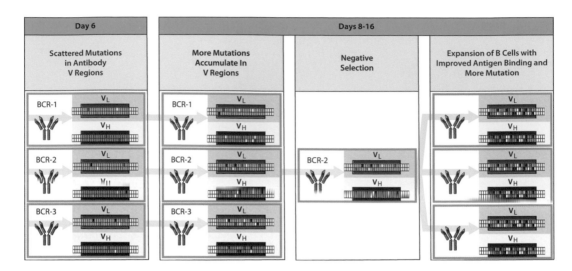

FIGURE 12.15. Somatic hypermutation

Late in primary immune responses and throughout secondary and subsequent immune responses against a given antigen, mutations (shown here as colored vertical bars) rapidly arise in B-cell genes encoding Ig molecules. These mutations fall mostly within the CDR1, CDR2, and CDR3 regions of the L and H chains.

B cell will not be able to reacquire antigen, and it will die (see Figure 12.16). Because most mutations would result in a BCR that has lower or the same affinity for the antigen, it is not surprising that many B cells die in this process of negative selection. Macrophages in the germinal centers remove dead B cells by phagocytosis. These macrophages are often referred to as tingible-body (stainable-body) macrophages because their cytoplasm contains B-cell chromatin fragments undergoing degradation and is characteristic of active germinal centers in a lymph node.

Some of these high-affinity B cells emigrate from the lymph nodes via the efferent lymphatics, enter the blood, and home back to the bone marrow. Along the way, these B cells differentiate into long-lived plasma cells and secrete higher-affinity antibody from the bone marrow (or sometimes from sites of inflammation) for months to years (see Figure 12.17).

Also in the germinal center, other B cells become long-lived memory B cells and remain in secondary lymphoid tissues. These cells persist for a long time and, after secondary infection or booster immunization, quickly differentiate into plasma cells producing isotypes other than M and very high-affinity antibody. These are the cells that dominate secondary and subsequent immune responses and, along with memory Th and Tc cells, are responsible for immunological memory. Figure 12.18 shows a summary of these processes and how they relate to the differences between primary and secondary responses that we discussed at the beginning of this chapter.

After primary immunization (or infection), naive B cells must acquire antigen, migrate to the secondary lymph nodes, and find T-cell help. Then, the first of these cells to be activated remains in the secondary lymphoid tissue and secretes IgM antibodies. These cells are usually short-lived. This process takes seven to ten days, and during that time antibody levels begin to rise in the serum. Late in the primary response, another group of B cells moves into the lymphoid follicles and, after interactions with Th cells and FDCs, undergoes isotype switch, somatic hypermutation, and selection.

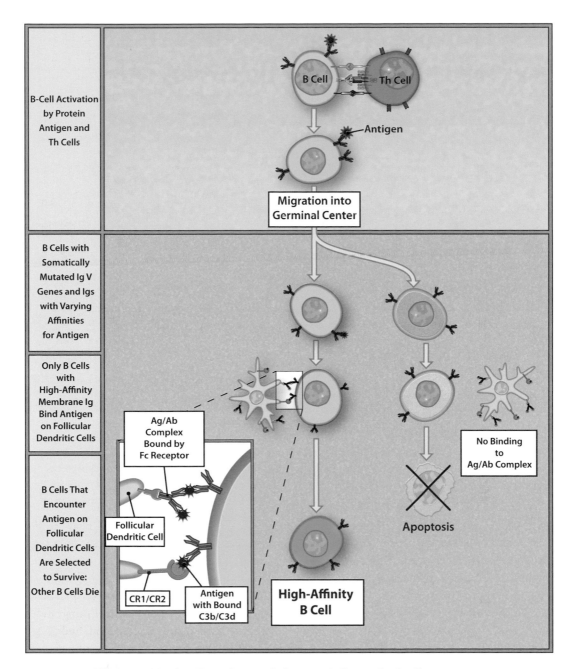

B-Cell Activation by Protein Antigen and Th Cells

B Cell

Th Cell

Antigen

Migration into Germinal Center

B Cells with Somatically Mutated Ig V Genes and Igs with Varying Affinities for Antigen

Only B Cells with High-Affinity Membrane Ig Bind Antigen on Follicular Dendritic Cells

Ag/Ab Complex Bound by Fc Receptor

B Cells That Encounter Antigen on Follicular Dendritic Cells Are Selected to Survive: Other B Cells Die

Follicular Dendritic Cell

CR1/CR2

Antigen with Bound C3b/C3d

High-Affinity B Cell

No Binding to Ag/Ab Complex

Apoptosis

FIGURE 12.16. Affinity maturation through somatic hypermutation and selection

Inside of lymph nodes, as they undergo the process of somatic hypermutation, B cells must repeatedly bind antigen through their BCRs to survive. The major source of antigen in germinal centers is in the form of antigen–antibody complexes bound directly or indirectly (through C3b and C3d receptors, CR1 and CR2) to FDCs. To bind that antigen, hypermutated BCRs must have greater affinity for antigen than the antibody on the FDCs. When this happens, B cells survive and continue as high-affinity B cells.

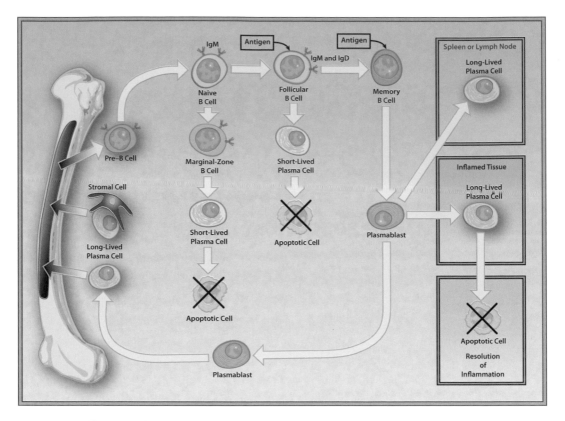

FIGURE 12.17. Life cycle of B cells

In most animals, B cells begin life in the bone marrow. They migrate from there, via the blood, to secondary lymphoid tissues, where they interact with Th cells. Some B cells immediately become plasma cells and secrete Ab from the medullary cords of the lymph nodes. Other B cells move to the lymphoid follicles and, after interactions with Th cells and FDCs, switch isotypes, undergo somatic hypermutation and selection, and become either long-lived memory B cells or antibody-secreting, long-lived plasma cells at sites of inflammation, in the bone marrow, or in secondary lymphoid tissue.

Some of these high-affinity B cells migrate to bone marrow. Along the way, they differentiate into long-lived plasma cells secreting high-affinity antibodies specific for the immunizing antigen. In the germinal centers of the lymph nodes, another group of high-affinity, isotype-switched B cells become long-lived memory B cells. After secondary immunization (or infection), memory B cells dominate the immune response. These B cells, again after interactions with Th and FDCs, generate mostly IgG or IgA of even higher affinity. From these B cells come more long-lived plasma cells secreting high-affinity antibody in the bone marrow. During the process, another group of long-lived memory B cells arises and remains in secondary lymphoid tissues awaiting another antigenic insult.

In species such as chickens, rabbits, and sheep, in which most B-cell development occurs in the GALT, the process is a little different (see Figure 12.19). Also, B-cell maturation does not involve germinal centers in all species, nor is it entirely clear whether all species are capable of somatic hypermutation (see Figure 12.20).

On the surface, these species' variations might suggest that some species would be at greater risk of infection because of lower potential antibody diversity. In fact, some scien-

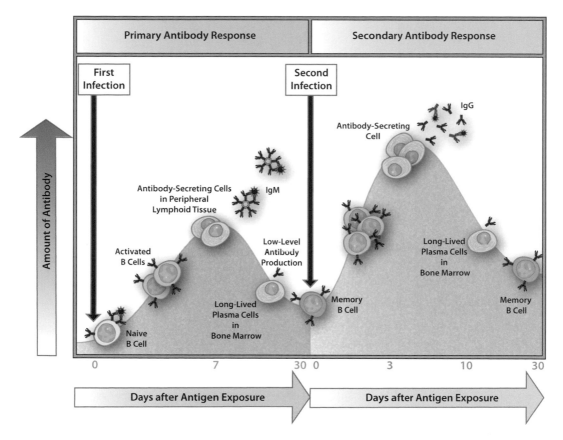

FIGURE 12.18. Primary versus secondary immune responses

tists have argued that the apparent low diversity among bony and cartilaginous fish might reflect the greater homogeneity of their environment compared with land species—a reduced need for highly diverse BCRs. No hard evidence exists for either fewer pathogenic threats or greater susceptibility to infection among these species. Regardless, it is apparent that at considerable energetic and genetic expense, all mammals and several other species have evolved very sophisticated means for generating astounding amounts of antibody diversity.

ANTIBODY EFFECTOR FUNCTIONS

Pathogen and Toxin Neutralization

During pathogenesis, viruses and bacterial toxins both bind to specific receptors (normal host-cell molecules co-opted by bacteria and viruses) on host cells and either destroy those host cells or pathologically alter host-cell functions. Antibodies bound either to the surfaces of viruses or to bacterial toxins prevent interaction with host-cell receptors (see Figure 12.21).

Opsonization and Activation of Complement

Antibodies can also bind to the surfaces of bacteria and coat them with antibody molecules, all with the C-termini of their H chains facing out. This process is opsonization, and the end result is more efficient destruction of bacterial pathogens (see Figure 12.21). Recall from chapter 6 that macrophages, neutrophils, and other cells have receptors, called Fc receptors, that

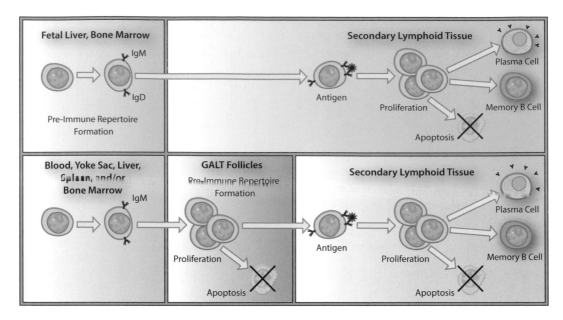

FIGURE 12.19. A comparison of B-cell development in species in which that development takes place in bone marrow (and often fetal liver) or GALT

In the so-called GALT species, such as rabbits, chickens, and sheep, Ig gene variability arises differently. Although the non-GALT species rely largely on genetic rearrangement and junctional diversification for generation of BCR diversity, GALT species use mechanisms such as gene conversion and somatic hypermutation before B-cell contact with antigen to generate Ig diversity. In both GALT and non-GALT species, final B-cell maturation occurs in secondary lymphoid tissues and involves somatic hypermutation, selection, and affinity maturation. GALT species may also use further gene conversion events and selection to enhance antibody affinity.

bind to the C-termini of Ig H chains. After binding antigens, the conformation of the C-termini of Ig H chains changes slightly. Aggregation of Ig adds to these changes and to the antibodies reactive with Fc receptors. As a result, once bacteria have been opsonized, macrophages, via Fc receptors, bind, phagocytose, and destroy these bacteria much more efficiently.

Similarly, after antigen binding, changes in the C-termini of the H chains of IgG and IgM molecules activate complement via the classical complement cascade (discussed in chapter 4). Complement activation results in the deposition of complement fragments, especially C3b, onto pathogen surfaces. Macrophages, neutrophils, and other phagocytic cells also have receptors for C3b. Thus, bound C3b also results

in more efficient interactions between phagocytic cell surfaces and pathogens and in turn leads to more rapid and more effective destructive of pathogens, especially bacteria. Activation of the terminal membrane attack pathway also leads to direct lysis of the pathogen.

Distribution and Function of Fc Receptors

Fc receptors actually appear on a variety of cells and perform several functions beyond simply enhancing phagocytosis. For example, Fc receptors on FDCs (FcγRIIB) capture antigen–antibody complexes for selection after somatic hypermutation. Also, mast cells, cells that play critical roles in inflammation and allergies, have

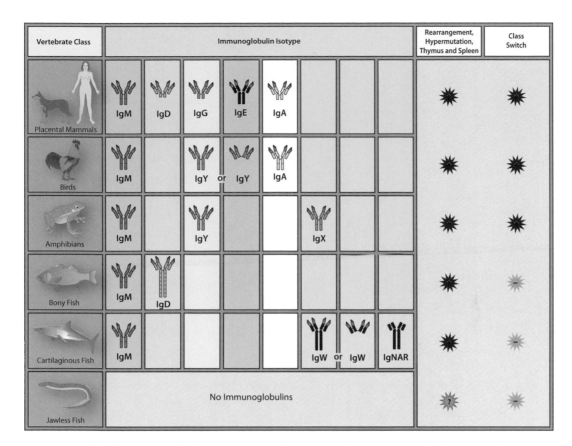

FIGURE 12.20. The forms of antibody and the use of hypermutation, Ig class switch, and germinal center formation in various classes of chordates

Fc receptors for IgE (Fcε). When the IgE bound to the Fc receptor interacts with antigen, the mast cell releases histamine and several of the mediators of inflammation. This inflammation is sometimes protective (perhaps in parasitic infections) and sometimes causes allergic reactions (see chapter 16).

Because of antibodies and Fc receptors, the humoral immune response is very effective at dealing with and defending against extracellular pathogens. Also, investigators have very recently found that some antibodies do get inside of cells as well. It still appears, however, that cellular immune responses and Tc cells deal most effectively with intracellular pathogens.

CLINICAL CORRELATION FOLLOW-UP

Student Considerations

Selective Ig deficiencies are the most common immune deficiencies of dogs. As mentioned at the outset of this chapter, as many as 80 percent of Chinese shar peis have selective IgA deficiencies. Their symptoms include recurrent dermatitises (staphylococcal), demodectic mange, otitis externa, flea allergies, cystitis, food intolerance, and bronchitis. On the basis of this chapter and the preceding one, you should be able to offer an explanation for why an animal with an IgA deficiency might have the symptoms seen in these dogs. You should also be able to offer one or more plausible

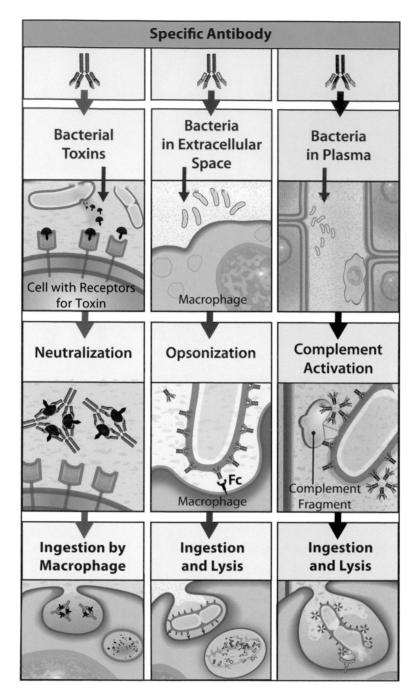

FIGURE 12.21. Effector mechanisms of antibodies

As shown in the left column, when antibodies bind to toxins (or viruses), the toxins can no longer bind to specific receptors on host cells and are neutralized. The center column shows how antibody binding to bacteria (a process called opsonization) allows macrophages to adhere more readily and facilitate phagocytosis. The right column shows a similar process. Once IgM or IgG antibodies have bound to a pathogen, the complexes activate complement. Macrophages and other phagocytic cells also have receptors for complement fragments.

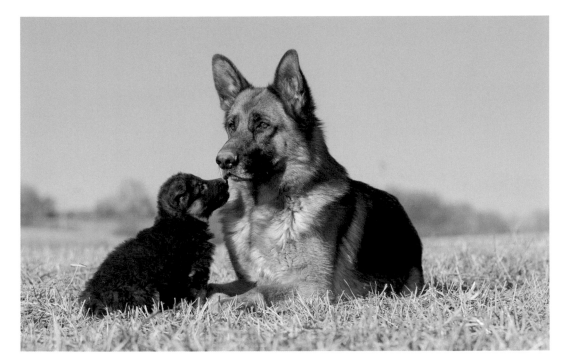

FIGURE 12.22. Adult German shepherd and puppy (© Lenkadan / Shutterstock)

Selective Ig deficiencies have also been reported in German shepherds.

explanations about how an IgA deficiency might arise and how it could produce the observed symptoms.

Possible Explanations

As the result of specific transport mechanisms that have evolved to deliver IgA antibodies to epithelial surfaces, as described in chapter 11, IgA—especially dimeric IgA—is the predominant antibody at body surfaces, including mucosal and other epithelia. No similar mechanism transports any other isotype across epithelial surfaces. Furthermore, infections that occur at epithelial surfaces induce primarily IgA antibody responses.

In the absence of normal levels of IgA, epithelia are at much greater risk of primary and recurrent infections such as dermatitis, demodectic mange, otitis externa, cystitis, and bronchitis and are unable to make protective IgA antibody responses against the infecting pathogens. It may also be that in the absence of IgA, responses dominated by IgE might be more common and lead to flea and food allergies. Clearly, the majority of the symptoms seen in these dogs result from a deficiency of IgA antibodies.

Just how an animal might come to have a selective IgA deficiency is less clear. Several possible explanations exist. It could be that these animals have an inherited genetic defect in the C-gene segment encoding IgA H chains. In this case, it would be impossible for B cells to switch from IgM to IgA under any circumstances. Also, as shown in Figure 12.14, Th-cell–derived cytokines (such as TGF-β) direct isotype switches, including the switch to IgA. A deficiency or defect in any one of these cytokines or their receptors on B cells could also lead to a selective IgA deficiency. Similarly, defects in the signal transduction machinery associated with any of these cytokine-specific receptors on B cells could lead to a selective IgA deficiency.

Gerald N. Callahan

Adaptive Immune Responses to Infections and Immunological Memory

Chapter 13

10.5876_9781607322184.c013

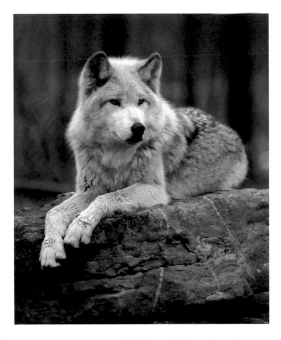

FIGURE 13.1. **Gray wolf (© Dennis Donohue / Shutterstock)**

CLINICAL CORRELATION: CANINE PARVOVIRUS AND THE WOLVES OF ISLE ROYALE

Isle Royale National Park is an island in Lake Superior. The island is roadless, covers about 544 square kilometers (338 square miles), and sits 25 kilometers (15.5 miles) from Ontario. Because of its usual isolation from the mainland, ecologists have studied the island for nearly a century to learn more about how ecosystems work and animal populations react to different stressors.

In about 1900, moose migrated across an ice bridge onto Isle Royale. Around 1940, a wolf (Figure 13.1) pack, also via an ice bridge, arrived on Isle Royale. Both wolves and moose prospered until the early 1970s (see Figure 13.2). About then, the wolf population began to deplete the moose herd.

And that was how things continued—increasing wolf population, decreasing moose population—until 1981. In that year, the wolf population fell precipitously, from nearly fifty wolves

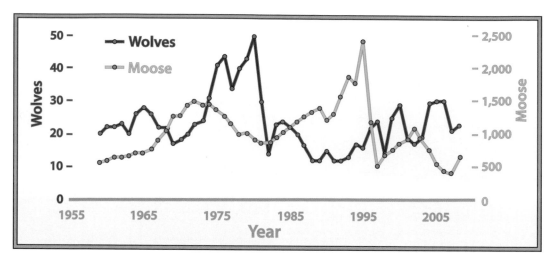

FIGURE 13.2. **Wolf and moose populations on Isle Royale, 1955–2010**

to fourteen, and the moose herd began to recover. By 1985, the moose population reached an all-time high, but the wolf population never fully recovered. Many people offered theories about the cause of the wolf population's crash, but nothing seemed consistent with all the facts. Then veterinarians completed a series of wolf necropsies in the early 1980s. Essentially, every necropsied wolf had died as a result of a parvovirus infection. Canine parvovirus was unknown until 1978. By 1979, the virus had spread around the globe and ravaged dog and coyote populations, especially pups. The virus is very similar to feline panleukopenia virus and some viruses of raccoons and foxes and may have evolved from one of them.

Isle Royale National Park was established in 1940, and among its regulations was the exclusion of domestic dogs (the most common reservoir for parvovirus). That means the only plausible explanations for the appearance of parvovirus on Isle Royale all involve humans. Among the possibilities, it seems most likely that this parvovirus outbreak originated when humans carried the virus onto Isle Royale, probably stuck to the soles of their boots. Because parvovirus is a nonenveloped virus that persists for long periods outside of host cells, this explanation seems entirely plausible.

Parvovirus infections occur most frequently when dogs ingest food or other things contaminated by feces from an infected animal. Figure 13.3 shows the pathogenesis of canine parvovirus.

Approximately 70 percent of dogs infected with canine parvovirus will die from their infections. At necropsy, these dogs exhibit leukopenia, extensive necrosis of the intestinal epithelium and secondary lymphoid tissues, and severe dehydration.

LEARNING OBJECTIVES

After reading this chapter, you should be able to

- describe mammalian adaptive immune responses from beginning to end;
- understand how the effectiveness of these responses may vary depending on the nature of the pathogen;
- understand how and why adaptive immune responses may fail to provide protection;
- describe the unique nature of adaptive immune responses that arise in the gut;
- understand the nature of immunological memory and describe the cells involved;
- describe how immunological memory arises and is maintained.

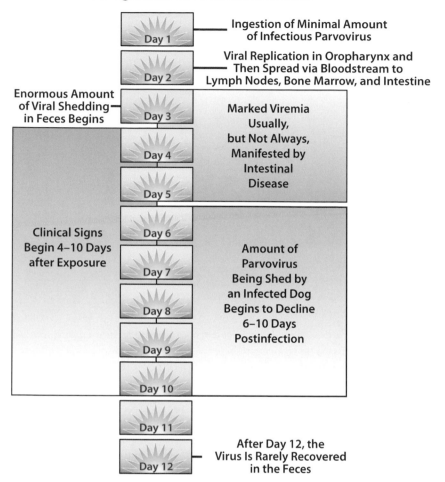

FIGURE 13.3. Pathogenesis of canine parvovirus

Canine parvovirus infections occur when canids (especially puppies) ingest food or other material contaminated with feces from another parvovirus-infected canid. The virus then spreads from the mouth to the lymph nodes and the gastrointestinal tract. Often, but not always, the virus then causes a massive bloody diarrhea, leucopenia, gastrointestinal necrosis, dehydration, and death.

ADAPTIVE IMMUNITY: THE BIG PICTURE—FROM INSULT TO RECOVERY

After most encounters with pathogens, a race ensues—a race between the host animal's defenses and the pathogen. The progress and the outcome of that competition determine which survives and which dies.

The race begins when the pathogen enters the host and triggers innate defense mecha-nisms. Until the past decade, most immunologists ignored the potential of these innate defenses and focused on adaptive immunity; however, outside of chordates, adaptive immune responses are nonexistent. Because most animals are not chordates (insects being the single largest population of animals), most animals, including humans, rely solely on innate defenses to survive the millions of daily pathogenic assaults they encounter.

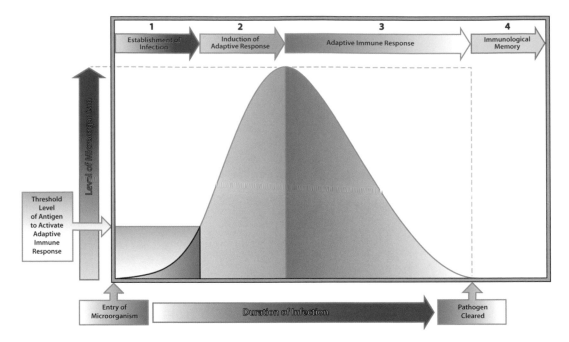

FIGURE 13.4. Acute infection

Infections always result in a race between the host defenses and the replicating pathogen. After initial contact with the pathogen, two things begin to happen: the host's innate responses engage and the pathogen begins to replicate. When numbers of pathogens exceed a certain threshold and move beyond the innate defenses, adaptive responses follow. Over a period of days to weeks, these adaptive responses usually reach protective levels, and the pathogen disappears from the infected animal.

Clearly, innate immunity can provide a powerful weapon against infectious agents, and even among animals that possess adaptive immune capabilities, innate defenses are terribly important. First, innate immune responses occur much more rapidly than adaptive responses. Because this is a race between pathogen and host defense, speed is of the essence. Second, few—if any—adaptive responses can develop without some assistance and direction from early innate responses.

Beginning with sharks, however, adaptive immune responses often dominate immune responses. An adaptive immune response provides some things innate immunity cannot, namely, specificity, memory, and affinity maturation. In a world of evolving pathogens, these aspects of adaptive immunity add a level of protection unattainable through innate immunity alone. Plus, adaptive immune responses make possible one of the greatest achievements in the battle against infectious diseases—vaccination.

It is likely that innate defensive responses to some pathogens fully control infections. Just how many is not known. First, innate responses occur so rapidly that clinical signs of infection may not appear before the pathogen is gone. Deficiencies in innate defense mechanisms are rarer (perhaps an indication of the animals' absolute dependence on them) than deficiencies in adaptive responses. So, fewer opportunities have arisen to directly assess the importance of innate defense to overall protection. Regardless, many pathogens multiply so rapidly that they outstrip innate defenses. When this happens, adaptive immune responses engage (see Figure 13.4).

Most immune responses appear to involve both innate and adaptive aspects, but all begin

Extracellular		Intracellular	
Interstitial Spaces, Blood, Lymph	**Epithelial Surfaces**	**Cytoplasmic**	**Vesicular**
Viruses, Bacteria, Protozoa, Fungi, Worms	Worms, Mycoplasma, *Streptococcus pneumoniae*, *Escherichia coli*, *Candida albicans*	Viruses, Chlamydia spp., Rickettsia, *Listeria monocytogenes*, Protozoa	Mycobacteria, *Salmonella typhimurium*, *Yersinia pestis*
Antibodies, Complement, Phagocytosis, Neutralization	Antibodies (Especially IgA) Antimicrobial Peptides	Cytotoxic T Cells, NK Cells	T-Cell– and NK-Cell– Dependent Macrophage Activation

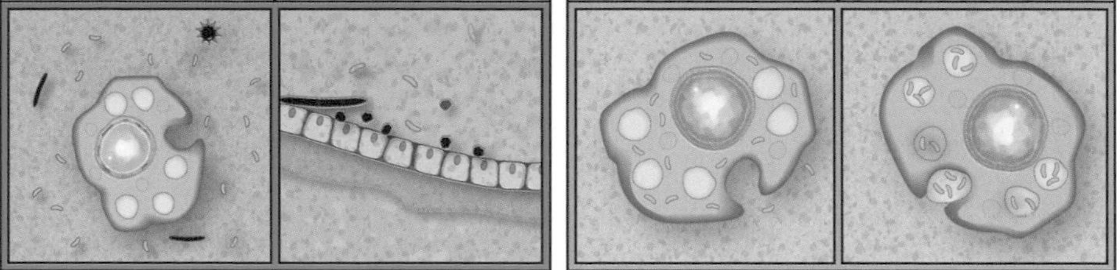

Row labels (left column): **Site of Infection**, **Organisms**, **Protective Immunity**

FIGURE 13.5. **Replication of pathogens in various compartments within animals**

Different pathogens thrive in different compartments inside of infected animals.

with innate responses. As shown in Figure 13.4, it appears that once a pathogen replicates beyond the defensive power of innate mechanisms, adaptive immunity becomes involved. Time frames may vary between species and among individuals, but innate mechanisms generally engage within seconds to hours, and the development of a primary, full-blown adaptive immune response takes a week or longer.

Routes of Infection

Infectious agents (i.e., prions, viruses, bacteria, fungi, and parasites) are also known as transmissible agents of disease because, when transmitted from an infected to an uninfected animal, these agents will again induce the same disease. The possible routes of transmission include inhalation, ingestion, and injection (by mosquitoes or other blood-sucking arthropods); during mating; and through wounds.

Mechanisms of Pathogenesis

Once pathogens gain access beyond the barriers of skin and mucosal epithelia, they can thrive and replicate in different compartments inside of animals (see Figure 13.5). All pathogens exist as either intracellular or extracellular infections. Extracellular infections may occur in any of the body fluids—blood, lymph, interstitial fluid, and urine. Bacteria, protozoa, fungi, and worms are the most common extracellular pathogens. Pathogenic microorganisms can

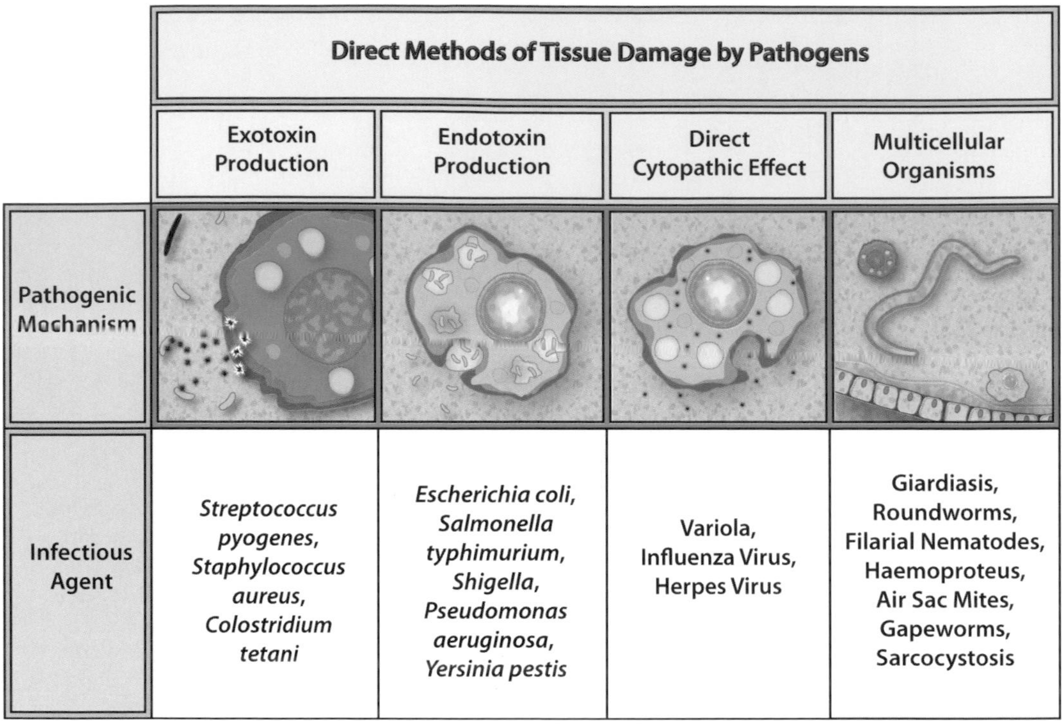

Direct Methods of Tissue Damage by Pathogens			
	Exotoxin Production	**Endotoxin Production**	**Direct Cytopathic Effect**	**Multicellular Organisms**
Pathogenic Mechanism				
Infectious Agent	*Streptococcus pyogenes, Staphylococcus aureus, Colostridium tetani*	*Escherichia coli, Salmonella typhimurium, Shigella, Pseudomonas aeruginosa, Yersinia pestis*	Variola, Influenza Virus, Herpes Virus	Giardiasis, Roundworms, Filarial Nematodes, Haemoproteus, Air Sac Mites, Gapeworms, Sarcocystosis

FIGURE 13.6. **Mechanisms of pathogenesis**

Various microorganisms cause diseases in various ways. Bacteria produce exotoxins and endotoxins as well as directly infect cells and alter normal cell function. Viruses infect cells and kill or interfere with normal host-cell activities. Fungi grow on tissue surfaces and can enzymatically degrade underlying cells. Protozoan parasites also often infect host cells and alter these cells' abilities to perform their normal functions. Worms can cause diseases in a variety of ways.

also grow intracellularly. Bacteria and viruses are the most common intracellular pathogens. Each of these different locations presents particular problems for immune systems. Transmissible agents also cause diseases in different ways (see Figure 13.6).

On the basis of their abilities to retain Gram stain, bacteria can be split into two large groups—Gram-negative and Gram-positive. Recall from chapter 3 that the defining feature of Gram-negative bacteria is that they have a thick outer coat of LPS—a powerful PAMP—on their cell walls. Gram-negative bacteria release LPS into their surroundings, particularly when they die. LPS is endotoxin, and endotoxin causes disease by activation of macrophages and inducing inflammation. When this same

LPS is present systemically (as in Gram-negative sepsis), however, it can cause endotoxic shock and death (described in chapter 3).

Both Gram-negative and Gram-positive bacteria can also produce other types of toxins called exotoxins. Living bacteria produce exotoxins, and unlike endotoxins, there are many types of exotoxins with very different sorts of effects on host animals. To exert their effects, exotoxins can bind directly to specific molecules on host cells.

For example, as they grow, *Clostridium botulinum* bacteria release botulinum toxin, possibly the most potent toxin known (a median lethal dose is about 1 ng/kg). When an animal ingests botulinum toxin, the toxin moves quickly into and out of the blood where it binds receptors in

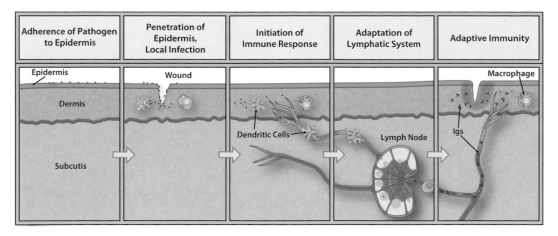

| Adherence of Pathogen to Epidermis | Penetration of Epidermis, Local Infection | Initiation of Immune Response | Adaptation of Lymphatic System | Adaptive Immunity |

FIGURE 13.7. Initiation of an adaptive immune response

Antigen gains access to host cells after a break in the skin. DCs ingest this antigen, process it, transport it to the nearest lymph node, and present the antigen to T cells. Adaptive immune responses begin here and eventually culminate at the site of infection.

neuromuscular junctions. There, it inhibits the release of acetylcholine from presynaptic nerve terminals. The neurotransmitter acetylcholine is essential for normal muscle activation. In the presence of botulinum toxin, muscle contraction becomes impossible, and respiratory and cardiovascular systems fail rapidly.

All viruses and some bacteria such as Chlamydia grow inside of host cells. The pathogenic effects of these infections result from the tissue tropism of the infectious agent and the damage these pathogens do to those host cells as well as from host inflammatory responses. For example, in infectious canine hepatitis, the virus enters the body through the mouth or nose, or both, and infects the tonsils and the cervical lymph nodes. From there, the virus moves into the blood and spreads to (among other places) the liver. Here, the virus infects hepatocytes. Some of these hepatocytes die, which stimulates a host inflammatory response that results in hepatitis.

Fungi cause diseases by attachment to host tissue surfaces and enzymatic degradation of the underlying host cells. Most often, this attachment and degradation occur on the skin.

Protozoan parasites commonly cause disease by infecting host cells and interfering with normal host-cell function. Multicellular parasites can cause disease in many different ways—from simple mechanical obstruction of fluid flow (as in canine heartworm) to inflammation (as in sarcoptic mange).

Innate Response Cells and Cytokines of Innate Responses Direct T-Cell Differentiation

Adaptive immune responses begin when professional (dedicated) APCs ingest antigens and transport them to secondary lymphoid tissues (see Figure 13.7). Along the way, these APCs process the acquired pathogen into pieces, insert those pieces into MHC class II and MHC class I molecules, and relocate these MHC–antigen complexes to the surface of the APCs, where they become available for interaction with T cells (see Figure 13.8A–B).

Circulating T cells arrive in lymph nodes via specific interactions with receptors on HEVs. Initially, in the medullary regions of the nodes, these T cells encounter APCs displaying anti-

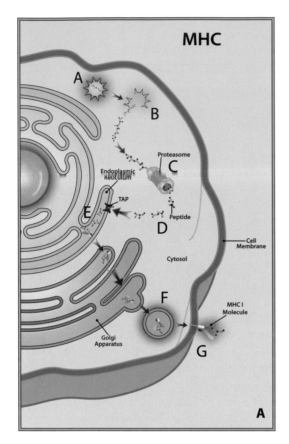

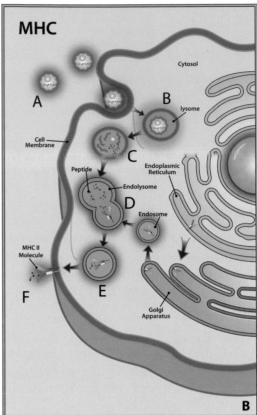

FIGURE 13.8A–B. **APC processing and presentation of antigen in MHC Class I molecules (panel A) and APC processing and presentation of antigen in MHC class II molecules (panel B)**

Panel A: A represents an infectious agent reproducing in the cytosol of the cell. B is antigen being synthesized in the cytosol of the cell. C is the proteosome where the protein products of A are digested into small peptides. D shows the peptides being transported into the lumen of the ER. E shows the peptides being bound by newly formed MHC class I molecules. F shows the movement of the MHC–Ag complexes inside an endosome. G shows the MHC–Ag complexes on the cell surface for presentation to T cells. Panel B: A represents exogenous antigen that is ingested by an APC via phagocytosis and confined inside of a phagosome (B and C). That phagosome then fuses with a lysosome to form a phagolysosome. D and E show how, inside of the phagolysosome, enzymes cleave antigenic proteins into small peptides that bind to MHC II molecules and return to the cell surface as Ag–MHC complexes (F) for presentation to T cells.

gens they have acquired locally or from remote sites. For a few days, antigen-specific T cells remain in the lymph node, where at least two types of interactions occur. Naive Tc cells interact with MHC class I–antigen complexes on APCs and, with or without Th-cell help, these naive Tc cells become antigen-activated effector Tc cells (see Figure 13.9A–B).

Effector T Cells Home to Sites of Infection and Inflammation

Tc effector cells express several different cell-surface markers. Among these are molecules that interact specifically with receptors on vascular endothelial cells at sites of infection and inflammation. Because of this, activated Tc cells home to sites where these cells are most

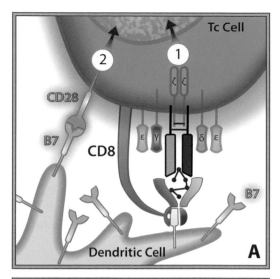

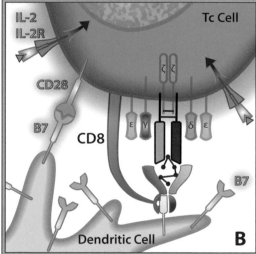

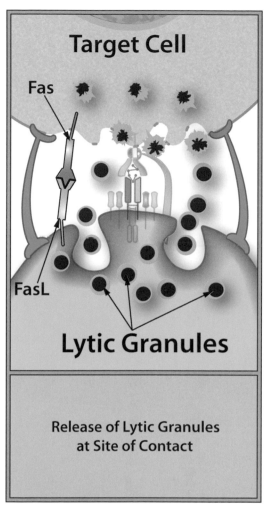

FIGURE 13.10. **Effector Tc-mediated destruction of pathogen-infected cells**

After specific recognition of MHC–antigen complexes, Tc cells release lytic granules that induce apoptosis in infected host cells.

FIGURE 13.9A–B. **Direct activation of Tc cells by highly effective APCs**

After exposure to PAMPs, DAMPs, or both, APCs (like DCs) will express high levels of MHC classes I and II as well as B7. This, along with processed antigen, can provide both the first (MHC–antigen) and the second (B7) signals to Tc cells (panel A). In response, the T cells begin to express the high-affinity receptor IL and produce IL-2 (panel B), which leads to activation.

likely to find pathogen-infected cells, especially virus-infected cells, and destroy them (see Figure 13.10).

Also, in secondary lymphoid tissues APCs present MHC class II–antigen complexes to Th cells. A combination of (1) the nature of the APC, (2) the nature of the innate responses, (3) the cytokines the APC produces, and (4) the affinity and frequency of TCR binding to the MHC–antigen complex determines what happens to the Th cell beyond this point (see Figure 13.11).

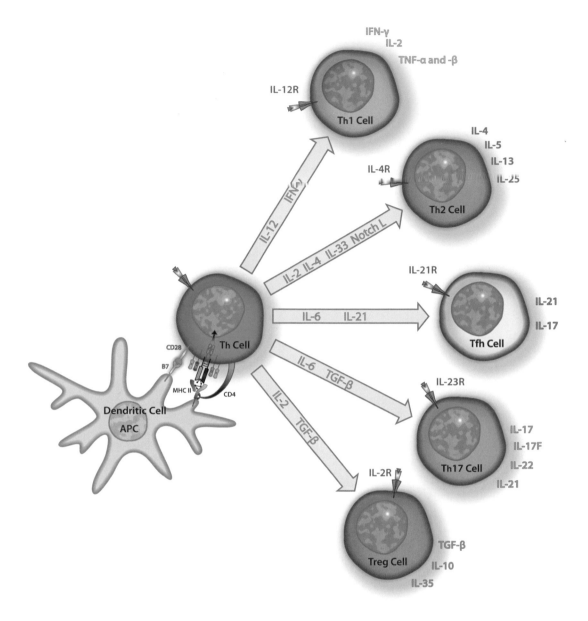

FIGURE 13.11. Alternative pathways of Th-cell differentiation

After interaction with an APC, Th cells may differentiate into several different cell types, including Th1, Th2, Tfh, Th17, Treg, Th3, and Tr1 cells. The pathway of Th-cell differentiation depends on what the cytokines produce during antigen presentation (arrows). Each Th cell type secretes a characteristic set of cytokines (far right) and participates in a unique way in the immune response.

Some of these Th effector cells, particularly Th1 and Th17 cells (because of cell-surface changes), also home to areas of infection and inflammation. They also bind to receptors on the vascular endothelium and engage in protective adaptive immune responses (as described in chapter 10), often enhancing inflammation and macrophage-mediated destruction of extracellular and intracellular pathogens. Other Th cells remain in the lymph nodes and

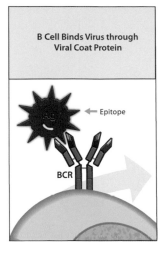
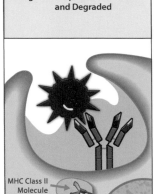
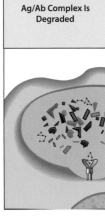
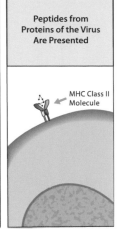

| B Cell Binds Virus through Viral Coat Protein | Ag/Ab Complex Is Internalized and Degraded | Ag/Ab Complex Is Degraded | Peptides from Proteins of the Virus Are Presented |

FIGURE 13.12. B cells as APCs

B cells acquire antigen through the immunoglobulin portion of their BCRs. After binding antigen and BCR cross-linking, B cells internalize the antigen–antibody (Ag–Ab) complexes and process both antigen and antibody into peptides. MHC class II molecules bind these peptides and present them on B-cell surfaces.

interact with B cells or aid in the activation of Tc cells.

Antibody Responses Develop in Secondary Lymphoid Tissues

B cells, usually after acquiring antigen, also arrive in the lymph nodes via the HEVs. B-cell interaction with antigen through the BCR and the B-cell coreceptor activates B cells. After activation, B cells express more MHC class II and B7 molecules. At the same time, BCR–antigen complexes enter B cells via receptor-mediated endocytosis, are processed, and are presented on the surfaces of the B cells in MHC class II molecules. All of this makes B cells very effective APCs (see Figure 13.12)

After interaction with Th cells, B cells follow one of three differentiation pathways. The first wave of B cells (all expressing IgM BCRs) migrates to the medullary cords, differentiates into plasma cells, and secretes pentameric IgM. A second set of activated B cells migrates to the lymphoid follicles, once again interacts with Th cells, and begins to divide, creating a germinal center. During these divisions, two things happen: isotype switching and somatic hypermutation.

Inside of lymphoid follicles, B cells undergo further genetic rearrangements that couple new H-chain constant-region genes with the variable regions generated in the bone marrow, which results in a switch from IgM to some other isotype, usually IgG or IgA but sometimes IgE (see Figure 13.13).

Also during B-cell division inside of lymphoid follicles, mutations rapidly accumulate in genes encoding L- and H-chain variable regions, a process called somatic hypermutation. With antibody H- and L-chain variable regions, most of the variability appears in three CDRs—CDR1, CDR2, and CDR3. Somatic hypermutation generates much of that hypervariability in these CDRs (see Figure 13.14).

When the B cell exits the cell cycle after somatic hypermutation, that B cell must again acquire antigen for presentation to another Th cell. If a B cell fails to once again bind antigen, that B cell dies. A ready source of antigen inside of lymph nodes is in the form of antigen–

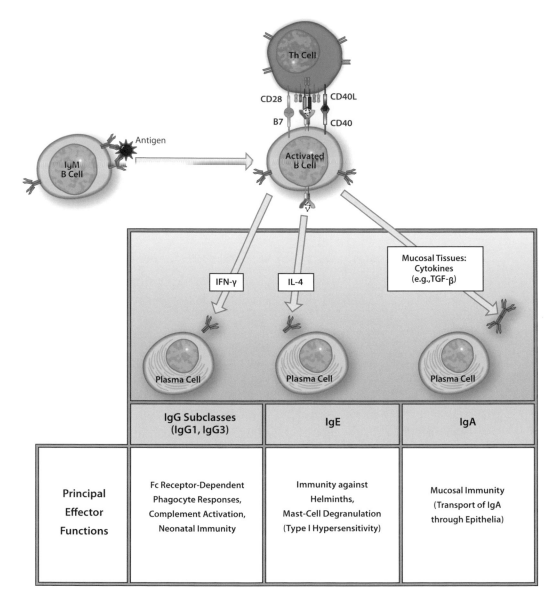

FIGURE 13.13. Cytokine control of isotype switching in germinal centers

In the upper left corner, a B cell first encounters antigen. Inside of a germinal center in secondary lymphoid tissue, this B cell interacts with a Th cell (upper right). Depending on the cytokines produced by the Th cell, the B cell switches from expressing IgM to expressing IgG, IgA, or IgE.

antibody complexes on the surface of FDCs. For the newly mutant B cell to acquire this antigen, its new BCR must have a higher affinity for antigen than the antibody on the FDC. So as the immune response progresses, only B cells with increasingly higher-affinity BCRs survive, resulting in affinity maturation: a continuing increase in antibody affinity for antigen during

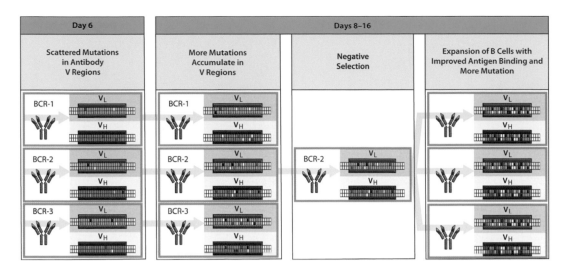

FIGURE 13.14. Somatic hypermutation during B-cell division inside of lymphoid germinal centers

Late in primary immune responses and throughout secondary and subsequent immune responses against a given antigen, mutations rapidly arise in B-cell genes encoding Ig molecules. These mutations fall mostly within the CDR1, CDR2, and CDR3 regions of the L and H chains, shown here as colored vertical bars.

secondary and subsequent immune responses (see Figure 13.15).

These newly formed isotype-switched, high-affinity B cells follow one of two paths. Some of them migrate out of the lymph nodes and eventually arrive in the bone marrow as long-lived plasma cells, where they secrete IgG, IgA, or IgE. Another group of isotype-switched, high-affinity B cells remain in the secondary lymphoid tissues as memory B cells (see Memory B Cells section).

Antibodies secreted by B cell–derived plasma cells enter the blood, the lymph, and interstitial tissues and arrive on epithelial surfaces to participate in several ways in adaptive immune responses against extracellular pathogens. In particular, IgM and IgG antibodies, after antigen binding, can activate complement. Complement components aid in protection in several ways, including the direct lysis of microbes, opsonization of pathogens—which enhances ingestion and destruction by macrophages and neutrophils—and enhancement of protective inflammatory responses. Also, IgM and IgG can

opsonize bacteria and enhance macrophage-mediated destruction of these bacteria. By blocking specific molecules, antibodies can also neutralize bacterial toxins as well as viruses. Antibodies also facilitate NK cell–mediated destruction of infected host cells via antibody-dependent cellular cytotoxicity. Finally, it appears that some antibodies can have effects inside of host cells.

By these means, adaptive immune responses have evolved to deal with each of the compartments mentioned at the outset of this chapter and provide protection from a variety of pathogens. The final results are primary, secondary, etc., adaptive immune responses. The unique features of those responses are their specificity, memory, and affinity maturation (see Figure 13.16).

Low-affinity IgM antibodies dominate the primary immune response, whereas high-affinity IgG antibodies derived from memory B cells dominate most secondary immune responses. After repeated exposures to antigen, the affinity of the antibody for its specific antigen continues

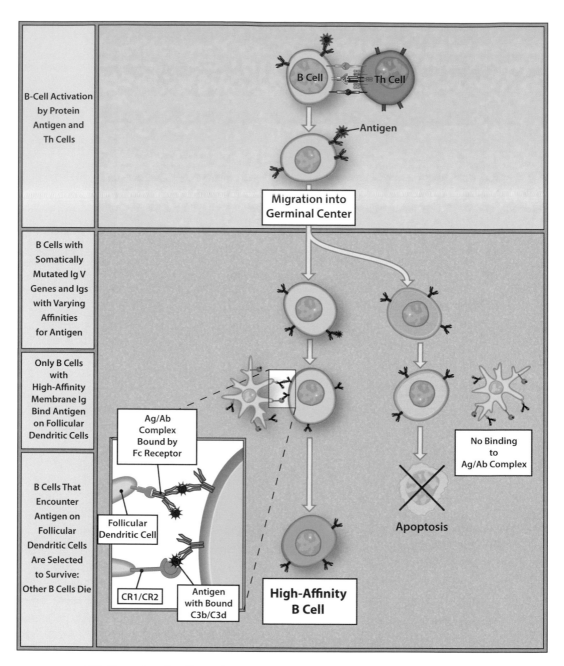

FIGURE 13.15. Affinity maturation through somatic hypermutation and selection

Inside of lymph nodes, as they undergo the process of somatic hypermutation, B cells must repeatedly bind antigen through their BCRs to survive. The major source of antigen in germinal centers is in the form of antigen–antibody (Ag–Ab) complexes bound directly or indirectly (through C3b and C3d receptors) to FDCs. To bind that antigen, hypermutated BCRs must have greater affinity for antigen than the antibody on the FDCs. When this happens, B cells survive as high-affinity B cells.

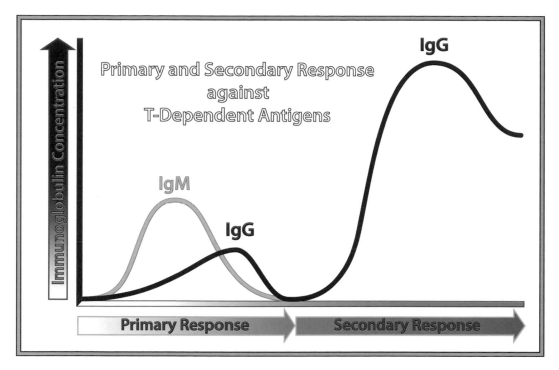

FIGURE 13.16. **Primary and secondary adaptive immune responses**

to increase. All of these arise because of the unique characteristics of B and T cells and their antigen-specific receptors.

Importance of Different Adaptive Responses to Clearance of Different Pathogens

As mentioned earlier, pathogens arrive inside animals via different routes, multiply in various spaces, and cause disease in various ways. Because of this, different classes of pathogens present different challenges to animals' immune systems, which is important for several reasons. First, understanding the process and outcome of infections depends on understanding how particular types of responses protect against or exacerbate diseases caused by different pathogens. Second, effective vaccination must elicit protective immune responses. With different pathogens, vaccines may have to induce very different types of immune responses to be pro-

tective. Generally, antibody responses are most effective against extracellular infections, and Th1 and Tc cells are most effective against intracellular infections (see Figure 13.17).

Different antibody isotypes may provide greater or lesser protection against a given pathogen. Also, antibodies can provide effective protection against intracellular pathogens by neutralizing the pathogens before they can infect their target cells.

Immune Responses in the Gut

All of the material presented so far in this chapter is most directly relevant to immune responses occurring in the lymph nodes and the spleen and, therefore, most relevant to antigens and pathogens in lymph, interstitial fluids, and blood. As mentioned at the outset, though, there are even larger spaces where animals regularly encounter pathogens—the epithelia and, specifically, the gut mucosa.

Infectious Agent	Disease	Humoral Immunity	Cell-Mediated Immunity	
		Ig	CD4 T Cells	CD8 T Cells
Viruses — Variola	Cowpox		+	+
Influenza Virus	Influenza	+		+
FIV	AIDS	+		+
SIV	AIDS	+		+
Bacteria — *Staphylococcus aureus*	Boils	+		
Streptococcus pneumoniae	Pneumonia	+		
Clostridium tetani	Tetanus	+		
Bacillus anthracis	Anthrax	+		
Mycobacteria	Tuberculosis, Leprosy		+	+
Fungi — *Candida albicans*	Candidiasis	+	+	
Protozoa — *Toxoplasma gondii*	Toxoplasmosis	+	+	
Trypanosoma spp.	Trypanosomiasis	+	+	
Leishmania spp.	Leshmaniasis		+	
Worms — Schistosome	Schistosomiasis		+	

FIGURE 13.17. Different types of immune effector mechanisms are effective against various pathogens

Plus signs indicate the probable importance of different effector mechanisms to protect immunity against viruses, bacteria, fungi, and parasites. In general, cellular mechanisms are most effective against intracellular pathogens, and antibodies are most effective against extracellular pathogens. FIV = feline immunodeficiency virus; SIV = simian immunodeficiency virus.

Scientists have estimated that there are approximately 10^{29} bacteria on this planet. The mass of that number of bacteria is equivalent to enough aircraft carriers to cover the United States three deep—that's seventy stories high. No living species exists because it has learned how to completely avoid infection. Instead, each species exists because life requires a compromise with bacteria in the form of commensal and mutualistic relationships. Bacteria, especially the gut bacteria, are essential to animal health. Interestingly, in some species (if not all)

FIGURE 13.18A–B. Mammalian Peyer's patches and lymphoid tissues in the small intestine

Panel A shows a diagram of a thin section of small intestine. Within this section, the dark purple–rimmed ovoid areas represent specialized lymphoid tissue called Peyer's patches— sites of immune responses in the intestine. Panel B shows a diagrammatic representation of the interaction between the cells of a Peyer's patch and an enteric pathogen. Multifenestrated or microfold (M) cells carry antigens from the gut lumen into the Peyer's patch, where DCs process and present these antigens to the immune system. As with splenic lymphoid tissues, the patches have discrete T-cell–rich and B-cell–rich areas.

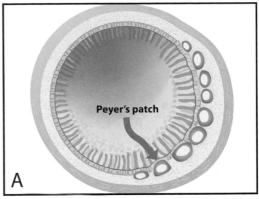

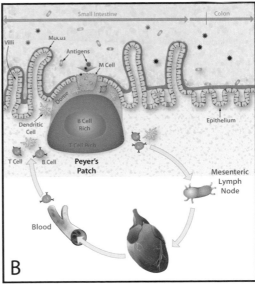

the composition of the normal flora is as distinctive as the animal itself. No two are alike.

The other consequence of the enormous biological success of bacteria is that all natural foods are teeming with bacteria and fungi as well as viruses and perhaps a parasite or two. One of the most important transitions a newly born animal makes is moving from a sterile gut to one carrying much of the normal flora. If an animal fails to acquire these bacteria, that animal fails to develop normal gastrointestinal and immune systems. For all animals, bacterial colonization is an essential part of early life. Somehow, the gut immune system, meaning GALT, must deal with all the potential threats and, at the same time, maintain healthy normal flora.

Because of this, gut immune mechanisms differ some from the immune mechanisms operative in lymph and spleen. Perhaps for different reasons, the same appears to be true of immune responses in or on respiratory epithelia and the epithelia lining the major body cavities.

The gut has several specialized lymphoid tissues, including tonsils and adenoids. At the moment, we focus on Peyer's patches, found mostly in animals' small intestines (see Figure 13.18A–B).

Specialized cells called multifenestrated or microfold (M) cells make up a significant part

of the follicle-associated epithelium of Peyer's patches. Unlike enterocytes, these cells have no glycocalyx and do not secrete mucus. Instead, M cells have evolved to interact directly with the antigens of the gut. Using phagocytosis and endocytosis, M cells take up antigens from the gut lumen and transfer these antigens across the gut epithelium and deliver them into the extracellular space on the opposite side of the epithelium. Here, APCs acquire these antigens, process them, and present them to T cells (see Figure 13.19). Beyond M cells, gut-associated DCs have evolved the ability to insert pseudopodia (or dendrites) between gut epithelial cells and sample the contents of the gut lumen.

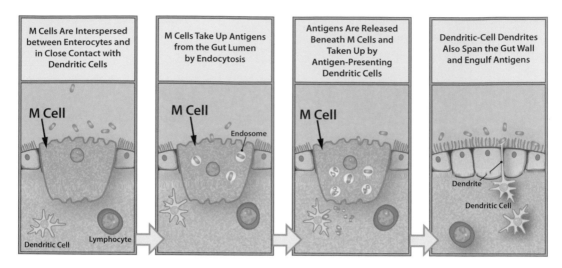

FIGURE 13.19. Antigen transfer across the gut epithelium by M cells

M cells acquire antigens by phagocytosis and endocytosis. The basal surfaces of M cells wrap around lymphocytes and DCs. As antigens cross the gut epithelia, DCs acquire them, process them, and present them as MHC–antigen complexes. DCs also extend long dendrites into the gut lumen to sample and present gut contents.

In addition to Peyer's patches, foci of plasma cells and lymphocytes appear scattered along the length of the small intestine. These are the effector cells of gut immunity. As with all T and B cells, these cells originate in the bone marrow and the thymus. Because of specific receptors on their surfaces, however, these B and T cells home to the gut mucosal epithelia and move into the Peyer's patches. Once there, if these cells find their specific antigens, the B and T cells become active effector cells and migrate—via the lymphatics—to the mesenteric lymph nodes, and from there to the thoracic duct and the blood. Using specialized blood vessels that line the MALT and specific surface receptors, these effector cells return from the blood to the lamina propria and the epithelium of the gut and other mucosa. As a result, an immune response that began in an isolated area of the intestine spreads to the mucosa, throughout the body, and back to the gut.

Similar processes occur within many epithelia, and specialized groups of lymphocytes have evolved specific cell-surface markers to target them to individual epithelia. In addition to the conventional α/β T cells expressing CD4$^+$ or CD8$^+$, MALTs contain type b lymphocytes, which include CD4$^-$, CD8$^-$ γ/δ T cells, T cells with γ/δ TCRs, T cells with α/β TCRs, and CD8$^+$ T cells with α:α TCRs. These unique T-cell subsets do not recognize conventional MHC–antigen complexes on APCs. Instead, these cells react with several different sorts of molecules and with MHC class IB molecules. MHC class IB molecules structurally resemble classical MHC class I molecules; however, MHC class IB molecules do not come from genes in the MHC.

Because several classes of type b lymphocytes are present in athymic mice, it is clear that these lymphocytes do not develop in the thymus. Also, type b lymphocytes exhibit little, if any, gene rearrangement. These cells may represent an aspect of innate immunity and not adaptive immunity, or they may function at the boundary of both.

A variety of unique cells and immune mechanisms have evolved to deal with the intimate and intricate relationship between the gut mucosa and the gut flora. As you will see, this relationship somehow makes possible normal gut activity and normal lives for most animals.

As we have explained, the predominant antibody found at mucosal surfaces in most mammals is IgA and in particular dimeric IgA. The variety of IgA isotypes can vary a lot, with rabbits expressing thirteen different subclasses of IgA. In amphibians, IgX appears to perform functions similar to IgA in mammals. Reptiles use a modified form of IgG at mucosal surfaces, and chicken IgA looks more like mammalian IgM than IgA. In spite of these variations, it is clear that all species have evolved special types of antibodies to deal with immunity at mucosal surfaces. This specialization is essential because each species faces the same dilemma—an absolute requirement for gut colonization and constant contact with gut microbes, some of which could be potential pathogens. In general, mucosal immunity is a complex mixture of innate and innate-like mechanisms along with adaptive immune responses and a touch of benign neglect.

The gut immune system, interestingly, not only fails to react to most ingested antigens, it often becomes permanently tolerant of those antigens—a thing called oral tolerance. For example, if one injects a rabbit with ovalbumin (the major protein in hen-egg whites), the rabbit will usually make a powerful adaptive immune response to the foreign antigen. However, if one first feeds a rabbit hen-egg whites for a period of time and then injects the animal with ovalbumin, the rabbit makes no response to the foreign protein. It appears that all animals have evolved means to suppress immune reactions to the food they eat. Biologically, this makes sense, because it allows for tolerance to most food.

Clearly, though, animals can make immune responses against gut pathogens, including ingested gut pathogens. How is this possible in the face of the overwhelming tendency toward tolerance? Infection of gut epithelial cells and inflammation appear to be key.

Intestinal epithelial cells have surface receptors for pathogens (e.g., TLRs), but only on their basal surfaces. For recognition to occur, the pathogen must somehow first breech the defense of the epithelium. In response to a detected infection, gut epithelial cells secrete several chemokines that attract a variety of immune cells (in particular, macrophages and neutrophils). These recruited cells, after activation by pathogen and cytokines, can stimulate inflammation, antigen presentation, and innate and adaptive immune responses.

Beyond that, it is also clear that the gut flora themselves provide protection from infection. For example, after treatment with wide-spectrum antibiotics, animals may succumb to serious infections with *Clostridium difficile*. *C. difficile* produces two exotoxins that interfere with normal water resorption in the gut, resulting in life-threatening diarrhea and sometimes death from hypovolemic shock. Usually, the normal flora occupy most of the available space in the gut and use most of the available nutrients in the gut, and some normal flora even produce antimicrobial compounds. So, even though *C. difficile* is a common inhabitant of animal gastrointestinal tracts, it usually causes no problem. When antibiotics strip the protective flora, however, the gut epithelia become very susceptible to colonization by the normally innocuous *C. difficile*.

IMMUNOLOGICAL MEMORY

Primary and Subsequent Immune Responses

One of the most remarkable features of adaptive immune responses is memory (see Figure 13.16). A second encounter with a pathogen is rarely as dangerous as the first. In secondary and subsequent infections or vaccinations, the immune system responds faster; produces higher-affinity, isotype-switched antibody; and maintains higher levels of antibodies and effector cells much longer. All of this is possible because of memory T and B cells. In essence, immune systems remember things they have seen before, and when those same things appear again, immune systems react very differently—memory.

Up to now, we have focused most closely on the nature and events of primary adaptive immune responses, and although memory cells do begin to appear during primary responses, their effects are most apparent in secondary and subsequent immune responses.

Memory cells arise as T and B cells undergo multiple divisions (clonal expansion) after antigen- and cytokine-driven activation. Just what makes a B or T cell a memory cell is unclear, but several changes occur as cells become memory cells. These changes are mostly very different between B and T cells. But one thing seems common to all memory lymphocytes: they have very long lives. Trying to explain this, scientists have proposed very long-lived memory cells, long-term persistence of antigen, regular reinfection with the same pathogen, regular reactivation by cross-reactive pathogens, and cross-activation by cytokines produced during unrelated primary and secondary immune responses.

Presently, the most likely explanations involve some aspects of the first and last of these hypotheses. Memory T and B cells do appear to have unusually long lives, but not as long as immunological memory may last—sometimes decades or more. Recent studies have shown that memory cells, though mostly found in resting states, do occasionally divide. Scientists do not understand the stimulus for these divisions, but certain cytokines, such as IL-15 and IL-7, seem to prolong memory. So it appears that, in addition to their very long lives, occasionally as cells respond to unrelated antigens, cytokine production may drive infrequent memory cell division and expansion.

Memory B Cells

In vitro, memory B cells differ both quantitatively and qualitatively from naive B cells. The

	Source of B Cells	
	Unimmunized Donor Primary Response	Immunized Donor Secondary Response
Frequency of Specific B Cells	$1:10^4$–$1:10^5$	$1:10^3$
Isotype of Antibody Produced	IgM > IgG	IgG, IgA
Affinity of Antibody	Low	High
Somatic Hypermutation	Low	High

FIGURE 13.20. **Comparison of B cells and antibody from naive and immunized animals (adapted from C. Janeway, P. Travers, M. Walport, and M. Shlomchik, 2001, *Immunobiology*, fig. 10.24)**

frequency of antigen-specific B cells in immunized animals increases between 10- and 100-fold (see Figure 13.20).

In addition, most B cells from immunized mice express isotypes other than IgM, and the antibodies they produce show evidence of hypermutation and selection, resulting in much higher affinities for antigen (see chapter 12). Generally, these cells seem to follow the same circulation patterns as naive B cells. That is, memory B cells travel throughout the circulation, the spleen, mucosal epithelia, and the lymphatics. When their antigens reappear, these B cells settle into lymph nodes and other secondary lymphoid tissues, where they undergo multiplication and differentiation inside of lymphoid follicles (see chapter 12).

Memory T Cells

During primary immune responses, after activation T cells follow two distinct pathways of differentiation. One group becomes effector T cells, and the other group becomes memory T cells (see Figure 13.21).

Several cell-surface changes accompany the transition from naive to memory T cell. It may be that among memory T-cell populations are several subpopulations. Because of that, al-

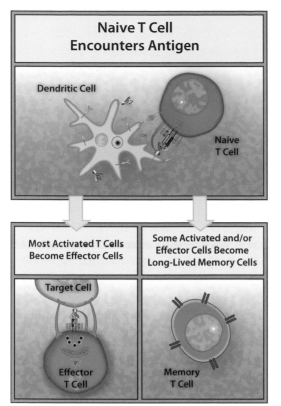

Naive T Cell Encounters Antigen

Dendritic Cell

Naive T Cell

Most Activated T Cells Become Effector Cells

Some Activated and/or Effector Cells Become Long-Lived Memory Cells

Target Cell

Effector T Cell

Memory T Cell

FIGURE 13.21. Encounter with specific MHC– antigen generates both effector T cells and memory T cells

though the changes described here seem to be characteristic of many memory T cells, they may not be characteristics of all of them.

The observed cell-surface changes include the loss of receptors for molecules present on HEVs and the acquisition of receptors for vascular endothelia in inflamed and infected areas of an animal's body. In addition, effector and memory T cells have reduced requirements for the second signal normally delivered through B7 to CD28. As a result, many memory T cells can respond more rapidly to a secondary infection, generate higher numbers of cells in shorter periods of time, and more quickly eliminate these secondary challenges.

Because of their characteristics, memory cells mediate almost all secondary and subsequent

immune responses. Memory B and T cells exist in much higher numbers in previously immunized or infected animals, memory B cells have higher affinities for antigen than naive B cells, and memory B and T cells respond faster than naive cells. For all of these (and probably a few other) reasons, naive T and B cells do not participate significantly after a primary response to their specific antigen.

CLINICAL CORRELATION FOLLOW-UP

Student Considerations

In 1981 and 1982, the wolf population on Isle Royale in Lake Superior fell from nearly fifty animals to fourteen. Parvovirus, carried in by humans, was the apparent cause. Canine parvovirus is highly contagious and often leads to severe diarrhea and fatal hypovolemic shock.

What aspects of these wolves' adaptive immune responses could have been relevant to survival? Why did fourteen animals survive? What factors may have contributed to the large die-off of wolves after exposure to canine parvovirus?

Possible Explanations

Because all of the wolves on Isle Royale were and are descendants of one wolf pack with few breeding pairs, it is likely that these wolves are highly inbred. As we discussed in chapter 8 regarding African cheetahs and Florida panthers, inbreeding may have dramatically reduced not only the MHC variety among these wolves (markedly limiting their antigen-presenting diversity) but also the amount of genetic variation available for the diversification of BCRs and TCRs. Any one or all of these might explain the large number of wolf deaths after exposure to parvovirus. However, death rates among domestic dogs are in the range of 70 percent, so it is difficult to evaluate the contribution of inbreeding to these wolf deaths.

As with most, if not all, viruses, parvoviruses are obligate intracellular parasites. To reproduce themselves, parvoviruses must enter the host cell. As discussed earlier, Tc cells deal with most intracellular parasites, especially viruses. Activation of T cells requires presentation of specific antigenic fragments inside of MHC class I molecules. To respond appropriately, a Tc cell must have a TCR reactive with that specific MHC class I–antigen combination.

For these reasons, MHC class I homogeneity could be a problem, as could relative TCR homogeneity. Because death rates in dogs are similar to those in the Isle Royale wolf population, though, it seems more probable that the difference between surviving and dead wolves was simple genetic variation. Survivors may have expressed MHC class I molecules that presented the critical parvovirus epitope, and the MHC molecules of the wolves that died could not. Alternatively, because of genetic differences, critical TCRs may have been present only among the survivors. Also, because antibodies likely play important roles in controlling the spread of viruses from cell to cell, critical

BCRs, isotype switch signals, or abnormalities in somatic hypermutation and selection might have prevented the development of specific antibodies to control the infection.

With viruses especially, all antiviral antibodies are not equal. Often, a single critical antigenic epitope is involved in virus attachment to host cells. When host animals produce antibodies to that critical epitope, they survive because their antibodies neutralize the virus's ability to infect host cells. Because of that, these antibodies are called "neutralizing" antibodies and are the most important target of vaccination.

The generation of a protective adaptive immune response is a complex process that depends, at many stages, on the genetic background of the infected animal. For this reason, the efficiency of these responses varies among individuals. Identifying the critical gene or genes is rarely possible, but understanding how adaptive immune responses develop and protect is a critical step in the process of understanding diseases and their therapies.

Fetal and Neonatal Immunity

Chapter 14

10.5876_9781607322184.c014

CLINICAL CORRELATION: FAILURE OF PASSIVE TRANSFER

Currently, veterinarians estimate that as many as 35 percent of dairy calves suffer from at least one serious and sometimes life-threatening bacterial infection during the neonatal period. Similar infections occur regularly, although less frequently, in beef calves, lambs, piglets, foals, and likely manatees (Figure 14.1), making these infections a major biological and economic issue for the livestock industry. In foals, the symptoms of these bacterial infections include infections of the navel, the joints, and the lungs and septicemia. Animals will also often have high fevers and be "off suck," and when the joints are involved, the animals suddenly become lame. Diarrhea is also common.

For all neonates, the routes of infection for bacterial invasion include ingestion, inhalation, umbilical infection, and in utero infection. The involved bacteria most commonly include *Escherichia coli* (most common), *Salmonella* spp., *Listeria monocytogenes*, *Pasturella* spp., *Streptococcus* spp., *Leptospira* spp., and *Actinobacillus* spp.

Untreated, many of these calves, foals, lambs, and piglets will die. In comparison, other animals from the same sire and dam will flourish and be infection free. What is the difference between the affected and unaffected animals?

LEARNING OBJECTIVES

After reading this chapter, you should be able to

- describe, in general terms, the fetal development of immune competence;
- describe species differences in maternal transfer of immunity and the underlying causes of these differences;
- describe the routes of maternal transfer of immunity;
- explain the rationale for neonatal vaccine protocols;
- understand how neonatal immunity is measured.

FETAL DEVELOPMENT OF THE IMMUNE SYSTEM

For many animals, immune system development is complete, or very nearly complete, at birth, but the prenatal times at which various aspects of immune systems mature vary considerably among species. However, some animals develop immune competence only after days or

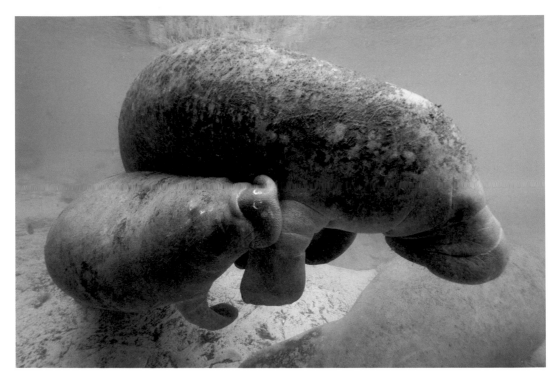

FIGURE 14.1. Nursing manatee calf (© Liquid Productions, LLC / Shutterstock)

Placentation in manatees, as with that in other sirenians, is endotheliochorial. As a result, transfer of antibodies across the placenta is limited, and the timely transfer of colostrum is essential for protection of the calf.

weeks of life. For example, opossums give birth to young after only fifteen days of gestation, and the newborn joeys have no functional immune tissues or organs. Only after seven days of life do these animals begin to make antibodies. The opossum is an example of surprisingly rapid immune development, but all of it occurs postpartum. As examples of fetal immune development, we focus on the calf and the chick. Other animals are generally similar, but time of appearances and completion dates can all vary considerably.

The gestation period in cattle is approximately 285 days, or about nine months. Figure 14.2 shows a general outline of immune development in calves. Sometime before birth, fetal calves acquire the ability to generate adaptive immune responses to antigens. This ability is apparent because some in utero infections by

agents such as bovine viral diarrhea virus do induce immune responses. Shortly before birth, as cortisol production rises, the cells of the adaptive immune system (including lymphocytes, macrophages, and neutrophils) decrease considerably.

Although immunocompetent, at birth calves are mostly protected by maternally transferred immunity and innate immune responses—rapid and effective reactions to environmental pathogens. Innate immunity in calves develops late during gestation, but just as with adults, it provides first-line, rapid responses to a variety of infectious agents, especially bacteria. Figure 14.3 shows a more detailed picture of immune development in cattle.

The thymus and bone marrow appear early, and lymphocytes and B cells are present after about sixty days of gestation. Granulocytes and

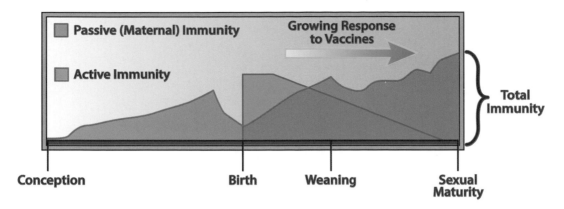

FIGURE 14.2. **The developing immune system of calves**

Passive immunity refers to immunity acquired from the mother. *Active immunity* refers to the calves' ability to develop adaptive humoral and cellular immune responses as well as memory cells. (Adapted from C. L. Christopher et al., 2008, *Veterinary Clinics of Northern America: Food Animal Practice*, 24: 87)

other cells of innate immunity do not appear until later. The mucosal lymphoid tissues are among the very last to appear and are not fully active until sometime after birth, which is also true of some of the other elements of innate immunity.

The process in chicks is quite different. Incubation time for domestic chicks is about twenty-one days. By five to seven days, stem cells have migrated to the thymus and the bursa. Lymphoid follicles appear in the bursa by about twelve days. IgM-positive B cells appear by about fourteen to sixteen days, and inoculated chick embryos can produce specific antibodies. *In ovo* vaccination for diseases such as Marek's disease is very effective by seventeen days. IgY-positive B cells appear at twenty-one days, but IgA-positive B cells appear in the gut only about a week after hatching. As with cattle, the innate immune functions of chicks are not fully active at birth. It is not until sometime after birth that calves and chickens attain immune competence levels approaching those of adult animals.

So in cattle and chickens, as in most other animals, neonates' immune systems are active but not yet fully protective. That leaves newly born animals at very high risk for infection between birth and full immune development. Because of this, animals have evolved means for transferring immune capacity from mother to offspring in utero, immediately after birth, or both.

MATERNAL TRANSFER OF IMMUNITY

The process of maternal transfer of immunity involves physical translocation of elements and products of the mother's immune system into the developing animal. This process varies considerably among species.

Prenatal Transfer of Immunity

In precocial chickens, maternal antibodies are transferred across the follicular epithelium into the yolk during oogenesis. As described earlier, chickens produce three classes of antibodies: IgY, IgM, and IgA. IgY (the equivalent of mammalian IgG) antibodies cross into the egg yolk at the highest concentrations. The egg white contains the greatest concentrations of IgA and IgM. Shortly before hatching, all maternal IgY and some IgM move into the embryonic circulation. There, they provide protection to the newborn (and immunologically immature) chick.

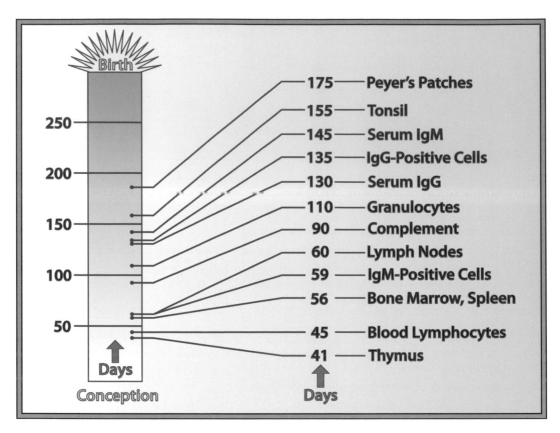

FIGURE 14.3. **Timeline for development of cells and organs of the immune system in neonatal calves**

Maternal antibodies persist in these chicks for fourteen to twenty-one days. During that time (by three to seven days), the newborns begin to produce their own antibodies. However, they do not achieve full immunological maturity until about the time maternal antibodies finally disappear from the chicks' circulation.

The timing varies considerably among bird species. For example, the half-life of maternal antibodies in precocial chickens is somewhere from three to ten days, whereas in altricial passerine birds, such as house sparrows, the reported half-life of maternal antibodies is closer to two days.

The optimum time for vaccinating embryonic chicks is when the stalk of the yolk sac begins its ascent into the abdomen and the head is nestled under the wing until external pipping (near hatching), which occurs at seventeen to

nineteen days. Studies have shown that immunization before day seventeen reduces viable hatching about 1 percent to 2 percent compared with vaccination on day eighteen. The site of vaccination is also important (see Figure 14.4). For embryonic turkey chicks, it appears that vaccine injection into the amniotic fluid is the most efficient route, but injection into the embryo itself is also very effective. Targeted *in ovo* vaccination might seem like a difficult and time-consuming approach to chicken protection, but in reality, machines routinely perform the task at rates exceeding 50,000 eggs per hour.

Placental mammals exhibit a range of anatomical relationships among the placenta, the mother, and the fetus. There are three types of mammalian placentas: endotheliochorial, epitheliochorial, and hemochorial (see Figure 14.5A–B). The character of the placenta

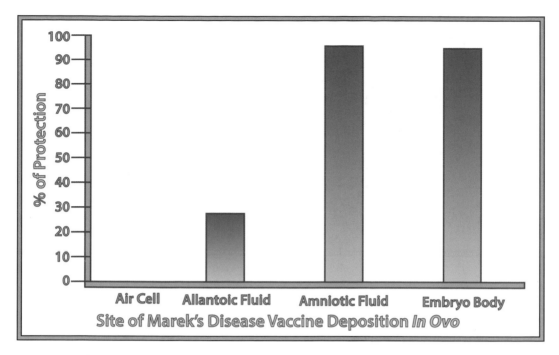

FIGURE 14.4. Effectiveness of vaccination of chick embryos at various sites

Marek's disease vaccine (a live, attenuated, viral vaccine) was injected into turkey embryos at the indicated sites on day seventeen or eighteen. At five days posthatch, the chicks were challenged with Marek's disease virus (based on data from P. Wakenell et al., 2002, *Avian Diseases*, 46: 274).

ultimately determines the routes of maternal transfer of immunity.

In primates and rodents—because the chorionic villi themselves have eroded through the maternal vascular endothelium—the fetal chorionic epithelium is in direct contact with maternal blood. As a result, IgG antibodies move freely from mother to fetus in these species. Therefore, in primates and rodents, much maternal transfer of immunity occurs before birth, but transfer of IgG and IgA continues after birth through the mother's milk.

Three layers of cells separate the maternal circulation in the fetuses of horses, cattle, pigs, and others. In these species, no cross-placental transfer of maternal immunity occurs. For this reason, all maternal transfer of immunity must occur during nursing.

In between these species are animals (such as cats and dogs) with epitheliochorial placentas.

Here, there is one less cell layer between the mother's circulation and the fetus's circulation than in animals with endotheliochorial placentas and one more cell layer than in animals with hemochorial placentas. In dogs and cats, some placental transfer of immunity occurs, but not as much as in primates. As with other species, in dogs and cats maternal transfer continues after birth through milk.

Postnatal Transfer of Immunity

Postnatal transfer of immunity occurs during nursing, first with colostrum and later with milk. Colostrum is the first milk that accumulates in the udder, and it is rich in proteins, fats, and carbohydrates. A few weeks before birth—as colostrum forms—antibodies begin moving from the blood into the cow's udder. At the same time, mammary-associated lymphoid tissues

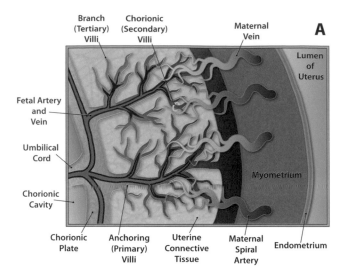

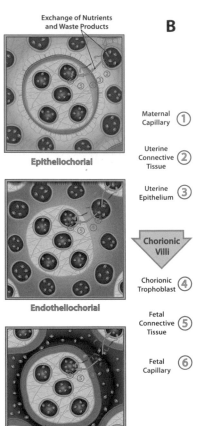

Maternal Capillary ①
Uterine Connective Tissue ②
Uterine Epithelium ③

Chorionic Villi

Chorionic Trophoblast ④
Fetal Connective Tissue ⑤
Fetal Capillary ⑥

Epitheliochorial

Endotheliochorial

Hemochorial

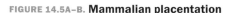

FIGURE 14.5A–B. Mammalian placentation

Scientists classify mammalian placentas on the basis of the number of maternal layers retained in the placenta. The more layers there are, the more restricted the movement of blood elements between mother and fetus. Panel A shows the general relationship between maternal and fetal circulation in the chorionic villi. Panel B shows cross-sections of the chorionic villi and the different layers between maternal and fetal blood.

also begin to add antibodies to the colostrum. Beyond Igs, bovine colostrum also contains neutrophils and macrophages that secrete several defensive proteins and cytokines, including antimicrobial proteins and peptides such as lactoferrin (a major antibacterial agent), complement, and lactoperoxidase (also an antibacterial agent), as well as defensins and cathelicidins, both of which are bactericidal. Mammary epithelial cells also secrete various immune-related effector compounds.

The agents of adaptive immunity include both antibodies and T cells. In ruminants, the primary antibody in colostrum is IgG1. In nonruminant animals, IgA often predominates in both colostrum and milk (see Figure 14.7). In addition to IgG, ruminant colostrum contains monomeric IgM, IgE, and dimeric IgA, although the amounts of these antibodies vary between species. The relative abundance of Igs drops dramatically in the milk of both ruminants and nonruminants, but IgG still predominates in ruminant milk, and IgA is the major Ig in nonruminant milk.

The antibodies that accumulate in colostrum reflect the cow's past and recent exposures to specific environmental agents (local bacteria, viruses, etc.), which are the same agents the cow's calf will face immediately after birth. These maternal antibodies offer the calf the same protection they offered the mother—opsonization, activation of complement, toxin neutralization, virus neutralization, and so forth. Furthermore, by vaccinating cows, veterinarians can manipu-

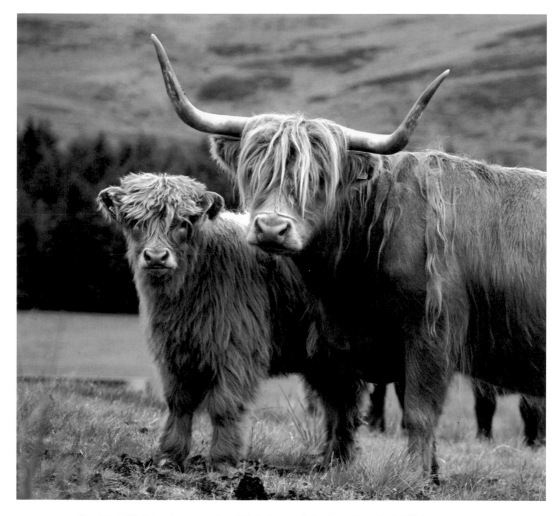

FIGURE 14.6. Scottish Highland cow and calf (photograph by Jonathan Sutcliffe)

In cattle, maternal immunity transfers solely via colostrum and milk.

late colostral antibodies. One example of this sort of manipulation involves vaccination of pregnant cows against rotoviruses and colostral transfer to calves of antirotovirus antibodies.

Newborn calves may ingest from two to more than six liters of colostrum. Two things help to prevent digestion of the ingested antibodies and other proteins. First, in the first hours after birth, the gastrointestinal tract of newborn calves has very low protease levels. Second, colostrum contains high levels of trypsin inhibitors. Both of these factors prevent immediate destruction of the transferred proteins.

Another mechanism ensures rapid transport of these Igs into the calf's blood and other body fluids. On the epithelial cells lining the surface of the gut are specialized Fc receptors that bind the ingested Igs. Intestinal epithelial cells endocytose the bound antibodies and move them from the gut and eventually to the blood and lymph. In cattle, essentially all colostral antibodies move quickly from the gut to the blood, but in other animals (horses and pigs, for example), most colostral IgA remains in the gut, providing protection against enteric pathogens.

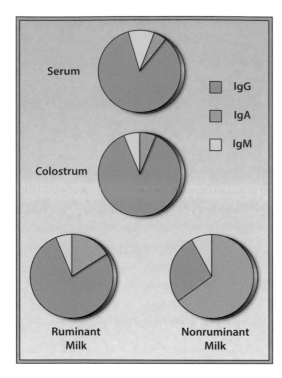

FIGURE 14.7. Antibodies in serum, colostrum, and milk

The predominant antibody in the serum and colostrum of most livestock is IgG (ranging from 60 to 90 percent). However, the transfer of IgA from serum to milk differs dramatically between ruminant and nonruminant animals. (Adapted from I. R. Tizard, 2009, *Veterinary Immunology*, 229)

Because in all placental animals the specialized Fc receptors are present for only a short period, successful maternal transfer of immunity must occur inside of a fairly narrow window. During the time the Fc receptors appear on the gut epithelium, the gut is permeable, and the duration of permeability varies some between species. In general, gut permeability is greatest immediately after birth, begins to decline by six hours, and ends by twenty-four hours. Colostrum itself appears to accelerate gut closure, because animals that fail to nurse immediately retain gut permeability for thirty-three hours or longer (as much as ninety-six hours in pigs).

After ingestion of colostrum, serum antibody levels peak between twelve and twenty-four hours. Because of normal metabolic breakdown, absorbed maternal antibodies have a fixed half-life. Different isotypes disappear at different rates, and the time at which any of the antibodies may fall below protective levels depends on the initial concentrations in the mother's colostrum and in the calf's serum (see Figure 14.8).

Once gut permeability reaches zero, further maternal transfer must occur through the mother's milk, which has proportionally more IgA than does colostrum. During this period, most of the antibodies in milk remain in the nursing animal's gut, providing longer protection against enteric pathogens.

In addition to antibodies, bovine colostrum contains about 1 million lymphocytes per milliliter, and nearly half of these are T cells. These cells may live as long as thirty-six hours in the calf's gut. Furthermore, in as little as two hours, some of these T cells cross the intestinal epithelium and reach the circulation. A variety of studies have shown that these T cells positively affect the immune status of the calf. Milk, however, contains very few or no lymphocytes. Thus, the transfer of cellular immunity continues only as long as the calf ingests colostrum.

Passive transfer failures may occur because the mother produced too little or antibody-depleted colostrum, because the newborn failed to ingest sufficient amounts of colostrum before gut closure, or because gut permeability was never high enough to allow for absorption of adequate amounts of antibody (which occurs in about 25 percent of newborn foals). Regardless of the cause, passive transfer failure is a life-threatening event and places the newborn animal at great risk.

NEONATAL ACQUISITION OF MEMORY AND IMMUNE CAPACITY

The earliest evidence of neonatal immunity is the appearance of pentameric IgM. Because of

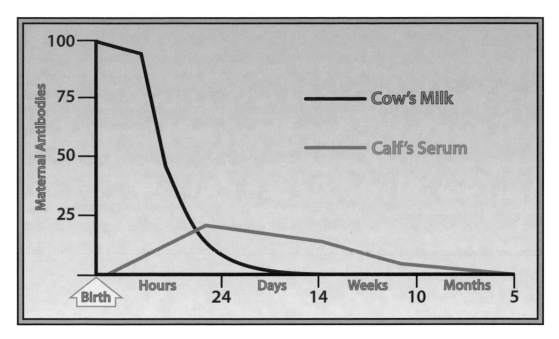

FIGURE 14.8. **Levels of maternal antibodies in the sera of cow and calf (Adapted from I. R. Tizard, 2009, *Veterinary Immunology*, 231)**

its considerable size, pentameric IgM can neither pass through the placenta nor find its way into colostrum or milk. So the appearance of this antibody in the neonate is definitive evidence of active calf immune responses.

As mentioned earlier, the production of IgM often begins before birth, declines briefly because of cortisol production, then rises as the newborn animal generates its first postnatal immune responses. Figure 14.9 shows an approximate time course for neonatal production of antibodies. Cattle usually achieve adult serum Ig levels of all isotypes before age six months. Production of the full range of isotypes requires fully functional B cells and Th cells and indicates the production of memory cells. Tc-cell activity follows a similar time course. GALT immunity and strong gastrointestinal immune responses are often demonstrable within a few days of birth and probably reach adult levels a little sooner than systemic immunity.

Again, things follow a similar order in chickens, but the timetables are very different. A group of protozoan parasites—*Eimeria*—causes coccidiosis in chickens. Coccidiosis is a disease of considerable economic importance, especially in broiler chickens. In one study, chicks were able to mount fully protective immune responses against three strains of *Eimeria* (*E. tenella, E. maxima,* and *E. acervulina*) by twenty-five, twenty-four, and twenty-six days, respectively. Parasite inoculations (in this case, *E. tenella*) began on the seventh day after hatching (postmaternal immunity). By day seven, dramatically fewer oocysts were detectable, and by day twenty-five, oocyst production ceased. As a result, functional immunity is present early, probably even before hatching, and chicks achieve a fully protective immune response within sixteen to twenty-five days.

VACCINATION OF NEONATES

Even though some neonates may be capable of many immune responses, the same maternal antibodies that protect neonates from lethal

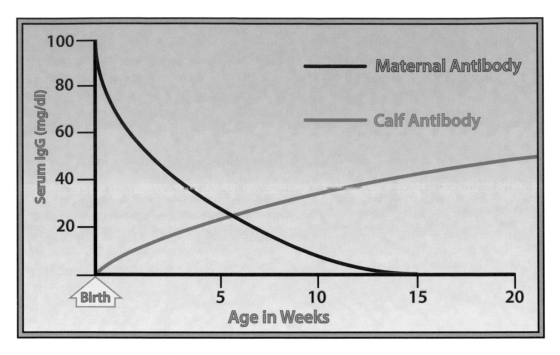

FIGURE 14.9. Maternal and calf antibody levels in newborn calves

For the first twelve weeks or so of calves' lives, they are protected by maternal antibodies transferred through colostrum. During that time, the calves' immune systems are beginning to produce their own antibodies. By week fifteen, calves' antibodies are all calf-derived and reach adult levels by about twenty weeks.

infections pose a formidable obstacle for vaccination. In at least two ways, maternal antibodies can interfere with vaccination (see Figure 14.10). Maternal antibodies may bind to injected pathogens or antigens and clear the inoculum before activation of enough cells to stimulate a new immune response. Because erythrocytes have Fc receptors, these cells bind small antigen–antibody complexes and very quickly clear such complexes from the blood, preventing effective antigen processing and presentation. Also, maternal antibodies may block essential BCR epitopes and prevent the formation of neutralizing antibodies.

Because of this, timing of vaccination and boosters in neonates has to be different from protocols for adult animals. As mentioned earlier, maternal antibodies absorbed from the gut reach peak levels within the first 24 hours. After

that, maternal antibodies begin to decline. The rate at which individual isotypes decline varies within and between species, and the rate of catabolism of antibodies against different antigens also varies. Therefore, determining an appropriate vaccination protocol for a given antigen must be an empirical process. For example, the half-life of maternally transferred antidistemper antibodies in dogs is about eight days and reaches negligible levels after about ten to twelve weeks. The half-life of maternally transferred rinderpest antibodies in cattle is about thirty-six days, and the antibody reaches negligible levels only after about eleven months.

As a result, neonatal vaccination is a trade-off between the ideal levels of maternal antibodies and the earliest possible protection for the young animal. For example, in puppies the ideal level of maternal antibodies (near zero) against

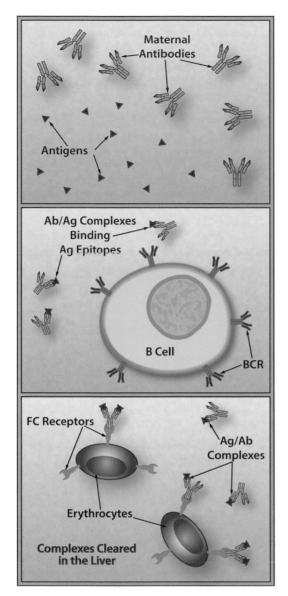

FIGURE 14.10. Maternal antibodies inhibit vaccination

Maternal antibodies may bind to injected antigens or pathogens and accelerate their clearance, or maternal antibodies may bind to critical antigen epitopes and prevent activation of B cells and antibody production. Also, RBCs bind antigen–antibody complexes and quickly remove those complexes from the blood. Ab = antibody; Ag = antigen.

canine distemper virus occurs between ten and twelve weeks. Considering only that data, it might make the most sense to wait until sometime after twelve weeks to vaccinate for canine distemper. However, the rate of maternal antibody decline varies a lot between puppies, and the consequence of distemper infection in unvaccinated animals can be catastrophic. In response (for mostly practical reasons, such as economics and convenience), veterinarians do not simply vaccinate puppies every week or so until immune protection is certain. As a compromise, canine distemper vaccination begins at six weeks and is repeated at nine, twelve, and fifteen weeks, usually as part of a five-way vaccine that also includes vaccines for adenovirus cough and hepatitis, canine distemper, parainfluenza, and parvovirus. Some combination vaccines may also include leptospirosis (seven-way vaccines), coronavirus, or both.

In calves, *Clostridium* infections cause a variety of very serious diseases, including blackleg, malignant edema, sord, black disease, red water, and three kinds of enterotoxemia. Early protection against *Clostridium* is essential. As in dogs, using a seven- or eight-way vaccine, calves may be vaccinated as early as one month, again four weeks later, and once more before weaning. The intent is the same as the vaccination protocol described earlier—immunize early and often to protect the maximum number of animals at the earliest possible date.

CLINICAL CORRELATION FOLLOW-UP

Student Considerations

As mentioned at the outset of this chapter, a significant percentage of dairy calves are unusually susceptible to early bacterial infections, especially *E. coli*. Grossly, these animals appear no different from healthy calves; however, blood work reveals that in comparison with healthy calves, the affected calves have near-normal levels of IgM but much lower levels of IgG. Similar

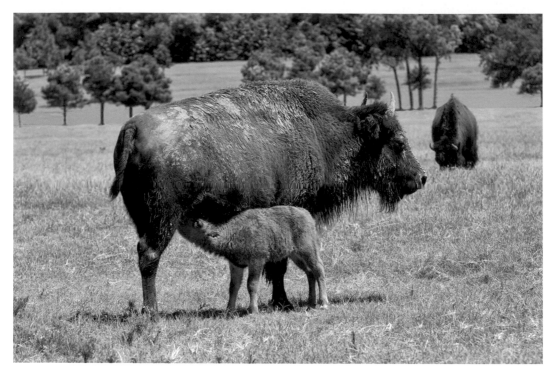

FIGURE 14.11 **Nursing bison calf (© Leena Robinson / Shutterstock)**

Bison, like other bovids, basically have an epitheliochorial placenta, but cells from the trophoblast invade the uterine epithelium, where they form binucleate giant cells. Thus, the ruminant placentation is most commonly called synepitheliochorial.

lesions likely occur in other ruminants (Figure 14.11)

Possible Explanations

The absence of IgG in the calves' blood could be due to several things, including immunodeficiency diseases, but the near-normal levels of IgM suggest something else—failure of passive transfer. Because the newborn calves have no memory cells and all initial immune responses will be primary immune responses, the presence of IgM is consistent with a normally functioning immune system. Calf-derived IgG will only reach normal levels weeks to months later as the animals' immune systems fully mature. Early calf IgG is all derived from the mother. Therefore, the finding of normal levels of IgM but low to no IgG suggests passive transfer failure.

As mentioned earlier in this chapter, passive-transfer failures may occur because the mother failed to produce sufficient colostrum, failed to incorporate sufficient Igs into her colostrum, or lost colostrum before the calf could nurse. The calf, in turn, may not have nursed long enough or failed to adequately absorb the Igs from the ingested colostrum.

Regardless of the reason, failure of passive transfer of immunity has placed these calves at great risk for life-threatening infections. Because of this risk, early identification of passive-transfer failure and immediate supplementation with stored colostrum are essential.

Gerald N. Callahan

Vaccination

Chapter 15

10.5876_9781607322184.c015

CLINICAL CORRELATION: ANIMAL VACCINES

Because of their lack of memory cells, puppies (Figure 15.1)—as with the young of most species—are especially susceptible to infectious diseases. Even in the developed world, infectious diseases are among the leading causes of death among puppies and kittens as well as livestock and among the leading causes of morbidity and mortality in feral animal populations. For this reason, people and their domestic animals receive a raft of immunizations to protect them from infectious diseases. Figure 15.2 shows the recommended schedule for dogs.

As we discussed in chapter 14, as soon as maternally transferred immunity begins to wane, young animals become susceptible to infection.

Remember, neonatal animals' immune systems contain mostly naive T and B cells. Because of that, in young animals all immune responses are primary responses, and those take time— sometimes too much time. Vaccination helps to shorten the time it normally takes to develop rapidly responding memory cells.

LEARNING OBJECTIVES

After reading this chapter, you should be able to

- describe the properties of effective vaccines and explain the reasons for each of them;
- describe the characteristics of the various forms of vaccines and explain the advantages and disadvantages of each;
- explain the need for as well as the chemistry and immunology of the most commonly used adjuvants;
- discuss the possible routes of vaccine administration and the advantages and disadvantages of each;
- discuss the reasoning behind vaccination schedules;
- explain the immunology behind specific issues for vaccines against specific pathogens.

VACCINES

Vaccine Characteristics

In 1796, Edward Jenner inoculated James Phipps with cowpox, and the modern era of vaccination was begun. Sarah Nelmes, a milk-

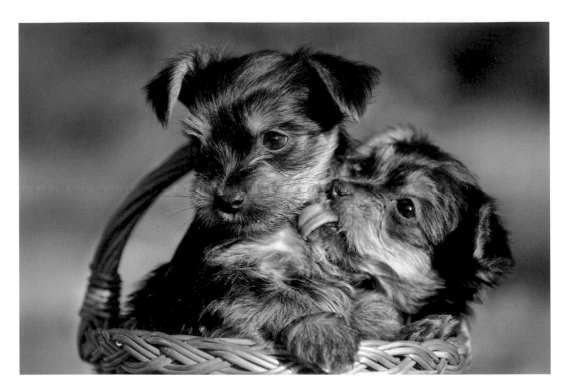

FIGURE 15.1. Puppies (© AnetaPics / Shutterstock)

maid, had contracted cowpox (variola virus) from Blossom, a dairy cow. Jenner had noticed that smallpox—then ravaging much of Europe—seemed rare among milkmaids. Jenner reasoned that infection with cowpox somehow prevented later infection with smallpox. To test his theory, he collected pus from the cowpox blisters on Nelmes. He then injected this pus repeatedly into James Phipps (the son of Jenner's gardener). Finally, Jenner injected young James with virulent smallpox from an infected person. The boy survived, and vaccination (from *vaccus,* Latin for cow) became widespread.

Although it would not be understood for more than a century, Jenner had taken advantage of the antigenic similarity between two viruses, cowpox or variola virus, only mildly pathogenic in humans, and smallpox virus, which causes a disfiguring and often fatal disease in humans. Because the two viruses have some antigenic epitopes in common, an immune response against cowpox virus generates

antibodies and T cells that react with similar antigens of smallpox virus. These anticowpox antibodies provide protection against the more virulent pathogen. However, an attempted immunization with even a few of the intact smallpox viruses would often be fatal.

This is true of many pathogens. As with smallpox virus in humans or parvovirus in dogs, inoculation of even a few virus particles is often enough to induce disease. The first requirement for a vaccine is safety in the majority of the target animals, which requires identification or creation of a less pathogenic or nonpathogenic form of the disease agent. Underlying this process is an attempt to copy what Jenner found fortuitously—a less dangerous microbe that shares antigenic epitopes with the virulent pathogen.

The other obvious issue for vaccine design is identifying the type of immunity most likely to be protective. In general, humoral immune responses are most effective against extracellular pathogens, and humoral plus cellular immune responses are most effective against intracellular pathogens. For example, many antiviral vaccines, such as canine parvovirus vaccines, by design induce both cellular immunity and powerful antibody responses.

The cellular immune response that parvovirus vaccines induce is essential to eliminate infected host cells. But cellular immunity alone is ineffective against free viruses (viruses as they enter the host are extracellular, as they are when they move between host cells). For this reason, the antibodies induced in response to parvovirus vaccines—because they help limit the number of cells infected after virus exposure and limit the spread of virus from cell to cell—are also essential for protection. Finally, because large numbers of animals will receive the vaccine, it must be immunogenic and nontoxic for most, if not all, recipients (see Table 15.1).

The route and frequency of administration are also important. Initially, we consider the composition of the vaccine. Generally, successful vaccines include

- live-attenuated pathogens;
- heat-killed or otherwise inactivated forms of the agent;
- subunit or component vaccines containing only pieces of the pathogen;
- toxoid (inactivated bacterial toxins) vaccines;
- conjugate vaccines using an immunostimulant to induce a response to a harmless piece of a pathogen;
- recombinant vaccines using a harmless virus expressing a gene product from the pathogen;
- naked DNA vaccines.

Live-Attenuated Vaccines

One approach to vaccine development is to produce a less virulent strain of a pathogenic agent. This technique has been used most often

TABLE 15.1. Essentials for useful vaccines

Safe	Does not cause illness or death in even a small percentage of recipients; minimal side effects
Protective	Prevents or reduces illness caused by pathogen
Provides long-lasting effects	Confers sustained resistance on vaccinated animals
Induces formation of protective antibodies	Stimulates production of antibodies reactive with appropriate antigenic epitopes
Induces formation of protective T cells	Stimulates production of cellular immunity; particularly important for intracellular pathogens
Other issues	Low cost, stable, easily administered

to produce antiviral vaccines, but live-attenuated vaccines are also used against bacterial agents, such as canine bordetella.

Live-virus vaccines are generally more effective and longer lasting than vaccines containing killed viruses, probably as a result of several factors. Live viruses continue to replicate inside of their hosts, which accomplishes two things: first, viral replication increases the time the immune system is exposed to antigen and the total antigen load. Also, because live viruses will replicate in the cytoplasm of infected cells, peptides from viruses are more efficiently presented inside of MHC class I molecules. Both of these factors enhance immunity, including production of $CD8^+$ T cells that are most effective in eliminating virus-infected cells and virus-neutralizing antibodies.

Again, the initial problem is the virulence of the unattenuated virus—the amount of virus necessary to induce an immune response is also often enough to induce disease and sometimes death. An attenuated virus retains many of the physical characteristics (especially antigenic epitopes) of the original virus but is less virulent. To achieve attenuation, vaccine makers usually grow viruses in cultured cells from another species. For example, canine parvoviruses

AVMA Vaccination Recommendations for Dogs			
Component	**Class**	**Efficacy**	**Length of Immunity**
Canine Distemper	Core	High	1 Year Modified Live Virus (MLV)
Parvovirus	Core	High	1 Year
Hepatitis	Core	High	1 Year
Rabies	Core	High	Dependent upon Type of Vaccine
Respiratory Disease from Canine Adenovirus-2 (CAV-2)	Noncore	Not Adequately Studied	Short
Parainfluenza	Noncore	Intranasal (MLV)— Moderate Injectable (MLV)— Low	Moderate
Bordetella	Noncore	Intranasal (MLV)— Moderate Injectable (MLV)— Low	Short
Leptospirosis	Noncore	Variable	Short
Coronavirus	Noncore	Low	Short
Lyme	Noncore	Variable— Appears to Be Limited to Previously Exposed Dogs	Revaccinate Annually

Dog Vaccination Schedule	
Age	**Vaccination**
5 Weeks	**Parvovirus:** For Puppies at High Risk of Exposure to Parvo
6 and 9 Weeks	**Combination Vaccine** without Leptospirosis **Coronavirus:** Where Coronavirus Is a Concern
12 Weeks or Older	Rabies
12 and 15 Weeks	**Combination Vaccine** **Leptospirosis:** Include Leptospirosis in the Combination Vaccine Where Leptospirosis Is a Concern
Adult (Boosters)	**Combination Vaccine** **Leptospirosis:** Include Leptospirosis in the Combination Vaccine Where Leptospirosis Is a Concern **Coronavirus:** Where Coronavirus Is a Concern **Borrelia:** Where Borrelia Is a Concern **Rabies:** Given by Your Local Veterinarian (Time Interval between Vaccinations May Vary According to Local Law)

FIGURE 15.2. **Canine vaccination schedule**

Core vaccines for dogs are those that should be given to every dog. Noncore vaccines are recommended only for certain dogs. Whether to vaccinate with noncore vaccines depends on a number of things, including the dog's age, breed, and health status; potential exposure to an animal with the disease; the type of vaccine; and how common the disease is in the area in which the dog lives or visits. *Source*: American Veterinary Medical Association.

have been attenuated by passage in insect cells. By selecting for the viruses that grow best in these insect cells, the investigators were able to isolate a strain of parvovirus that had a lower capacity for infection of canine cells (see Figure 15.3). When the virus was repeatedly cultured on insect cells, mutations began to accumulate, and these mutations allowed the virus to more efficiently infect insect cells. These same mutations generally reduced the virus's ability to infect canine cells. In essence, these virions experience accelerated evolution in an unnatural

host, and that evolution reduces the virus's ability to effect disease in its natural host.

When we vaccinate dogs with these live-attenuated virus vaccines, the attenuated infection induces sufficient levels of danger signals (particularly DAMPs) to activate APCs. This combination induces a protective immune response, but the attenuated viruses infect far fewer dog cells and—because of that—induce milder or no symptoms. Because the attenuated virus retains essential antigenic epitopes, the immune response to the attenuated parvovirus

FIGURE 15.3. **Production of a live-attenuated virus vaccine**

To produce a live-attenuated virus, vaccine manufacturers grow cultured dog cells along with virus from an infected dog to produce large numbers of the virus. They then transfer this virus to insect cells. Over time, mutations accumulate in the viral genome. These mutations make the virus more efficient at infecting insect cells and less efficient at infecting dog cells. Vaccinating dogs with these viruses may induce immunity without widespread infection and disease. Because the attenuated virus retains essential antigenic epitopes, the immune response to the attenuated parvovirus induces cross-protection against live, virulent parvovirus.

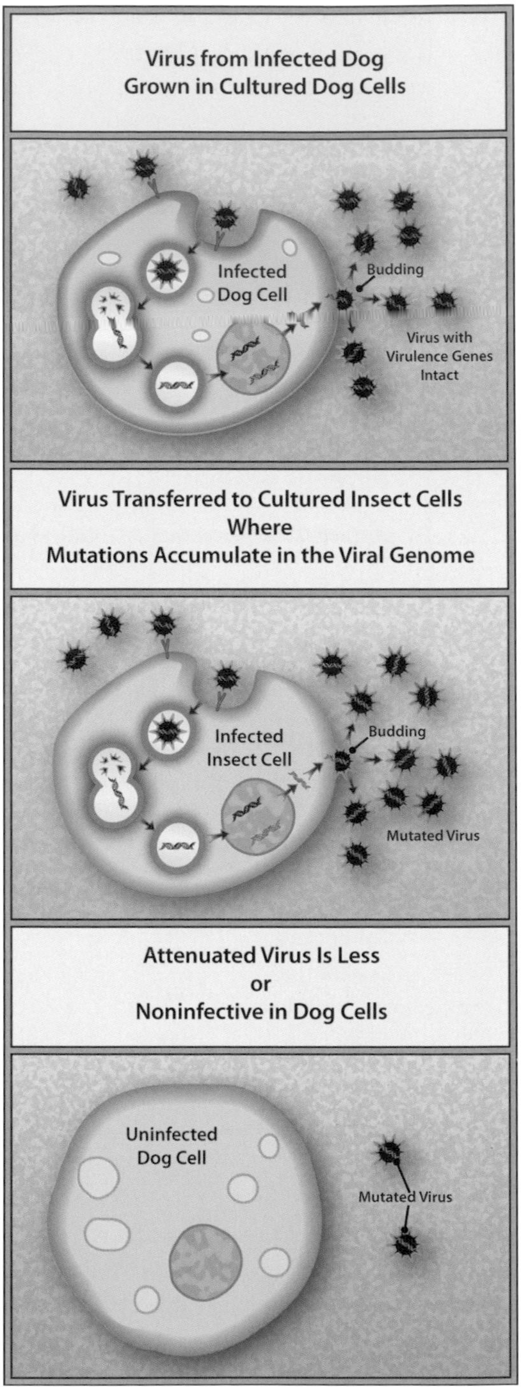

Virus from Infected Dog Grown in Cultured Dog Cells

Virus Transferred to Cultured Insect Cells Where Mutations Accumulate in the Viral Genome

Attenuated Virus Is Less or Noninfective in Dog Cells

induces cross-protection against live, virulent parvovirus.

Advances in molecular genetics now allow for precisely directed gene modification—an ideal approach to the generation of specifically engineered, attenuated viruses. Viruses produce disease by affecting essential functions of specific host cells. Scientists sometimes call the genes that allow viruses to do this "virulence" genes. Equipped with molecular techniques and some knowledge of the pathogenicity factors of a given virus or bacterium, site-directed mutagenesis within the virulence genes or complete removal of the virulence genes from a viral genome can generate attenuated strains of these agents. These viruses may remain highly infective for host cells and induce very effective host immunity but have little potential for pathogenicity. Because attenuated virus retains the majority of the components present in the native virus, the vaccine-induced immunity is also protective against the native virus. Because of rapid progress in the realm of genetic manipulation of transmissible agents, vaccine manufacturers either now use or will soon use these techniques to generate the majority of live-attenuated vaccines. Examples of live-attenuated vaccines for dogs include the trivalent vaccine for herpes virus, calcivirus, and parvovirus; distemper vaccines; and bordetella vaccines.

Live-attenuated vaccines, in spite of their huge successes, have risks. The catch is that completely avirulent strains do not make good vaccines, so the level of attenuation has to be titrated to achieve enough disease to elicit a strong immune response, but not enough for it to be clinically apparent. However, if an animal's immune system is somehow compromised (e.g., an immunodeficient animal), the virus, even in its attenuated form, can cause severe, sometimes fatal disease. Also, the low potential for virulence of a live-attenuated virus depends on the mutations accumulated during the attenuation process. As these viruses divide inside of the vaccinated animal, in rare cases additional mutations can alter the infectivity of the virus in host cells. Because of this, live-attenuated vaccines may still cause severe and sometimes fatal disease in immunized animals. However, because they are among the best at meeting all of the criteria listed in Table 15.1, live-attenuated virus vaccines are among the most common and most effective vaccines in all species.

Killed Vaccines

Obviously, inactivated viruses, dead bacteria, or other killed pathogens cannot cause disease or death (except through allergic responses). Because of this, one of the earliest methods for vaccine preparation involved using chemical or physical (particularly heat) means to kill bacteria or inactivate viruses. Pasteur's rabies vaccine is one example.

In addition to heat, killing or inactivating microorganisms for vaccine preparation has involved radiation, chemicals, and antibiotics. The target is, of course, dead but immunogenic microorganisms. That's the key. Heating, radiation, and these other procedures are most effective at killing microorganisms, but not without immunogenic consequences. All of these procedures result in dramatic alterations in the microorganisms' proteins through denaturation. For T cells, denaturation generally has few if

any consequences. After all, T cells can only "see" protein antigens after these molecules have been chopped into pieces and presented inside of MHC molecules. Not so for B cells. B cells' BCRs bind intact antigens, and this binding often depends absolutely on the structure of the antigenic proteins. When an animal receives a killed vaccine, most of the activated B cells bind the denatured form of the protein, and ultimately these B cells will produce antibodies that react only with denatured proteins. Such antibodies are likely to be of little use when the animal later encounters the native pathogen.

Furthermore, as mentioned earlier in this chapter, killed pathogens do not replicate inside of host cells. Although some crossover between antigen presentation pathways occurs, MHC class I presentation of the antigens from these killed pathogens is not as efficient as with live pathogens. Last, killed microorganisms do not persist for as long nor do they multiply inside the vaccinated animal.

For these reasons, killed vaccines are generally not as effective as live-attenuated vaccines. Regardless, many effective killed vaccines exist, including some canine, feline, and equine rabies vaccines.

One major plus for killed vaccines is that the immune status of the animal is less critical. Even among immune-compromised animals, there is essentially no possibility of causing microorganism-induced disease. But, as with live vaccines, because killed vaccines contain many potential allergens, there is the danger of allergic responses and anaphylaxis.

Component, Toxoid, Conjugate, Recombinant, and Naked DNA Vaccines

Obviously, immune responses against all components of a microorganism are not necessary for protection. For example, swine and avian influenza A viruses use only two molecules to infect host cells—hemagglutinin and neuraminidase. Vaccination with influenza A virus will produce antibodies against many components of the virus, but only when an animal's immune system produces antibodies against hemagglutinin and neuraminidase will the animal be protected against subsequent infection. Vaccination with intact live virus is always potentially dangerous. So why not simply vaccinate with hemagglutinin and neuraminidase molecules, that is, create a vaccine that contains only components of the virus—a component vaccine? Then there would be no risk of inducing influenza with the vaccine.

It turns out that immune systems do not handle isolated proteins very well. Immune responses that occur after vaccination with individual proteins are weak, include only poor cellular immunity, and are often ineffective against intact microorganisms. So until recently, very few effective component vaccines existed. However, one very effective approach uses components of pathogens: toxoid vaccines. Many Gram-negative and Gram-positive bacteria (such as *Clostridium tetani*) produce exotoxins that damage host animals. Toxoid vaccines contain inactivated bacterial toxins. For example, tetanus toxoid vaccine contains formaldehyde-denatured tetanus toxin. In this case, formaldehyde denaturation inactivates the toxin but leaves behind enough antigenic epitopes to induce an immune response, especially antibodies reactive with the native toxin. Vaccinated animals respond very quickly to subsequent exposure to tetanus and rapidly neutralize the otherwise fatal neurotoxin.

Because of new understanding about how immune systems work, it is now also possible to make effective conjugate vaccines using microorganism components linked (conjugated) to other T-cell–activating molecules. Vaccines against encapsulated bacterial pathogens are examples of this technology.

Several pathogenic bacteria contain polysaccharide capsules surrounding their cell walls. These capsules interfere with phagocytosis. The most effective immunity against encapsulated bacteria involves opsonizing antibodies that aid macrophages in phagocytosis and destruction of the encapsulated bacteria. However, under normal circumstances in adult mammals, the polysaccharides of bacterial capsules, even though they bind to some B-2 or regular B cells, directly activate only B-1 B cells. Th cells do not recognize and respond to polysaccharide antigens; thus, there are no antigen-specific T cells to help polysaccharide-specific B-2 B cells.

Sometimes, IgM antibodies derived from B-1 B cells are protective, but activation of B-1 B cells does not result in memory. Moreover, young animals have relatively fewer B-1 B cells and are at much greater risk for disease. The major aim of vaccination is immunological memory—a faster and more specific secondary response. So, under normal circumstances, vaccination for protective immunity is impossible, but conjugate vaccines circumvent this major block (see Figure 15.4).

As mentioned earlier, even though B-2 B cells bind some polysaccharide antigens, because there are no specific Th cells, B-2 B cells do not respond further. APCs effectively process and present only proteins, which means that although many polysaccharide antigens possess epitopes reactive with BCRs (B-cell epitopes), these antigens lack epitopes reactive with T cells (T-cell epitopes). To change the immunogenicity of bacterial-capsular polysaccharides, vaccinologists attached an immunogenic protein, tetanus toxoid, to provide a T-cell epitope—a protein portion that APCs can process and present to Th cells. When vaccinologists injected the conjugate into animals, it bound to BCRs through its polysaccharide portion, was internalized, and was processed. Then the B cell presented tetanus toxoid-derived peptides to Th cells. The Th cells produced the requisite cytokines, and the B cells divided and eventually differentiated into both B memory cells and plasma cells expressing antibodies specific for the bacterial polysaccharide. The resultant antibodies effectively opsonized the encapsulated bacteria, preventing disease. At the same time,

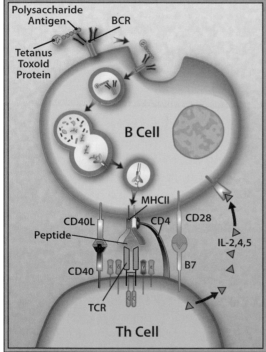

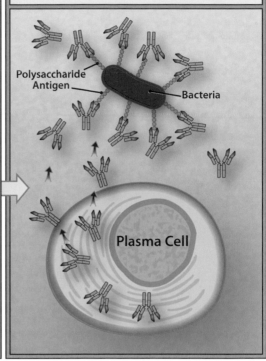

FIGURE 15.4. A conjugate vaccine against capsular polysaccharide

Under normal circumstances, bacterial polysaccharides fail to activate B-2 B cells, primarily because these polysaccharides do not contain T-cell–activating epitopes. Conjugation of an immunogenic protein (tetanus toxoid) to the polysaccharide provides the needed T-cell epitope. This conjugate activates toxoid-specific Th cells and polysaccharide-specific B cells. The end results are production of protective antipolysaccharide antibodies and memory T and B cells.

memory cells offered vaccinated animals protection in future encounters with the bacteria.

Similarly, scientists have identified many other T-cell epitopes—portions of proteins that bind to MHC molecules and are recognized by TCRs. As described earlier, when coupled with these molecules, antigens or pieces of antigens that bind to BCRs but normally fail to stimulate antibody production can effectively immunize animals and elicit memory cells.

Another approach to vaccine preparation has been to insert genes from pathogens into relatively innocuous viruses and use this recombinant vector for vaccination. Called recombinant vaccines, these constructs have had great success in treating important veterinary diseases. Most notable among these is rabies in wild animals. In 1984, workers at the Wistar Institute in Philadelphia isolated the gene that encoded the essential coat glycoprotein of the

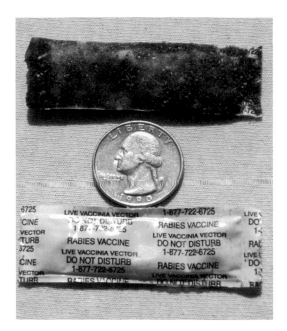

FIGURE 15.5. Oral rabies vaccine

Packets such as this one contain live recombinant rabies vaccines. Dropped from aircraft, the packets were very effective in controlling rabies in wild animal populations.

rabies virus. They then inserted this gene into the genome of vaccinia virus. Vaccinia virus is closely related to cowpox virus (remember Sarah Nelmes) and was first widely used as a vaccine for smallpox. By itself, vaccinia has very low potential for virulence.

Vaccinia virus does, however, infect animals and induce a strong immune response. By inserting the rabies glycoprotein gene into vaccinia, the scientists created a relatively innocuous virus that expressed an essential rabies glycoprotein. Once the vaccinia virus infected host cells, it produced not only vaccinia components, but the rabies glycoprotein as well.

When APCs phagocytosed these infected cells, the rabies glycoprotein entered the MHC class II pathway and, through cross-presentation, the MHC class I pathway, inducing strong antibody and T-cell responses. Even when administered orally, that recombinant vaccine

proved very effective in stimulating immunity against rabies virus.

Traditionally, because of the large wild animal reservoir, control of rabies in domestic animals had never been very effective. The availability of a potent oral vaccine offered a new avenue to rabies control (see Figure 15.5). Dropped from aircraft, these vaccines dramatically lowered the incidence of fulminant rabies in wild foxes in Europe and raccoons, coyotes, and foxes in the United States, and resulted in a much lower incidence of rabies in general.

Another vaccine approach uses structures called immune-stimulatory complexes (or IS-COMs). By themselves, many peptides are poor immunogens. At least one reason for this is that these peptides do not often enough get inside of APCs and into both MHC class I and class II molecules. One approach to solving this problem is to incorporate peptide antigens into lipid micelles (see Figure 15.6).

The lipids serve multiple purposes. They provide a carrier for the antigenic peptides and stimulate innate immune responses (see Adjuvants section). Finally, lipids easily fuse with APC cell membranes, delivering the peptides into MHC class I pathways of presentation. Because some of the micelles are also acquired by endocytosis, the peptides also arrive in MHC class II antigen-presentation pathways.

One of the most unusual approaches to vaccine development involves the use of naked protein-encoding DNA. Today, it is often easy to identify the portions of a microorganism's DNA that encode essential antigenic proteins or epitopes. In some cases, after injection of this DNA into muscle, injected animals make antibodies against peptides encoded by the DNA. The underlying mechanisms are not entirely clear but, within host cells, the injected DNA generates RNA and proteins that APCs eventually engulf, process, and present to T cells. Presently, naked DNA vaccines are few, but in the near future these vaccines may become more common.

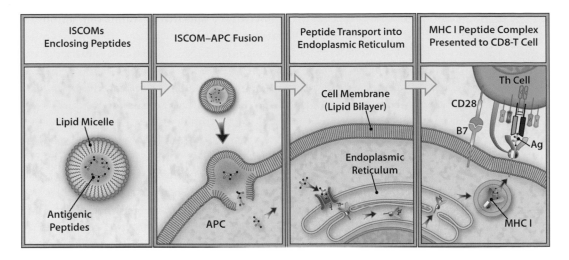

| ISCOMs Enclosing Peptides | ISCOM–APC Fusion | Peptide Transport into Endoplasmic Reticulum | MHC I Peptide Complex Presented to CD8-T Cell |

FIGURE 15.6. The use of ISCOMs as vaccines

Combining poorly immunogenic peptides with lipid micelles generates more immunogenic complexes. When injected, these micelles fuse with membranes of APCs, effectively delivering the antigen in both MHC class I and class II pathways.

In the end, regardless of the approach, the purpose of vaccination is to place the immunogens where they will interact with components of both innate and adaptive immunity, especially aspects of both sorts of immunity most critical to protective immunity.

Adjuvants

Immunologists have known for decades that antigens alone were often not enough to induce protective immune responses. Good vaccines usually required the addition of an adjuvant—a substance that enhanced the immunogenicity of an antigen without altering the specificity of the immune response. The most common early adjuvants included oil, emulsifiers, and bacterial cell-wall components, with or without aluminum salts. At first, no one knew much about what adjuvants did, but vaccine makers understood their necessity. This consensual ignorance once led Charles Janeway, a famous immunologist, to refer to adjuvants as "our dirty little secret." In the past few years, attitudes about adjuvants have changed. Particularly as vaccines have become more refined and less pathogenic, the need for adjuvants and understanding about how they work has become essential.

It is often true that the more refined an antigen is, the less immunogenic it is. For example, effective live-attenuated vaccines may require no adjuvant at all, but killed and component vaccines usually do. As you learned in chapter 10, APCs present normal host antigens all the time but do so in an unactivated state (low expression of costimulatory molecules and proinflammatory cytokines). Administration of large doses of antigen without proinflammatory stimuli (e.g., PAMPs, DAMPs, and activating cytokines) may actually have the opposite effect—T-cell anergy and tolerance to the antigen. As a result, just delivering the antigen is not enough; the APCs must also receive signals that the administered antigen is potentially hazardous.

The primary goals of vaccine design are to stimulate a strong immune response of the appropriate type (cellular, humoral, or both) inexpensively and with minimum toxicity. Adjuvants can have major effects on all of these aspects of vaccination. And because of their importance to vaccine efficacy, the components of adjuvants are among the most closely guarded secrets of the vaccine industry.

Most adjuvants help to stimulate more aggressive innate immune responses. As mentioned earlier, innate immune responses play major roles in initiating and directing the adaptive immune response. In general, adjuvants affect the immune response in one of three ways. First, some adjuvants—such as aluminum salts—act by creating a depot effect. That is, some adjuvant–antigen combinations dissipate very slowly from the site of injection. Without such an adjuvant, injected antigens spread very quickly in lymph or blood. Because many important APCs are almost exclusively outside of lymph and blood, the immunogenic effects of the vaccine are thus dramatically reduced. Second, many adjuvants (particularly liposomes) act as carriers, effectively delivering antigen into APCs. Last, some adjuvants have immunostimulating properties (see Figure 15.7).

The most commonly used adjuvants include liposomes, microspheres, ISCOMs, minerals (particularly aluminum salts such as alum), water-in-oil emulsions and oil-in-water emulsions, and agonists for PRRs (such as TLRs). All of these act by one (or more) of three means: antigen-depot formation, antigen-carrier effects, or immune stimulation.

Antigen-depot effects result from introducing antigens in a form that does not quickly dissipate into intravascular fluids. Neutral liposomes do this because they are large, remain at the injection site, and can fuse with and introduce antigens into APCs. Similarly, attaching antigens to relatively inert microspheres or other particles slows dissipation and enhances phagoctyosis. Antigens adsorbed onto mineral salts, especially alum, not only dissipate slowly from the injection site but also stimulate the eventual development of Th2 cells and antibody responses. Aluminum salts (especially alum), perhaps the most commonly used adjuvant, are among the best at creating an antigen-depot effect (but the effects of aluminum salts are likely more complex). With these ad-

juvants, the adsorbed antigens remain mostly at the site of injections and are phagocytosed more efficiently, considerably enhancing immune responses.

Immunostimulatory and carrier effects result when adjuvants more specifically affect cells of the innate immune system. Most cell membranes, including those of APCs, have a net-negative charge. The net-positive charge of cationic liposomes attracts them to APCs and other cells. When cationic liposomes fuse with APCs, incorporated antigens readily move into antigen-presentation pathways, enhancing immune responses. Also, adjuvants containing antigens in oil-in-water or water-in-oil emulsions enhance interactions between immune cells and stimulate either Th1- or Th2-directed immune responses. Again, macrophages more effectively ingest and process emulsified antigens, and the emulsions persist longer than simple aqueous solutions.

Some of the most potent adjuvants contain immunostimulating compounds derived from pathogens. These adjuvants include agonist to PRR, such as the TLR agonists. These molecules mimic PAMPs or DAMPs that bind to PRRs and activate APCs. These synthetic copies of pathogen-derived molecules activate mast cells and APCs, enhance antigen presentation, stimulate inflammation, and initiate specific sorts of Th cells and immune responses. Because of improved understanding of the innate response, many of these sorts of immune stimulants already exist, and many more are likely to be available soon.

Other sorts of immune stimulants include cytokines, such as IL-2 and IL-12, that stimulate Th1 cells. These sorts of stimulants favor very specific responses in immunized animals, responses that help to push immunity toward antibody and T-cell responses. For this reason, these immune stimulants may one day allow veterinarians to direct immune response along the most effective pathways.

In general, adjuvants include a variety of antigen-unrelated compounds that act to non-

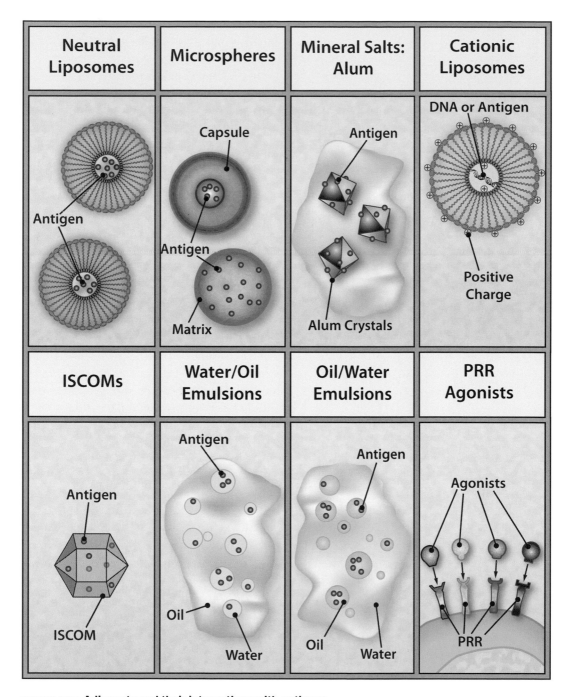

FIGURE 15.7. Adjuvants and their interactions with antigens

specifically enhance the immune response, often through enhancement of aspects of innate immunity. As understanding of the innate immune response and its interactions with the adaptive immune response grows, it seems clear that immunological adjuvants will come to play an even greater role in vaccination and the direction of the immune response.

Administration

In some cases, the route of vaccine administration may make little difference. For example, *Vibrio anguillarum* is a Gram-negative bacterium that infects many fish, but especially intensively farmed fish, such as salmon. In one study involving trout and immunity to *V. anguillarum*, investigators found that whether they administered the vaccine orally, by immersion, or via intramuscular injection, the vaccinated fish produced similar amounts of antibody that reacted, for the most part, with the same antigenic epitopes on the bacterium.

This is not always the case. Often, the route of immunization is very important to the induction of protection. Routes of vaccination include some surprising options, such as intraocular, intraperitoneal, intrathecal, intracranial, intravenous, and immersion (as in the preceding example). In practice, however, the most commonly used routes are intramuscular (IM), subcutaneous (SC, although sometimes Sub Q), oral, and intranasal (IN).

Among these, IM and SC are the most common. These routes offer several immunological advantages. First, after IM or SC injection, the inocula tend to form small depots of antigen that slowly leak into the surroundings. Second, muscles and, especially, subcutaneous tissues contain large numbers of mast cells and APCs, including DCs. When properly stimulated, mast cells help to induce innate immune responses that are essential to the development of adaptive immune responses. The inflammation that ensues draws macrophages and neutrophils and sends DCs to the secondary lymphoid tissues. These all help to stimulate robust immune responses.

Some vaccines, such as the IN canine pertussis vaccine, do not necessarily induce as much inflammation, but they do immediately engage the mucosal immune system, including mucosal B cells. As a result of activation, some B cells ultimately isotype switch and begin producing pathogen-specific IgA, and IgA, in its dimeric form, returns to mucosal surfaces, where the vaccinated animal is most likely to again encounter *Bordetella bronchiseptica,* one bacterium responsible for pertussis.

Oral vaccines offer especially attractive advantages—they involve a painless procedure for the patient and are easy to administer. As with IN vaccines, oral vaccines directly engage the mucosal immune system and are effective at inducing protective mucosal immunity. The Sabin polio vaccine is a good example. One major polio transmission route is through feces left in places such as public swimming pools (fecal–oral transmission). The virus then enters the host via the gastrointestinal system. For this reason, mucosal immunity is key in defense against polio. Again, because of the predominance of the mucosal response, the oral vaccine has proven very effective. Similarly, the oral rabies vaccine is especially effective because it induces a mucosal immunity that helps to neutralize the virus at epithelial surfaces. It is likely that many more ways exist in which vaccines might take advantage of mucosal immune systems, but a necessary first step will be greater understanding of how mucosal immunity works.

Frequency

Frequency of administration is another major issue with any vaccine. In general, immunity induced with live vaccines lasts longer than immunity induced by killed vaccines. Two factors play major roles in veterinary vaccination: the status of the animal's immune system and the longevity of the immune response.

As discussed in chapter 14, the blood and other fluids of neonatal animals often contain large amounts of maternal antibodies, perhaps even some maternal T cells. The presence of these antibodies makes effective immunization impossible. That is why, under normal circumstances, veterinarians give no vaccines before four to five weeks of age. But even then—because the exact point at which maternal antibodies become few enough to allow for vaccination varies from animal to animal and species

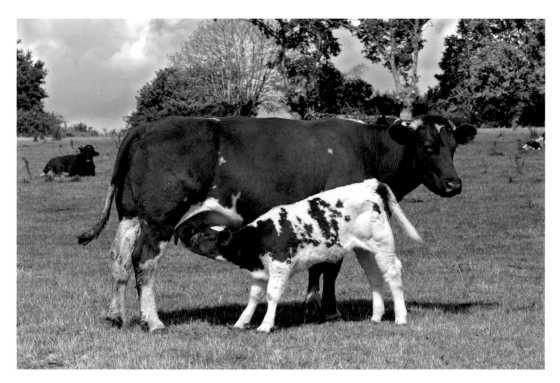

FIGURE 15.8. **Cow–calf pair (© Christian Musat / Shutterstock)**

to species—the results of early vaccination are difficult to predict. For this reason, veterinarians give most early vaccines repeatedly and at relatively short intervals. The aim is to provide protection as soon as possible after the maternal antibodies disappear.

Beyond this, efficacy studies should determine the frequency of administration of any vaccine. Efficacy studies, over long periods of time, measure the levels of antibodies (antibody titers) in vaccinated animals and establish when antibody levels fall so low they are no longer protective. Regardless of the nature of the vaccine, there is simply no other way to establish the necessary frequency of revaccination. Unfortunately, vaccination regimens are not always determined this way, and recommended frequencies may be unnecessarily high. For this reason, with animals at risk for problems because of excessive vaccinations, practitioners often measure antibody titers before revaccinating.

PASSIVE IMMUNOTHERAPY

The intent of passive immunotherapy is to inject enough preformed antibodies to bind and neutralize antigen (commonly toxins) and protect the host animal. Immunologists call it passive immunotherapy or passive transfer (sometimes even passive immunization) because the host animal plays no active role in the development of immunity against the toxins. Passive transfer induces no host immunity against the toxins, produces no memory cells, and lasts only as long as the antibodies persist in the injected animal (usually a matter of weeks), just as with the passive transfer of maternal immunity discussed in chapter 14.

Regardless of its shortcomings, passive immunotherapy can be a powerful aid in the treatment of several diseases, including those induced by toxins (such as tetanus toxin), inhalation of anthrax, and even animal cancers. As we have described, antibodies have a wide range of effects, and their sudden introduction

TABLE 15.2. Recommended vaccination schedule for cattle

Timing and goal	Vaccination
Prebreeding: The goal is to provide protection against pathogens of general health concern and those that may increase pregnancy wastage. These vaccines should be completed 30 days before breeding.	IBR, BVDV, PI-3, BRSV (MLV preferred) Leptospirosis (five strains; two doses); may also consider *L. hardjo* vaccine Campylobacter fetus (vibrio) if using bulls Clostridium (seven-way)
Precalving: The goal with precalving vaccinations is to enhance colostral antibodies and protect against early lactation pathogens.	Rotavirus, Coronavirus, *E. coli* (for calf scours)
Four to six months—weaning. The goal is to provide protection against common pathogens that may cause problems when colostral antibodies begin to fall off.	IBR, BVDV, PI-3, BRSV (MLV preferred) Clostridium (seven-way) Mannheimia / Pasteurella (vaccine needs to contain toxoid component)

Note: IBR = infectious bovine rhinotracheitis; BVDV = bovine viral diarrhea virus; PI-3 = parainfluenza virus; BRSV = bovine respiratory syncytial virus; MLV = modified live vaccine.

into an animal can dramatically change the course of some diseases. Possible risks always include type III hypersensitivities and anaphylactic shock, but prophylactic treatments such as anti-inflammatory and immunosuppressive drugs can greatly reduce these risks.

CLINICAL CORRELATION FOLLOW-UP

Student Considerations

Obviously, calves and adult cattle (Figure 15.8) face many infectious challenges. To help protect cattle, clinical researchers recommend a series of vaccinations throughout the lives of these animals. (Table 15.2 shows the recommended vaccination schedule for cattle.) Each infectious agent presents a particular set of challenges, and the vaccines for each agent must address those immunological issues. For this reason, each vaccine is different in essential ways.

At least one parainfluenza virus (PI-3) vaccine contains live-attenuated virus and is administered IN. The virus in this vaccine is a temperature-sensitive mutant of the pathogenic parainfluenza virus. This mutant will grow only in the relatively cooler respiratory tissues of cattle. Most leptospirosis vaccines contain inactivated virus and are administered IM or SC, and most

contain adjuvants. The recommended vaccine for pasteurella contains a toxoid.

On the basis of the material in this chapter, you should be able to offer plausible explanations for the differences in the composition and routes of administration of these vaccines.

Possible Explanations

Each potential cattle pathogen presents a unique set of problems to the animals' immune system and to vaccine designers. Cattle will most likely encounter parainfluenza virus at the respiratory mucosa. Protective immune responses against parainfluenza virus will likely require both cellular and humoral immune responses—antibodies to slow or prevent virus from infecting epithelial cells and Tc cells to destroy virus-infected cells. Furthermore, the best antibodies for the job are IgA antibodies because of their presence and actions at mucosal surfaces. For these reasons, the vaccine contains live virus to stimulate both T-cell and humoral responses. Because the viruses are live, no adjuvant is needed, and by administering the vaccine IN, the potential for production of IgA antibodies is greater.

Leptospirosis, however, is caused by a spirochete, *Leptospira interrogans*. The bacterium grows extracellularly and moves from animal to animal through urine, milk, aborted fetuses, and contaminated water. The most effective immune responses against extracellular bacteria include antibodies, primarily IgG and IgM, because both can opsonize bacteria and both can activate complement—essential elements of antibacterial immune responses. The vaccine includes an adjuvant as well, most likely one that activates macrophages and helps to induce both Th1 and Th2 responses—important for antibody production, activation of macrophages, and inflammation, and all essential in antibacterial immune responses.

Finally, the pasteurella vaccine contains a toxoid. *Pasteurella multocida,* the Gram-negative organism responsible for pasteurellosis, produces an exotoxin that interferes with aspects of signal transduction and causes a severe respiratory syndrome in cattle. Effective vaccination for pasteurellosis requires the inclusion of the toxoid (inactivated *Pasteurella multocida* toxin) to provide toxin-neutralizing antibodies.

Because each organism challenges animals' immune systems in particular ways, so must each vaccine engage animals' immune systems in correspondingly specific ways.

Gerald N. Callahan

Immune Deficiencies and Immune-Mediated Diseases

Chapter 16

10.5876_9781607322184.c016

CLINICAL CORRELATION: FELINE IMMUNODEFICIENCY VIRUS

Feline immunodeficiency virus (FIV) infects about 2 percent of domestic cats in the United States. Infection rates are higher among free-roaming and feral cats—around 8 percent (see Figure 16.1). FIV is also enzootic in some large cats, such as snow leopards, tigers, Florida panthers, bobcats, and African lions. The effects of FIV infection on these wild populations are mostly unknown, but the virus appears to have much less impact in the wild.

Like HIV, FIV is a retrovirus—an RNA virus that uses reverse transcriptase to generate a DNA copy of its RNA and inserts that copy into the host's genome. Unlike feline leukemia virus, transmission of FIV does not result sim-ply from prolonged contact. Instead, cats shed FIV in saliva and transmit the virus through bite wounds. Vertical transmission appears rare.

FIV infects, among others, $CD4^+$ T cells—Th cells. As with HIV, FIV-induced disease progresses through five stages:

1. acute infection (four to sixteen weeks);

2. asymptomatic carrier (months to years);

3. persistent generalized lymphadenopathy (usually very short and sometimes missed by cat owners);

4. AIDS-related complex (including chronic oral fungal infections and gastrointestinal and respiratory disease);

5. AIDS, including respiratory infections (canine herpes and calciviruses); oral infections (mostly fungal); ocular disease, including glaucoma; chronic diarrhea (bacterial, parasitic, malignant); and skin and ear infections (parasites, yeasts, and bacteria). After the development of AIDS-related complex or AIDS, infected cats survive less than one year.

LEARNING OBJECTIVES

After reading this chapter, you should be able to

- describe the nature and possible causes of congenital immune deficiencies;
- describe the nature and possible causes of acquired immune deficiencies;
- classify and explain the bases of types I, III, and IV immune-mediated hypersensitivities;
- understand the nature of autoimmune diseases, including type II hypersensitivities.

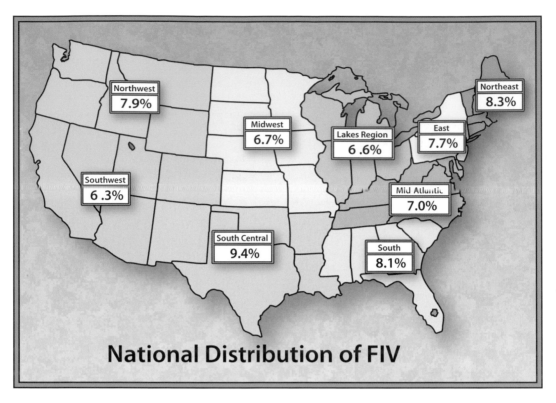

National Distribution of FIV

FIGURE 16.1. Impact of feline immunodeficiency virus in the United States

Infection rates among symptomatic and high-risk cats. (Data from the National FeLV/FIV Awareness Project, sponsored by the IDEXX Corporation.)

IMMUNE DEFICIENCIES

Perhaps the most familiar immune deficiencies are acquired immune deficiencies (AIDS) induced by retroviral infections in some mammals. However, immune deficiency disorders come in many forms.

Congenital Immune Deficiencies

Congenital immune deficiencies are those present at birth. These deficiencies may result from the mother's exposure to environmental agents such as over vaccination, vaccinating during the mother's heat cycle or pregnancy, antibiotics, steroids, protein malnutrition, too few calories, vitamin or mineral insufficiencies, hormones, and viruses and other infectious agents, as well as other drugs. Exposure of mother or fetus to any of these agents can lead to suppression of the maternal and fetal immune systems, which can result in severe immune deficiencies in the neonate. In general, these environmental agents damage immune systems through interference with or destruction of essential elements of the innate or adaptive immune responses. For example, steroids (especially glucocorticoids) suppress production of several important cytokines, including IL-1, IL-2, IL-4, IL-6, and gamma IFN. All of these play critical roles in the development of innate (especially inflammatory) and adaptive immune responses. Glucocorticoids also induce apoptosis in some T-cell populations and directly affect B cells. The result is a pronounced immune suppression. Sex hormones may also have similar effects on immunity, as can malnutrition.

The most common causes of congenital immune deficiencies, though, are genetic mutations. We have already described several of these diseases, including SCID in Arabian foals, XLSCID in basset hounds, and IgA deficiencies affecting several dog breeds.

Each of these diseases results from a mutation that affects a gene critical to the development of immune responses. Foals with SCID lack a functional DNA-dependent protein kinase; dogs with XLCID lack the γc chain, an essential component of receptors for IL-2, IL-4, IL-7, IL-9, IL-15, and IL-21; and IgA-deficient dogs lack the genes necessary for functional isotype switches to IgA and effective mucosal immunity. Each of these diseases results in reduced or no ability to defend against infections, sometimes resulting in premature death.

These examples are probably just the tip of the iceberg. Effective immune responses rely on complex series of genes, cytokines, receptors, MHC molecules, cells, tissues, and organs. A defect in any element of the series can diminish an animal's ability to generate effect defensive responses.

Sometimes these defects are subtle, and sometimes not. Recognizing something such as SCID in Arabian foals is easy because of the dramatic recurrent infections and deaths among affected animals. Detecting minor changes is much harder. Animals' abilities to respond to infectious threats vary considerably, even within a single species or within a single litter. Some of this variation reflects subtle differences in immune competence, changes that can range from undetectable to fatal. The same can be said about animals' responses to vaccination; individual animals can show great variation in immunity after vaccination. Although this variation is not usually considered to reflect underlying congenital immune deficiencies, to some extent it clearly does.

Acquired Immune Deficiencies

Acquired immune deficiencies arise later in life, sometime after birth. Some of the best-known immune deficiencies result from viral infections, such as AIDS, but animals can acquire immune deficiencies in a variety of ways. The most common causes include

- nutritional deficiencies;
- drugs;
- stress;
- aging;
- microbes.

As we have described, clonal expansions among both T and B cells are essential parts of immune responses, as are multiple rounds of T- and B-cell division that generate effector populations essential for defense against infection, which takes a lot of ATP and a lot of nutrients. As a result, immune systems have high nutritional requirements. Because of these requirements, what might seem like a relatively minor nutritional deficiency can result in a significant immune deficiency that manifests as repeated infections or lack of response to vaccination.

Glucocorticoids such as hydrocortisone, prednisone, and dexamethasone are strongly immune suppressive and anti-inflammatory. In addition, both chemotherapeutic and radiotherapeutic cancer drugs, such as methotrexate and cisplatin, are immunosuppressive. Methotrexate prevents the normal synthesis of thymidine, a base essential for DNA replication. Cisplatin causes cross-linking of DNA, which leads to apoptosis. Both chemicals are effective against cancers because these drugs have their greatest impact on the DNA of rapidly dividing cells, as does radiation therapy. Immune responses also depend on rapid cell division, and for that reason, these drugs are often powerful immune suppressants.

In animals as divergent as horses and eels, cortisol is a major adrenal glucocorticoid. When an animal is stressed (ranging from perceived dangers to prolonged and repeated physical stress), the adrenal glands produce higher levels of cortisol. Through its actions on T and B cells, cortisol, like other glucocorticoids, suppresses the immune system. Under normal circumstances, this suppression may offer important protection against autoimmunity, but in repetitive stressful situations, cortisol can lead to pronounced immune suppression.

Also, as all animals age, they experience a progressive decrease in immune capacities. The exact rate of decline and character of these decreases can be hard to predict. In general, older animals are less responsive to vaccination and more susceptible to infections.

Finally, infectious agents cause acquired immune deficiencies. The most familiar of these is virus-induced AIDS, such as the feline AIDS that arises after infection with FIV (discussed at the beginning and end of this chapter). But with the apparent exception of prions, immunosuppressive examples are found among every class of transmissible agent.

For example, after infection with viruses, such as canine parvovirus, animals often become more susceptible to bacterial infections. This increase in susceptibility is the result of the immunosuppressive effects of the virus. In truth, many infections result in varying levels of immune suppression; the ones bearing the acronym AIDS simply represent the most severe of these syndromes.

IMMUNE-MEDIATED DISEASES

Immune responses are, of necessity, toxic. Immune responses have evolved to destroy things: bacteria, viruses, fungi, parasites, infected host cells, perhaps even tumor cells. Because of that, all animals have evolved sophisticated means for controlling immune responses—Treg cells, cytokines, receptors and their ligands, apoptosis, the thymus itself, positive selection, negative selection, central tolerance, and peripheral tolerance all help to control immune responses and try to limit the opportunities for animals' immune systems to turn against their hosts.

In spite of all the checks and balances and all of the selections that occur, immune systems sometimes overreact to innocuous agents and sometimes turn on self. The diseases that result are immune-mediated diseases or hypersensitivities (see Figure 16.2).

Although several immune-mediated diseases do not fall neatly into any one category, immunologists have divided hypersensitivity reactions into four major categories—types I–IV. Types I–III are the immediate-type hypersensitivities, all of which involve antibodies. After initial exposures, these antibodies reach high levels in sera and tissues and initiate responses very rapidly (immediate type). T cells mediate type IV responses, and even after initial exposures, it takes time to generate sufficient T cells to mount an apparent response. For this reason, immunologists also call type IV hypersensitivities delayed-type hypersensitivities (DTHs).

Type I hypersensitivities are true allergies and involve IgE antibodies. Type II hypersensitivities involve antibodies produced against self components and are autoimmune diseases. Type III hypersensitivities, also known as immune complex diseases, often arise when large amounts of preformed antibodies encounter large amounts of antigens and form immune complexes too large to remain soluble in plasma.

Hypersensitivities Type I, III, and IV

TYPE I HYPERSENSITIVITIES

As we have discussed, type I hypersensitivities are the true allergies, marked by the involvement of IgE, mast cells, and sometimes basophils and eosinophils. Signs of allergies can range from corn-induced gastritis and vomiting in dogs to toe tapping in parrots, from an annoying dermatitis to a fatal anaphylactic shock, but the underlying immune mechanisms are alike, and all involve IgE.

Antigens that cause allergies are called allergens. When an animal encounters an allergen

	Type I	Type II	Type III	Type IV	
Immune Reactant	IgE	IgG	IgG	Th1 Cells	CTL
Antigen	Soluble Antigen	Self Antigen	Soluble Antigen	Soluble Antigen	Cell-Associated Antigen
Effector Mechanism	Mast-Cell Activation	FcR+ Cells, (Phagocytes' NK cells)	FcR+ Cells, Complement	Macrophage Activation	Cytotoxicity
Example of Reaction	Allergic Rhinitis, Asthma, Systemic Anaphylaxis	Autoimmune Diseases	Serum Sickness, Arthus Reaction	DTH	Contact Dermatitis

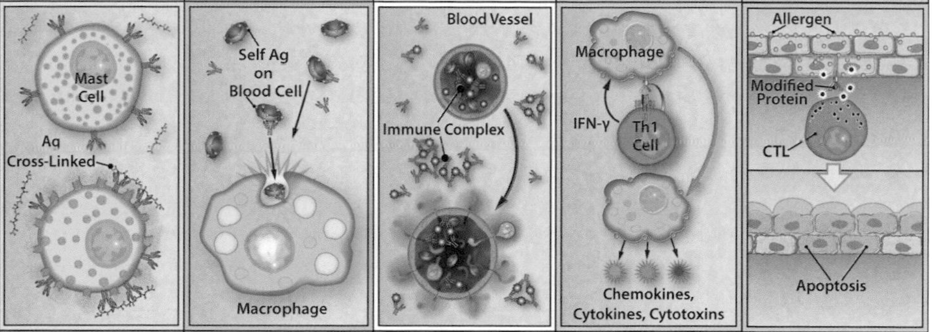

FIGURE 16.2. Immune hypersensitivities

Immune-mediated diseases fall into four major categories, types I–IV. Antibodies mediate the first three of these categories, and they are immediate-type hypersensitivities. T cells mediate type IV responses, including delayed-type hypersensitivities (DTHs). Ag = antigen; CTL = Tc cells.

for the first time, no grossly observable response occurs. However, inside of an allergy-prone animal, much is happening. First, APCs process and present the allergen to Th cells (in particular Th2 cells), which in turn interact with antigen-presenting B cells. Those B cells then undergo an isotype switch from IgM to IgE (see Figure 16.3), which is key. Clearly, some nonallergic animals also make antibody responses against allergens, but they do not make IgE responses.

The IgE produced in the primary exposure moves from the blood into the perivascular spaces, where it binds to specific Fc receptors on mast cells. These specialized Fc receptors (named FcεRs) have a very high affinity for IgE and stably maintain IgE on the surface of mast cells for long periods, essentially acting as an allergen-specific mast-cell receptor. This point is essentially where the primary response ends, with thousands upon thousands of armed mast cells and probably also basophils and eosinophils.

On secondary and later exposures, the allergen binds directly to the IgE on the mast cells, which causes the cells to degranulate, releasing large amounts of histamine and other mediators. After this, the mast cells begin to synthesize and secrete more proinflammatory mediators—such as prostaglandins and leukotrienes—just as they do during other inflammatory responses (see Figure 16.4 and chapter 5).

The release of these factors leads to vasodilation, increases in vascular permeability, swelling, smooth-muscle contraction plus bronchospasm, and recruitment and activation of

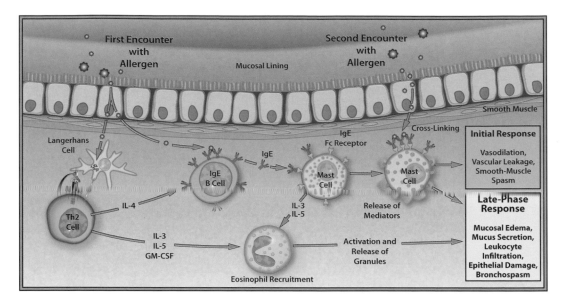

FIGURE 16.3. Type I hypersensitivity

On first encounter (upper left), APCs acquire the allergen, process it, and present it to CD4$^+$ T cells that eventually differentiate into Th2 cells. In response, the Th2 cells interact with and activate B cells. In the presence of IL-4, these B cells switch from IgM to IgE production. The IgE antibodies migrate from the blood into surrounding tissues, where they bind to specific Fc receptors on mast cells. On the second encounter, the allergen binds to the IgE on mast cells and induces mast-cell degranulation, which leads to inflammation, swelling, smooth-muscle contraction, and recruitment and activation of leukocytes.

leukocytes. These cells further enhance the ongoing inflammation (see Figure 16.5).

The results of this process can be annoying things such as flea allergies or the following scenario:

> On a routine well visit for a six-year-old indoor–outdoor cat, the veterinarian administered a vaccination for rabies and decided, as long as the cat was in, to give it a feline leukemia virus vaccination a couple of months early. Ten minutes later, the cat was lying flat, purple, struggling to breathe, with no detectable blood pressure.

It was not the first time the cat had received either vaccine, but it was the first time the animal had ever reacted this way. After earlier vaccinations, the cat had formed IgE antibodies with one or more of the components of the vaccines. When the veterinarian adminis-

tered this current vaccine, the cat's mast cells were armed with IgE. The antigens in the vaccines bound to the IgE on the cat's mast cells and caused the release of large amounts of histamine, prostaglandins, and leukotrienes and other proinflammatory cytokines, which caused systemic vasodilation and increased vascular permeability. Because the volume of the circulatory system had suddenly increased dramatically, the cat's blood pressure crashed, leading to anaphylactic shock. Fortunately, the veterinarian recognized this as an allergic response, implemented critical care measures, and saved the cat's life.

Why the cat responded this way is unclear. Although clear genetic predispositions to allergies exist, allergies may arise suddenly at any time, and many animals acquire them later in life. At some point, this cat switched from making IgG to making IgE in response to the vaccines, and

Class of Product	Examples	Biological Effects
Enzyme	Tryptase, Chymase, Cathepsin G., Carboxypeptidase	Remodels Connective Tissue Matrix
Toxic Mediator	Histamine, Heparin	Toxic to Parasites, Increases Vascular Permeability, Causes Smooth-Muscle Contraction
Cytokine	IL-4, IL-13	Stimulate and Amplify Th2-Cell Response
	IL-3, IL-5, GM-CSF	Promotes Eosinophil Activation and Production
	TNF-α (Some Stored Preformed in Granules)	Promotes Inflammation, Stimulates Cytokine Production by Many Cell Types, Activates Endothelium
Chemokine	MIP-1α	Attracts Monocytes, Macrophages, and Neutrophils
Lipid Mediator	Leukotrines Prostaglandins	Cause Smooth-Muscle Contraction, Increase Vascular Permeability, Stimulate Mucus Secretion
	Platelet-Activating Factor	Attracts Leukocytes, Activates Neutrophils, Eosinophils, and Platelets

FIGURE 16.4. **Products of activated mast cells**

After antigen binds to and cross-links IgE molecules on the surface of mast cells, the cells release their stored granules. The first two rows show the contents of these granules. The bottom three rows show synthesized mast-cell products. The net effect is to initiate and maintain inflammation. MIP = macrophage inflammatory protein.

at this same point, the animal became at risk for vaccination-induced anaphylactic shock.

Clearly, the manifestations of allergic responses can vary dramatically. The eventual outcome of an exposure to an allergen depends on the immune status of the animal, the dose of the allergen, and the route of exposure (see Figure 16.6A–B).

Intravenous exposure to large amounts of antigen holds the greatest risk for sudden,

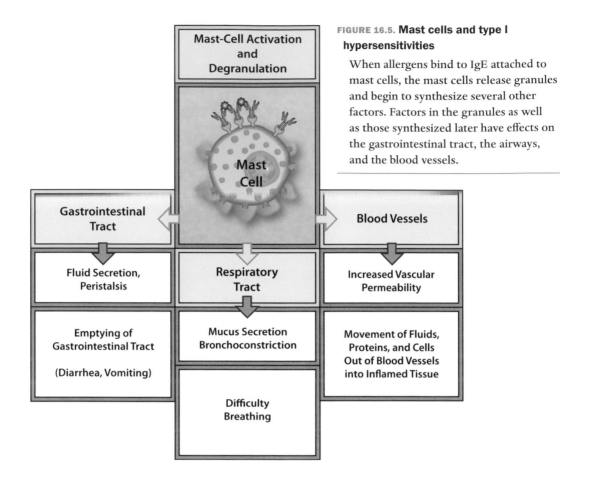

FIGURE 16.5. **Mast cells and type I hypersensitivities**

When allergens bind to IgE attached to mast cells, the mast cells release granules and begin to synthesize several other factors. Factors in the granules as well as those synthesized later have effects on the gastrointestinal tract, the airways, and the blood vessels.

Mast-Cell Activation and Degranulation

Mast Cell

Gastrointestinal Tract

Blood Vessels

Fluid Secretion, Peristalsis

Respiratory Tract

Increased Vascular Permeability

Emptying of Gastrointestinal Tract

(Diarrhea, Vomiting)

Mucus Secretion Bronchoconstriction

Movement of Fluids, Proteins, and Cells Out of Blood Vessels into Inflamed Tissue

Difficulty Breathing

systemic anaphylaxis. Generally, subcutaneous exposure poses less of a threat. Inhaled and ingested allergens can induce widely varying responses—from rhinitis and diarrhea to anaphylactic shock—depending on the amount of allergen and the immune status of the host animal.

Why some animals produce IgE in response to certain antigens and other animals do not is not clear. Two things favor IgE production: differentiation of Th0 cells into Th2 cells and the actions and products of those Th2 cells.

Factors important to the production of Th2 cells include the cytokines produced during antigen presentation and during the subsequent development of those Th2 cells, the intrinsic properties of the antigen, the dose of antigen, and the route of exposure to antigen. The presence of IL-4, IL-5, IL-9, IL-10, and IL-13 favors Th2-cell development, and Th2 cells are essential for the isotype switching of B cells to IgE. Also important are the cytokines produced during interactions between Th2 cells and antigen-presenting B cells. Again, no way currently exists to predict the antibody isotype an animal will produce after exposure to an antigen.

Beyond allergies, it seems that IgE antibodies must have a more productive role in defense. Evidence suggests that IgE antibodies are important elements for defense against infections by multicellular parasites (such as insects and helminths). As a result of their interactions with Fc receptors on mast cells, IgE antibodies end up distributed at the sites where animals are most likely to encounter such parasites—skin, lung, and gut epithelia. Another important factor seems to be inflammation. In the presence of inflammation, Th1-cell development pre-

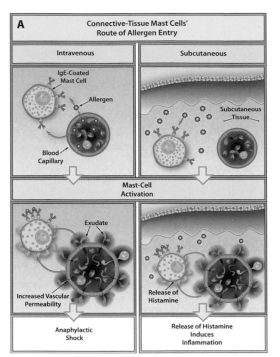

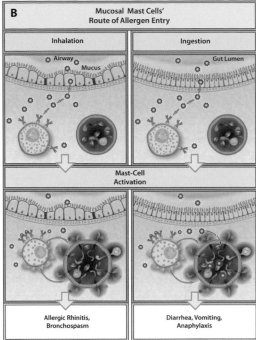

FIGURE 16.6A–B. The route of allergen exposure affects the clinical manifestation of the allergy

Mast cells appear in large numbers in two places in an animal's body: in the connective tissues surrounding blood vessels (panel A) and in the mucosa of the gut and airways (panel B). The severity of the response to an allergen depends on which and how many mast cells are activated.

dominates; without inflammation, Th2-cell development is most common. The fact that most allergens appear at epithelial surfaces and are unlikely to initiate inflammation may help to explain allergic responses. However, by themselves, these observations are not enough to explain allergic reactions because these factors often do not differ between allergic and nonallergic animals. Mast cells and basophil products also enhance IgE production, but again there are no observable differences between afflicted and unaffected animals.

Some animals have clear genetic predispositions. Offspring of allergic animals are more likely to develop allergies themselves. But because so many factors are involved in immune responses, just what those genetic variations might be remains largely unknown. Environmental factors also contribute to the risk of allergies.

Currently, among several animal populations the incidence of allergies is increasing significantly. In the developed world, the most affected populations are house pets and humans. This observation prompted several studies, and together they suggest that early exposure to some infectious agents, particularly bacteria, is essential for normal immune development. Animals intentionally shielded from infections do not develop normal immune or gastrointestinal systems. People's inclination toward sterilizing their and their pets' environments may be having pathological consequences.

TYPE III HYPERSENSITIVITIES

Type III hypersensitivities are also known as immune complex diseases because the underlying cause of type III hypersensitivities is antigen–antibody complexes. Here is a hypothetical

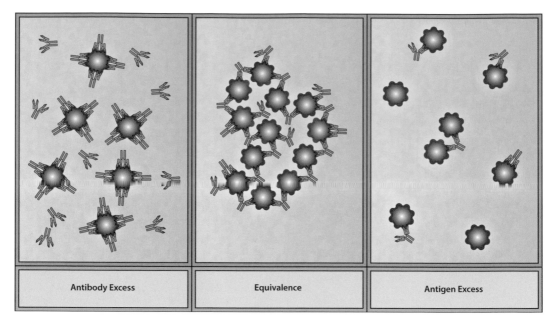

| Antibody Excess | Equivalence | Antigen Excess |

FIGURE 16.7. Type III hypersensitivities and immune complexes

When an excess of antibodies exists, each antigen is completely coated with antibodies and not accessible for binding into large complexes (left panel). When an excess of antigens exists, one or no antibodies bind most antigens and no large complexes form (right panel). When antibodies and antigens are equal or nearly so, these molecules can link together to form large complexes (center panel).

scenario (based on an actual scenario) that involves a type III hypersensitivity and a veterinarian's major oversight:

You regularly take your dog into the foothills for long, uneventful (except for the occasional rabbit) walks, but today is different. Today, your dog spooks up a rattlesnake and gets bitten. You pick up the dog and carry her to your car, cover her with blankets, and head to the nearest emergency veterinary clinic. There, the veterinarian begins therapy for the snakebite and administers antivenin, a concoction containing antibodies to the snake venom antigen. After a few days in the hospital, your dog seems to have shaken off the snakebite.

You move to another town and several months later you are out walking with your dog again. Again, she rouses an angry rattler and gets bitten. Again, you gather up the dog and rush to the emergency veterinary clinic. Again the veterinarian begins therapy and supportive care for the snakebite and initiates antivenin therapy. The next morning the dog seems fine, and the veterinarian discontinues antivenin treatment. Several hours later, the dog's temperature rises, her blood pressure crashes, she goes into kidney failure, and her breathing becomes very labored.

This scenario describes a type III hypersensitivity called serum sickness. Type III hypersensitivities occur when large and roughly equivalent amounts of antibody and antigen abruptly come together. Because antibodies are multivalent, each antibody molecule can bind multiple antigens, and because most natural antigens are also multivalent, each antigen can bind to antibody at multiple positions, meaning that, under the right conditions, antibodies can link multiple antigens together into massive chains of antigen–antibody complexes (see Figure 16.7).

These complexes quickly become insoluble because of their size. They then fall out of solution in the blood and deposit onto the vascular endothelium, where they activate complement. As a result, C3b fragments appear and attach to the endothelium. Neutrophils, via their Fc and C3b receptors, bind to the IgG and C3b of the complexes, which, in turn, stimulates release of enzymes that damage vessel walls (see Figure 16.8).

In addition to C3b, complement activation results in the formation of C5a, a powerful anaphylatoxin (inducer of anaphylaxis; see Figure 16.9). C5a acts in several ways to enhance inflammation, up to and including anaphylactic shock. C5a induces blood vessel dilation and increased vascular permeability, activates macrophages and epithelial cells to produce TNF (another major proinflammatory cytokine), and activates neutrophils, all of which combine to produce the outcome in the hypothetical case described earlier.

Most antivenins are not simply antivenoms. Most are horse sera containing antivenom antibodies. Administration of antivenin after the first snakebite not only blocked the effects of the snake venom, but also induced immune responses to all of the protein components of the horse serum. At the time of the second antivenin treatment, the possibility of a type III hypersensitivity reaction was high—lots of preformed antibodies and lots of antigens. As the antibody levels rise and the serum protein antigens wane (see Figure 16.10), however, serum sickness can occur even on a dog's first exposure to horse serum.

Once the veterinarian discontinued the antivenin in this dog, antigen levels began to fall. When the serum antigen and antibody levels reached the point of equivalence, large immune complexes formed and precipitated onto blood vessel endothelia, which triggered complement activation, neutrophil-induced blood vessel damage (leading to glomerulo-

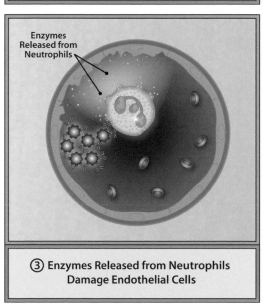

FIGURE 16.8. Immune complexes and blood vessel damage

Large immune complexes are insoluble and, as they form, deposit onto blood vessel walls. There, these complexes activate complement, which results in the appearance of C3b. Neutrophils bind to IgG and C3b and release destructive enzymes.

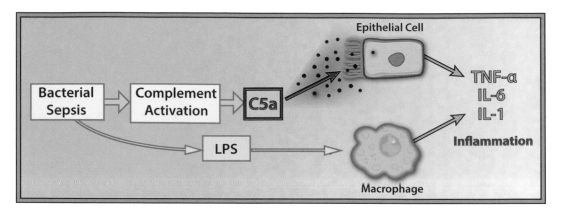

FIGURE 16.9. Actions of C5a

The C5a fragment of C5 stimulates a variety of cells, including epithelial cells, endothelial cells, macrophages, and neutrophils. The net result is a dramatic increase in inflammation. Both antigen–antibody complexes and Gram-negative sepsis activate complement and release C5a.

nephritis), and systemic anaphylaxis, including bronchospasms.

Because of this possibility, veterinarians routinely scratch-test animals to assess sensitivity before initiating antivenin therapy. Even after negative scratch testing, therapy with immunosuppressive drugs often accompanies antivenin therapy.

Type IV hypersensitivities

Type IV hypersensitivities are unique among the hypersensitivities, because T cells, not antibodies, are the underlying causes of the clinical manifestations. Because of this, type IV hypersensitivities take longer to develop. Type IV hypersensitivities have two major forms: DTHs and contact hypersensitivities. Clinically, contact hypersensitivities are the most relevant.

Th1 cells mediate DTH responses. A classic example is a positive response to tuberculin skin testing. CD8[+] Tc cells cause contact hypersensitivities, and the classic example is poison ivy dermatitis. In this case, oils (catechols) on the poison ivy leaf surface absorb into animal skin and attach to host proteins. Dogs' fur helps to protect them from this phase, but hairless areas, such as the abdomen, are very sus-

ceptible to poison ivy dermatitis. APCs ingest, process, and present the catechol-modified proteins to Th1 and Tc cells. Once they emigrate from the secondary lymphoid tissues, effector T cells migrate to the affected skin. On secondary exposure, local Th1 cells induce inflammation, and newly created Tc cells migrate to the inflamed areas to induce apoptosis in cells presenting catechol-modified peptides in MHC class I molecules.

In this case, the results are the classic rash, itching, and pain of poison ivy, but a number of other agents can—using the same means—also induce contact hypersensitivities. These agents include

- insecticides (flea collars, sprays, and dips);
- wood preservatives;
- carpet dyes;
- dermatology creams and ointments;
- leather;
- paints;
- some house plants.

Essentially, anything that contains chemicals capable of binding to and modifying skin proteins is a potential cause of a contact hypersensitivity.

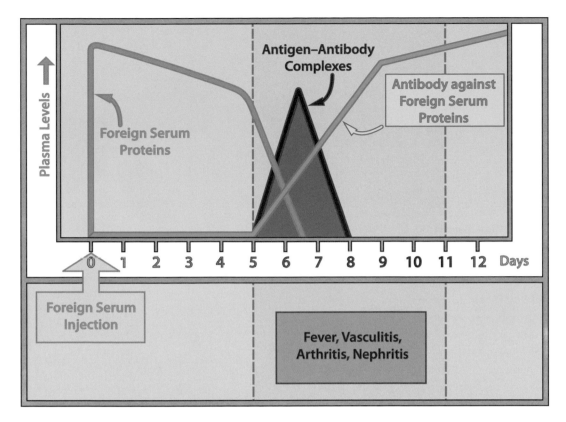

FIGURE 16.10. **Serum sickness**

After a first or subsequent injection of foreign serum, the host animal begins to make antibody to serum components. When, during the course of treatment, the antigens and antibodies reach the point of equivalence, large immune complexes form and precipitate onto blood vessel walls.

Type II Hypersensitivities and Autoimmune Diseases

Antibodies also mediate type II hypersensitivities, but these antibodies are different from those described earlier. The antibodies of type II hypersensitivities are anti-self antibodies, which makes most type II hypersensitivities autoimmune diseases. For example, immune-mediated hemolytic anemia (IMHA) is a relatively common disorder of dogs, especially in cocker spaniels, old English sheepdogs, poodles, and Irish setters. Its most common symptom is severe anemia. During IMHA, these animals' immune systems are making antibodies against their own RBCs. When those antibodies bind to their antigens, complement activates, enhancing both inflammation and phagocytosis by macrophages. Under these conditions, erythropoiesis cannot keep pace, and the red cell count drops dramatically.

As is the case with all autoimmune diseases, scientists do not know why animals with IMHA produce self-reactive antibodies. A complete list of animal autoimmune diseases would fill a page or two, and although some of these diseases are not antibody mediated (type II hypersensitivities), many are. Some examples include diabetes in dogs, cats, gorillas, horses, and others; systemic lupus erythematosus (SLE) and thyroiditis in dogs; and immune-mediated arthritis in many species.

Obviously, antibody-mediated autoimmune diseases come in many forms and are far from rare in animals. It is clear that both environmental and genetic factors (as demonstrated by breed predispositions in dogs) contribute to these diseases. In most cases, the essential genetic factors remain unknown. Also, with one exception (celiac disease), the environmental factors for autoimmune diseases of animals are unknown.

Other autoimmune diseases result from the actions of self-reactive T cells and still others from the combination of self-reactive antibodies and T cells. At the root of them all, though, are self-reactive Th or Tc cells. Self-reactive B cells by themselves do not pose an equivalent risk, because most B cells cannot proliferate or differentiate into antibody-secreting plasma cells without the aid of Th cells.

In chapter 9, we discussed central and peripheral means for maintaining tolerance. Obviously, these processes are inadequate to eliminate all autoimmune responses in animals. Recent evidence has suggested that certain types of self-recognition may even be essential for the maintenance of normal populations of T and other cells. Regardless of the mechanisms, some animals clearly retain the ability to respond to their own tissues.

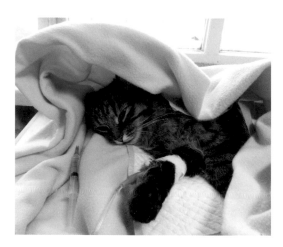

FIGURE 16.11. **Affected cat**

CLINICAL CORRELATION FOLLOW-UP

Student Considerations

FIV is a retrovirus that infects CD4⁺ T cells (Th cells). Months to years after exposure, most cats infected with FIV will develop chronic infections—fungal, bacterial, or viral infections. Eventually, these cats succumb to their infections (Figure 16.11). In effect, after FIV infection, the cats disappear and are replaced by a host of other living organisms. After reading this and preceding chapters, you should be able to explain the cause and results of this immunodeficiency disease.

Possible Explanations

FIV resides, among other places, inside the host cat's Th cells. After infection, the virus uses reverse transcriptase to make a DNA copy of the viral RNA. That DNA inserts itself into the nuclear genome inside of the infected cell, where it resides until an APC or some other factor activates that Th cell. After activation, using host ribosomes, bases, amino acids, and enzymes, viral DNA transcribes and new viruses assemble.

FIV is an enveloped virus, so it exits the cell along with a bleb of host-cell membrane and seeks other cells to infect. Cats' immune systems do respond to FIV infections, but during those responses, many Th cells die because infecting viruses have depleted essential factors. In addition, reverse transcriptase (unlike other polymerases) has no editing function, so mutations accumulate rapidly. As a result, an animal's immune system is aiming at a constantly moving target. Over time, FIV outstrips its host's immune system and destroys most of the CD4⁺ Th cells, and the cat becomes severely immune deficient. That acquired immunodeficiency leaves the cat at considerable risk. Opportunistic infections usually follow, and eventually the cat dies. Immune deficiencies, both congenital and acquired, put animals at great risk for debilitating and often fatal infections. Moreover, although FIV causes a pronounced immunodeficiency that results in major clinical symptoms, all immunodeficiencies are not so obvious. Because of the complexity of immune systems, even under the best of circumstances, immune competence varies among individual animals. Some of that variance is likely due to subclinical immunodeficiencies. The veterinarian's challenge is to be aware of that as part of diagnosis and therapy.

Gerald N. Callahan

The Immune System and Cancer

Chapter 17

10.5876_9781607322184.c017

CLINICAL CORRELATION: CANINE CANCER

In 2009, Hiroshi Ito and colleagues carried out a study of 65 dogs of various breeds, including Irish wolfhounds (Figure 17.1). Nineteen of the dogs were healthy, and the rest had tumors of various cell origins. During the course of the study, Ito collected blood from both normal and tumor-bearing dogs and analyzed his samples for several markers of immune status. Here is part of his description of his findings:

> We found that tumor-bearing dogs had higher leukocyte counts than normal dogs, and that the counts increased as the tumors became more advanced. In addition, tumor-bearing dogs had higher differential counts of leukocytes and ratios of inflammatory cells such as neutrophils, acidophils and monocytes. This finding was suggestive of an inflammatory reaction at sites of tumor development and infection resulting from decreased immunity. We also found that tumor-bearing dogs had lower counts of lymphocytes, CD3$^+$ T cells and CD4$^+$ T cells, than normal dogs, and that these counts became much lower as the tumor stage progressed.

> (Itoh et al., 2009, *Journal of Veterinary Immunology and Immunopathology,* 132: 85)

Clearly, tumor progression correlated with substantial changes in the immune status of these dogs. Why?

LEARNING OBJECTIVES

After reading this chapter, you should be able to

- understand the concept of immune surveillance;
- explain why tumor cells might trigger host immune responses;
- describe several ways in which host animals' immune systems may limit tumor-cell growth;
- describe several ways in which tumor cells may interfere with the development of host immune responses;
- explain the relationships between host animals and their tumors;
- describe the possible outcomes of host–tumor interactions.

BACKGROUND

In the early 1900s, Paul Ehrlich first proposed the idea that immune systems help to eliminate cancer cells. In fact, Ehrlich even went so far as

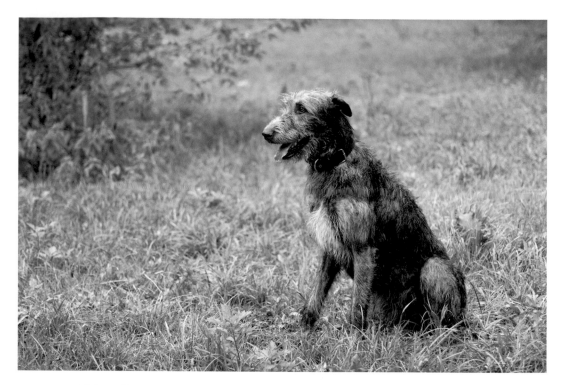

FIGURE 17.1. Irish wolfhound (© foaloce / Shutterstock)

Irish wolfhounds have an increased risk of developing osteosarcoma, the most common bone tumor in dogs.

to propose that cancer might have provided a part of the selective force that led to the evolution of modern mammalian immune systems. About sixty years later, Lewis Thomas and Sir MacFarlane Burnett formalized these concepts under the title "immune surveillance"—the idea that many tumors never fully mature into life-threatening cancers because of immune-mediated destruction of nascent malignancies.

The basic idea behind the theory of immune surveillance was the recognition that the driving force behind malignant transformation—the conversion of a normal host cell into one with the potential to invade and metastasize—is genetic mutation. At its root, cancer results from imbalances in the rates of cell division and cell death. When cells divide more rapidly than they die, tumors arise.

Decades ago, research on cancer cells demonstrated that it was possible to transfer some genes from cancer cells to normal cells and cause the normal cells to behave more like cancer cells. Because of their apparent role in the malignant phenotype, these genes came to be called oncogenes, after the process of oncogenesis (tumorigenesis). Other researchers found that some genes from normal cells could cause cancer cells to behave a little more like their normal-cell counterparts. These genes were named tumor-suppressor genes because of their ability to suppress the malignant phenotype.

It is now clear that all oncogenes have their counterparts in normal cells, and all tumor-suppressor genes have their counterparts in cancer cells. The normal-cell versions of oncogenes are called proto-oncogenes. The differences between proto-oncogenes and oncogenes are mutations that alter the amino acid sequences and functions of the protein products of these genes. Similarly, the tumor-suppressor genes of tumor cells no longer suppress malignancy because of mutations that produce proteins with altered amino acid sequences and altered function.

This is important for two reasons. In general, proto-oncogenes are genes that regulate cell division—genes that produce cell growth factors, receptors for growth factors, second messenger system proteins, and so forth—and tumor-suppressor genes, in general, are genes whose products are involved in regulating cell death and DNA repair. So, first of all, mutations in proto-oncogenes and tumor-suppressor genes provide the basis for the observed imbalance in the rates of cell division and cell death among tumor cells. Second, these genetic changes should produce altered self proteins—proteins with distinct amino acid sequences recognizably different from the corresponding normal cellular proteins. Also, these proteins arise in ways that potentially circumvent all of the normal means for generating self tolerance. There is, then, every reason to imagine that these altered proteins could potentially trigger protective immune responses, responses that could slow the division of or eliminate the newly transformed malignant cells.

These ideas suggested a most attractive new approach to cancer therapy. Most cancer therapies are relatively indiscriminate, killing many host cells as well as tumor cells. Immune attacks, however, are specifically focused on foreign elements of invading pathogens and do relatively minor damage to host cells. The combination of foreign proteins on and in tumor cells, coupled with the specificity and efficiency of immune responses, made cancer immunology a particularly attractive approach to tumor therapy.

This new approach, along with President Richard Nixon's declaration of the war on cancer in 1971 and the passage of the National Cancer Act, launched nearly innumerable research projects based on identifying and exploiting mutations in proto-oncogenes and tumor-suppressor genes as well as changes arising from any other sorts of mutations in cancer cells, with the hope that these proteins might provide new avenues for cancer diagnosis and therapy. Among all the research ignited by the National Cancer Act, cancer immunology became one of the fastest-growing fields.

By the early 1990s, though, little had come from this massive effort. In addition, the available evidence indicated that humans and other mammals with severe immune deficiencies, such as AIDS, developed only a few tumors during the course of their diseases, and those tumors were virus-induced tumors, such as Kaposi's sarcoma. These data did not fit very well with the idea of immune surveillance.

EVIDENCE THAT MAMMALIAN IMMUNE SYSTEMS AFFECT TUMORS

As a result, some tumor immunologists began to believe that, under normal circumstances, mammalian immune systems had little or no effect on developing tumors. However, by the mid-1990s, some investigators found that transplanted tumors grew more aggressively in mice treated with antibodies against IFN-γ. Similarly, mice that lacked parts of the IFN-γ receptor developed more tumors after exposure to chemical carcinogens. However, because these studies focused on chemical carcinogenesis, the relevance of immunity to spontaneously arising tumors remained open to question. To address this issue, other investigators showed that mice lacking either IFN-γ responsiveness or *RAG2* genes (which results in the absence of T, B, and NK T cells) developed more spontaneous tumors and more aggressive chemically induced tumors.

But what about therapy? Could the power and specificity of mammalian immune systems be exploited to change the course of developed cancers? In support of this idea, humans treated with immune stimulants, such as antibodies that block CTLA-4 (a receptor on T cells that, when coupled to its ligand, slows T-cell division), have been shown to have improved prognoses and fewer tumor recurrences.

The reality of tumor immunity seemed clear. How, then, were many tumors regularly avoiding host immune responses? It is now clear that some tumors actively subvert a host immune response. For example, at least some tumor cells are very poor presenters of endogenous antigens. The evidence for this came from experiments in which tumor cells transfected with a gene encoding a TAP were used to effectively immunize host animals against their own tumors, suggesting that recognizable tumor antigens (i.e., modified self proteins) were present all along but were not effectively presented in MHC class I molecules on the tumor cells.

Also, certain groups of γ/δ T cells have recently been shown to recognize and respond to proteins expressed by some tumor cells. These T cells not only bind to tumor-specific proteins and peptides but also can express MHC class II molecules and act as professional APCs in antitumor immune responses.

For decades, it had been apparent that many intrinsic factors acted to limit the development and spread of cancer cells. These factors included tumor-suppressor genes, proto-oncogenes, and the general processes of cellular senescence and apoptosis. But these studies of mice and humans with modified immune systems were among the first to demonstrate that host immune systems might produce tumor cell–extrinsic factors that limited the formation, proliferation, and spread of malignant cells.

Currently, most of the evidence in support of immune surveillance comes from studies on mice and humans. Therefore, the immediate relevance of these findings to veterinary medicine remains unclear. However, the general significance of these findings to cancer biology and therapy seems apparent, as does the possibility that, in the near future, these findings will affect both human and veterinary practices.

FIGURE 17.2. Effects of innate and adaptive immunity on tumor cells

TRAIL—TNF-related apoptosis-inducing ligand—is produced by neutrophils and stimulates apoptosis in tumor cells; NKG2D is an activating receptor on NK cells, powerful elements of innate and adaptive immunity; during tumor progression; TGF-β induces proliferation, angiogenesis, invasion, and metastasis and suppresses the antitumor immune response; indoleamine 2,3-dioxygenase (IDO) is produced by DCs and inhibits T-cell proliferation; galectin-1, produced by a variety of cells, inhibits T-cell activation; vascular endothelial cell growth factor (VEGF) is produced by some tumor cells and stimulates angiogenesis; programmed cell death ligand 1 (PD-L1), a B7 analogue produced by some macrophages, binds to a death receptor on T cells; myeloid-derived suppressor cells (MDSCs) are induced by tumor-secreted and host-secreted factors, many of which are proinflammatory molecules and inhibit both adaptive and innate immunity. (Adapted from Vesley et al., 2011, *Annual Review of Immunology,* 29: 235)

TUMOR–HOST INTERACTIONS

A general model of how host immunity may limit or even promote the development, proliferation, and spread of malignant cells is shown in Figure 17.2.

As shown in Figure 17.2, after malignant transformation many tumors may be eliminated by intrinsic mechanisms, but some are not. One of the roles of the immune system is to deal with these transformed and potentially deadly cells. These host responses involve a variety of both innate and adaptive mechanisms. Neutrophils, major elements of the innate immune response, produce TNF-related apoptosis-inducing ligand, which stimulates apoptosis in tumor cells; NK cells, important factors in both innate and adaptive immunity, have a cell-surface receptor called NKG2D. When bound to its ligand, this receptor stimulates strong NK-

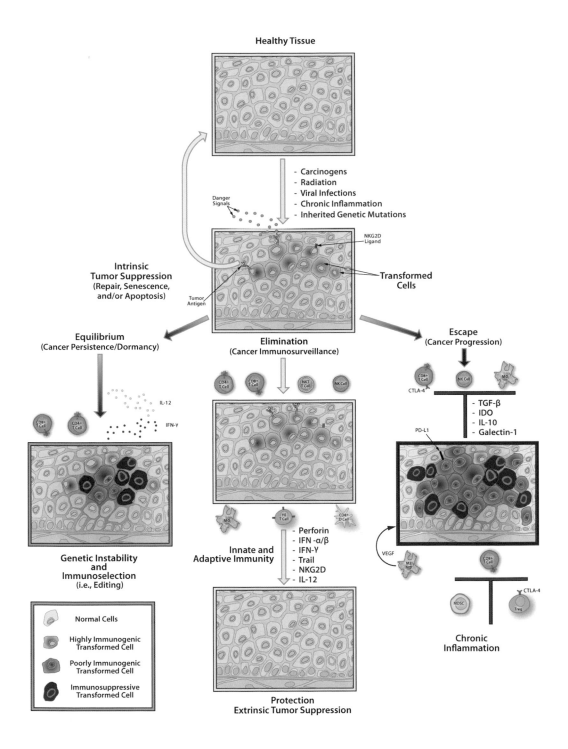

cell activation. Two NKG2D ligands, MICA and MICB, appear on many tumor cells.

Also as shown in Figure 17.2, CD8+ T cells (activated by tumor-specific peptides presented in MHC class I molecules on tumor cells) can, using perforins and granzymes, directly lyse tumor cells. Also, CD4+ T cells may be activated by APCs presenting tumor-specific antigens, and these T cells may give rise to any or all of the types of T cells and responses described in chapter 10. The activation of these cells may, then, lead directly or indirectly to destruction of the tumor. Particularly important among these T-cell effector functions is production of IFN-γ (also produced by NK cells), which is a potent stimulator of macrophages and immune functions in general. NK T cells are a heterogeneous group of T cells that recognize (among other things) modified self antigens presented by nonclassical MHC class I molecules on tumor and other cells. This aspect of innate immunity appears to be particularly important during tumor progression. CD8+ DCs cross-prime for presentations of endogenously derived peptides in MHC class II molecules, ensuring activation of a full range of adaptive immune responses against tumor cells.

Although an impressive arsenal of weapons may be activated by tumor cells, it is now clear that some tumor cells actively suppress host immune responses. TGF-β, produced during tumor progression, induces tumor cell proliferation and angiogenesis (providing essential blood vessels for tumor growth) and accelerates tumor invasion and metastasis. TGF-β also suppresses elements of the host antitumor immune response. Tumor-activated DCs, in nearby lymph nodes, secrete indoleamine 2,3-dioxygenase, which suppresses T-cell proliferation. Tumor cells also often secrete galectin-1, which stimulates angiogenesis, again causing nourishing blood vessels to grow into the developing tumor. In addition, some tumor cells secrete vascular endothelial cell growth factor, another stimulator of angiogenesis. Inhibitory factors, such as programmed cell death ligand 1, secreted by tumor cells may dramatically slow immune responses. Programmed cell death ligand 1 is an analogue of B7 and binds to CD28, but instead of stimulating proliferation as B7 sometimes does, PD-L1 induces T-cell apoptosis. Last, myeloid-derived suppressor cells, induced by some tumor cells as well as some host-derived inflammatory factors, suppress aspects of both innate and adaptive host immune responses.

OUTCOMES

In one sense, then, the relationship between host and tumor may be thought of as a competition in which the power and specificity of host immune mechanisms are pitted against the evasive tactics of the tumor cells. In some cases, host immunity may triumph and eliminate the tumor. In other instances, all the immune system can throw at tumors is only enough to maintain a sort of equilibrium, or steady state, in which tumor cells remain but do not progress. In these cases, tumor cells are not completely eliminated, but neither do they proliferate—unless something happens to alter the immune competence of the host animal or the nature of the tumor cells. Evidence of this steady-state situation comes from newer studies of longer-living AIDS patients in whom the frequency of spontaneous tumors is higher.

In still other instances, all the potential innate and adaptive mechanisms the immune system can muster are not sufficient to prevent tumor cell proliferation. In one sense, developing tumor cells are evolving. As immune mechanisms eliminate some tumor cells, others undergo mutations that allow them to escape both adaptive and innate responses either directly (e.g., by preventing tumor antigen presentation) or indirectly through production of factors that suppress immunity. These tumor cells, even in the face of a host immune response, may progress to local invasion and metastasis.

Under still other conditions, it appears that immune mechanisms, especially inflammation, may not only fail to prevent tumor cell growth and proliferation but actually, through the effects of proinflammatory factors (as described earlier), promote both. Here again, the outcome is progressively growing, potentially fatal tumors.

At this point, immunotherapy—with exogenous agents such as cells, antibodies, and immunoactivating cytokines—is the only option. Immunotherapy is the area in which cancer immunology is undergoing some of its most promising developments. Also, although most laboratory and clinical trials of immunotherapies have been limited to mice and humans, immunotherapy is the area of cancer biology most likely to affect veterinary practitioners soonest.

Currently, immunotherapy appears to be most effective in combination with chemotherapies and radiation therapies. Positive effects have been found using adoptively transferred tumor-specific T cells as well as passively transferred antibodies. Antibodies against immunosuppressive agents, such as CTLA-4 (mentioned earlier) are also improving prognoses, and tumor-specific vaccines, prepared from host tumor cells themselves, have slowed development of and in some cases eliminated established tumors. Thus, as of now, immunotherapy, especially in combination with other antitumor therapies, offers considerable promise. The potential outcomes of the interactions between developing tumors and host immune systems are shown in Figure 17.3.

That developing tumors face a variety of immune attacks now seems evident. Just how those immune mechanisms may be manipulated to change cancer prognoses for veterinary patients remains to be clarified, but the potential seems enormous.

CLINICAL CORRELATION: FOLLOW-UP

Student Considerations

We found that tumor-bearing dogs had higher leukocyte counts than normal dogs, and that the counts increased as the tumors became more advanced. In addition, tumor-bearing dogs had higher differential counts of leukocytes and ratios of inflammatory cells such as neutrophils, acidophils and monocytes. This finding was suggestive of an inflammatory reaction at sites of tumor development and

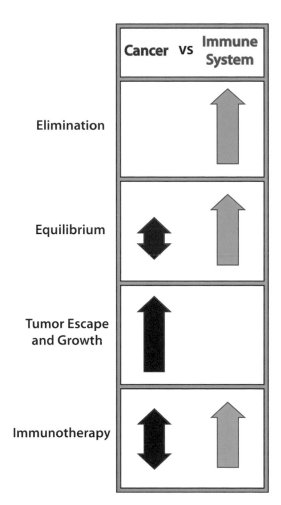

FIGURE 17.3. **Immunity and cancer**

Interactions between tumor cells and mammalian immune systems can have several outcomes. Immune attack may result in complete elimination of tumor cells (elimination) or an equilibrium state in which tumor cells remain but cannot proliferate (equilibrium), or in some cases, immune mechanisms, such as inflammation, may promote changes that favor tumor cell proliferation. Either because of such an immune assist or through mutation and evolution, the tumor cells may escape innate and adaptive immune responses and proliferate and metastasize (tumor escape and growth). Even after escape from immune surveillance, immunotherapeutic interventions may stimulate a new set of effective immune responses that eliminates the tumor.

infection resulting from decreased immunity. We also found that tumor-bearing dogs had lower counts of lymphocytes, CD3$^+$ T cells, and CD4$^+$ T cells than normal dogs and that these counts became much lower as the tumor stage progressed.

(Itoh et al., 2009, *Journal of Veterinary Immunology and Immunopathology*, 132: 85)

The important elements in the tumor-bearing dogs here are the elevated white cell counts and the increase in these counts as the tumors progressed. Also, the increases in neutrophils and acidophils over the course of the study are noteworthy. Finally, the decreases in CD3- and CD4-bearing lymphocytes are important to consider. Also, not included in this excerpt, Itoh et al. described elevations in the levels of TGF-β in the tumor-bearing dogs.

Possible Explanations

The results of the study described at the beginning of this chapter are clouded by the fact that the tumor-bearing dogs were receiving antitumor therapy throughout the course of the study. Those therapies might have been responsible for some of the observed differences in immune status between the experimental and control groups. Regardless, on the basis of the material presented in this chapter, several intrinsic factors may have played a role in generating the observed changes.

The elevated white cell counts and the increase in those elevations over the course of the study suggest inflammation. As the authors suggested, some of the elevation might be due to infections as a result of tumor-induced immune suppression. Tumors themselves, however, are also often inflammatory, and that inflammation may serve to promote tumor cell proliferation. Elevated neutrophil and monocyte counts are also compatible with increased inflammation. CD3 is present on all T cells, and CD4 is characteristic of Th cells. Decreases in T-cell numbers during tumor progression fit with tumor cell production of T-cell toxins, such as PD-L1 (mentioned earlier). Last, elevations in TGF-β could be both immunosuppressive (because of the known roles of TGF-β in establishing immune tolerance) and supportive of angiogenesis (providing additional blood vessels to support continued tumor growth and accelerating tumor invasion and metastasis).

The host–tumor relationship is complex, and the role of host immunity in tumor progression is still unfolding. It is clear, though, that a full understanding of veterinary oncology must include an appreciation of the role and nature of host antitumor immune responses as well as the means by which tumor cells may manipulate those antitumor responses.

CLINICAL CORRELATION: TRANSFUSION REACTIONS

In several clinical situations, the transfusion of blood or blood products is critical to saving the life of an animal (Figure 18.1). Most of these situations involve the loss of one of the major blood components (RBCs, platelets, or clotting factors), either directly by hemorrhage or indirectly in an immune-mediated process (such as IMHA or immune-mediated thrombocytopenia). In the case of anemia, the animal presents with hypoxia. Animals with thrombocytopenia and coagulation factor deficiencies typically present with bleeding, either as microhemorrhages (petechiae) or overt hemorrhages.

One of the most direct ways to restore normal blood oxygen levels and coagulation factors is to transfer blood from another animal. However, as we have discussed, several factors, including MHC molecules, present immunological barriers to tissue (including blood) transfer between individuals.

Even though RBCs do not express either MHC I or MHC II molecules, they do express a less diverse group of potentially antigenic molecules called erythrocyte or red blood cell (RBC) antigens, which are genetically determined immunogenic markers on the surface of erythrocytes. If an animal with a particular (RBC antigen) blood type is transfused with blood of a different type, a severe immune transfusion reaction can develop.

Each species has several defined groups of erythrocyte antigens, and these groups differ in

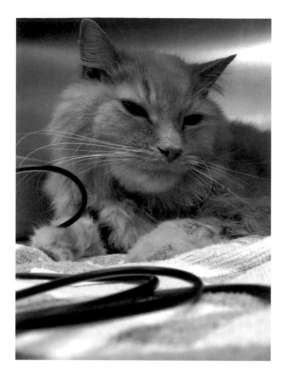

FIGURE 18.1. **Domestic short hair cat receiving a blood transfusion (photograph courtesy of Dr. Josiane Houle)**

their antigenicity. In light of all we have covered in this book, one would anticipate that, once an animal is transfused with foreign RBCs, the transfused animal would produce antibodies against the foreign RBC antigens.

Because of this, one might also expect that animals receiving their second or third transfusion would be at greater risk of a transfusion reaction—antibodies binding to RBC antigens, destruction of RBCs, and inflammation (much as in hypersensitivity reactions). That certainly does happen, but surprisingly many animals are at considerable risk of transfusion reactions even when they receive blood for the first time. These adverse reactions happen because many animals have naturally occurring antibodies to RBC antigens called alloantibodies, which are literally antibodies of one individual that react against the alloantigens (homologous molecules) of another individual of the same

species. During transfusions, these alloantibodies attack the donor's RBCs and also initiate inflammatory and other reactions.

In dogs, the most important antigens involved in blood group incompatibility are the dog erythrocyte antigen 1 (DEA-1) group. Untransfused dogs do not have immunologically significant amounts of naturally occurring alloantibodies to DEA-1, but when exposed to DEA 1.1–positive blood cells, dogs lacking DEA 1.1 will produce large amounts of anti–DEA 1.1 antibodies, which on secondary challenge will agglutinate and lyse RBCs. Other blood groups exist in dogs but are less commonly implicated in clinical disease (Table 18.1).

In cats, there are three main blood groups, types A, B, and AB, and a newly recognized group, Mik (Table 18.1). Unlike dogs, some untransfused cats have naturally occurring anti–blood group antibodies. Specifically, even before a primary transfusion, cats that have type B blood produce high titers of anti-A antibodies. For this reason, cats with type B blood will have a strong transfusion reaction to type A blood on the first transfusion, reportedly with as little as 1 ml of type A blood. Why type B cats naturally produce anti-A antibodies is unknown.

Horses have a number of different erythrocyte antigens, with types Aa, Qa, and to a lesser degree Ca being the most clinically important (Table 18.1). Unlike dogs and cats, blood transfusion of horses is less common. The most important disease process that arises from blood group–antigen incompatibilities in horses is neonatal isoerythrolysis. During delivery of a first blood group–incompatible foal, some of the foal's blood enters the maternal circulation and induces an immune response that produces anti–blood group antibodies. After a second pregnancy with an additional blood group–incompatible foal, the mare's colostrum will contain large amounts of anti–blood group antibodies. After nursing, those antibodies can enter the foals' circulation and induce what is essentially a transfusion reaction that is potentially life threatening.

TABLE 18.1. Major known blood groups in dogs, cats, and horses

Blood groups	Genetics	Naturally occurring alloantibodies	Special considerations
Dog			
DEA 1.1, DEA 1.2	Codominant RBC positive or negative for each 1.1 and 1.2	None	Most important group in transfusions as causes acute hemolytic reaction
DEA 3	DEA 3 (dominant) and null	In some DEA-3 negative, but results in delayed RBC survival	Rare 23% of greyhounds are DEA 3–positive
DEA 4	DEA 4 (dominant) and null	None	~98% of dogs in the United States are DEA 4–positive
DEA 5	DEA 5 (dominant) and null	In some DEA-5 negative, but results in delayed RBC survival	10% of dogs; as many as 30% of grey hounds are DEA 5–positive
DEA 7	DEA 7 (dominant) and null	None	99% of dogs in the United States are DEA 6–positive
Dal		None	100% of the general dog population; absent from Dalmatians
Cat			
A	AA, Aa^{ab}, or Ab*	Low anti-B titer	~90% of cats are A positive
B	Bb	High anti-A titer	Agglutinins and hemolysins resulting in severe transfusion reaction
AB	a^{ab}b or a^{ab}a^{ab}	Most have no alloantibodies	Rare
Mik		Mik-negative cats might have alloantibodies to Mik	Most type A cats are Mik-positive
Horse			
EAA group Aa most important		Minute amounts	Aa important in neonatal isoerythrolysis
EAC group		Anti-Ca in horses that are C-negative	
EAQ group Qa most important		Minute amounts	Qa important in neonatal isoerythrolysis

*The A allele in cats is dominant to b and a^{ab} (Bighignoli et al., 2007, *BMC Genetics* 8: 27).

Cattle, sheep, and pigs have a wide variety of erythrocyte antigens, so many that blood typing and transfusions are rarely practical. Because of the nature of veterinary care in these species, transfusions are rare anyway, so transfusion reactions are generally not an issue. If a transfusion is warranted, cross-matching is a more practical way to avoid transfusion reactions.

LEARNING OBJECTIVES

After reading this and the preceding chapters, you should be able to

- describe the immunological principles underlying antibody-based tests;

- list and describe different examples of antibody-based tests used in veterinary diagnostics;

- describe and explain blood typing and cross-matching;

- describe the diagnostic tests available for diagnosing immunodeficiencies;

- describe the diagnostic tests available for diagnosing autoimmune diseases.

PRINCIPLES OF ANTIBODY-BASED TECHNIQUES

As discussed in previous chapters, the humoral immune response generates antibodies (Igs) that bind to antigens with great specificity. Aside from protecting animals from invading microbes, the humoral immune systems of domestic species can be exploited to produce antibodies for laboratory research and diagnostic tests. Indeed, many of the immunologic techniques used in diagnostic veterinary medicine use antibodies purposefully raised against particular antigens.

Because it is easy to collect and often contains disease-defining antibodies and antigens, serum is the most common diagnostic sample used. Serum is the portion of the blood left after clotting (which removes platelets, white blood cells, RBCs, and clotting factors). For the most part, antibody-based diagnostic tests either directly detect antigens of infectious agents (bacteria, virus, or parasite) or detect the presence of antibodies that recognize a particular antigen (such antibodies are evidence of a previous exposure to the relevant antigen or pathogen).

Many different types of antibody-based diagnostic tests are available, but they all require two components: (1) antibodies that are specifically generated to detect a particular antigen (e.g., antibodies may be generated that recognize the Fc portion of a dog Ig [antiglobulins], which are useful when one is trying to detect dog Ig in serum) and (2) a method of "visualizing" the antibody–antigen reactions. For visualization, radioisotopes, fluorescent dyes, or enzymes are commonly coupled to the diagnostic antibodies, or the precipitation of antibody–antigen complexes is observed.

Generating Antibodies: Polyclonal and Monoclonal Antibodies

Two common methods are used to generate antibodies for research and diagnostic purposes.

Both begin with inoculation of animals with the antigen of interest. The simplest method produces a mixture of Igs that detect multiple epitopes of an antigen. This mixture is often referred to as polyclonal antibodies (usually antisera; *anti* for antibodies in *sera*). The term *polyclonal* means that these preparations contain antibodies derived from many different clones of B cells. The alternative method uses cell-culture techniques to propagate a single B cell clone from an immunized animal. These monoclonal antibodies are homogeneous and react strongly with only a single antigenic epitope.

PRODUCTION OF POLYCLONAL ANTIBODIES

Polyclonal antibodies are sera from animals immunized with a relevant antigen (e.g., a molecule from distemper virus) plus an adjuvant (Figure 18.2). Beyond their diagnostic potential, antisera are also important in a process known as passive transfer. In certain situations (e.g., after a snakebite), an animal may have an immediate need for antibodies (in this case, antivenom antibodies). Infusion of antisera can provide a source for these antibodies. In some cases, antisera can be used directly as diagnostic tools.

Because raw serum is full of antibodies directed against hundreds of different antigens (not just the immunizing antigen), an additional purification step is often used to purify only antigen-specific antibodies from antisera. This purification step involves passing the serum through a solid-matrix column with linked specific antigen molecules. Under these conditions, the unwanted serum products, including the nonspecific antibodies, pass freely through the column. However, the antibodies that bind the specific antigen remain in the column. Using a variety of techniques, the antigen-specific antibodies can then be recovered as purified polyclonal antibodies. Such antigen-specific, polyclonal antibodies usually still contain a mixture of different Ig isotypes that bind multiple antigenic epitopes.

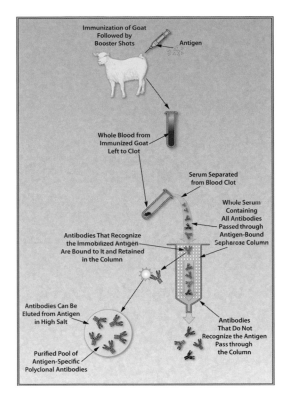

FIGURE 18.2. Production and purification of polyclonal antibodies

After injection of canine distemper virus antigen, a goat mounts an adaptive humoral immune response. The polyclonal antibodies produced are then harvested from the goat's serum as an antiserum and purified using antigen–matrix columns. These antibodies can then be used in diagnostic tests for canine distemper virus infections.

Although the production of polyclonal antibodies is relatively simple and cheap, it requires the continued use of animals and, because of animal-to-animal and batch-to-batch variations, the products are not always predictable. However, many antigen-specific reagents (especially anti-Igs) are still produced this way.

PRODUCTION OF MONOCLONAL ANTIBODIES

Monoclonal antibodies are products of a single B-cell clone (hence the term *monoclonal*) and thus contain only a single type of antibody

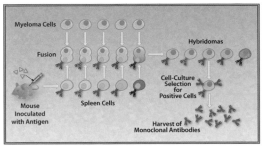

FIGURE 18.3. Production of monoclonal antibodies

A mouse is inoculated with an antigen and mounts an acquired humoral immune response. B cells from the mouse's spleen and lymph node are harvested and fused with immortal neoplastic plasma cells (myeloma cells), which produces an immortal B cell that produces an antibody directed against a single antigen epitope.

---

strongly reactive with a single antigenic epitope. Monoclonal antibodies provide a consistent and predictable source of antibodies for antibody–antigen assays.

As with the production of antisera, the generation of monoclonal antibodies starts with the inoculation of an animal (typically a mouse, rat, or rabbit) with a specific antigen along with an adjuvant (Figure 18.3). After the animal mounts a humoral immune response to the antigen, B cells are isolated from the lymph nodes, spleen, or both. In tissue culture, these B cells are fused with myeloma cells (an immortal neoplastic plasma cell line) to produce antibody-secreting, hybrid, immortalized cells called hybridomas. Hundreds, sometimes thousands, of these hybridomas must be screened to identify the ones that secrete antibodies reactive with the antigen of interest. Once one such hybridoma is identified, this immortalized plasma cell can be propagated and grown in cell-culture media indefinitely, producing copious quantities of a monoclonal antibody. This process produces antibodies of a particular isotype directed toward a single epitope of one antigen, and the process does not require the continuing use of animals.

Detecting Antibody–Antigen Reactions

Generating polyclonal or monoclonal antibodies reactive with specific antigens is only half the battle when designing antibody-based diagnostic tests. The other half involves designing a means to detect these antibodies when bound to their specific antigens. Tests that exploit antigen–antibody reactions can either directly detect the bound antibody or indirectly detect it through the use of secondary antibodies. In both direct and indirect reactions, labels such as enzymes (including horseradish peroxidase or alkaline phosphatase) or fluorescent or radioactive chemicals allow for detection of the specific antigen–antibody interaction.

Antibody–enzyme complexes typically react with a substrate to produce a detectable color change or chemiluminescence detectable using either photometric methods or photographic film. When illuminated, fluorescent chemicals attached to antibodies produce a specific wavelength of light observable with a fluorescent microscope or fluorometer. Because of the dangers of working with radioactive chemicals, radioactive labeling has become less common.

Specific Techniques

Enzyme-linked immunosorbent assays

Enzyme-linked immunosorbent assays (ELISAs) use antibodies or antigens labeled with an enzyme that, when combined with a substrate, causes a detectable color change. The color change is typically measured using a spectrophotometer. In recent years, fluorescent labels have also been used in ELISAs. ELISAs are typically performed in multiwell plates (Figure 18.4), allowing for multiple simultaneous assays.

In veterinary diagnostics, ELISAs are most commonly used to detect antibodies in the serum of an animal to quantitate that animal's immune response to a given pathogen. Usually, a variant of the ELISA known as the indirect ELISA is involved. Several other varia-

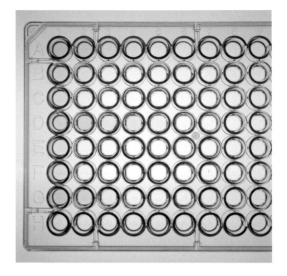

FIGURE 18.4. A multiwell plate for ELISA

The wells that are yellow have detectable antibody; wells that are clear do not. The yellow color is produced by an enzymatic reaction mediated by the enzyme attached to the binding antibody.

tions of ELISA are also available, including a sandwich ELISA (so named because it features an antigen sandwiched between two different antibodies).

Indirect ELISAs detect antibodies in the serum of an animal. For example, if a veterinarian wanted to know whether a dog has Lyme disease, he or she could use an ELISA to detect serum antibodies against the Lyme disease bacterium *Borrelia burgdorferi*. In this example, antigens of *B. burgdorferi* are bound to the base of the microwells. The dog's serum is then added to the wells, and if the dog has antibodies against *B. burgdorferi*, those antibodies will bind to the bacterial antigens. Unbound antibodies are washed away, and the bound antibodies are detected using a second antibody labeled with a marker, such as the fluorescent streptavidin phycoerythrin. The amount of fluorescence emitted from the well reflects the amount of specific antibody in the dog's serum (Figure 18.5). ELISA tests are available for a multitude of different infectious agents important in vet-

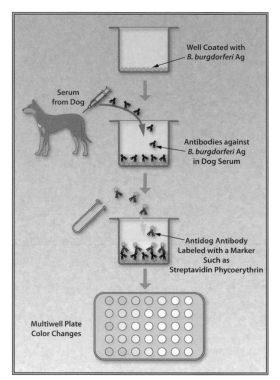

FIGURE 18.5. **Indirect ELISA to detect serum antibodies against *B. burgdorferi* (Lyme disease)**

B. burgdorferi antigen is coated on the bottom of a well. The dog's serum is added, and if the dog has antibodies against *B. burgdorferi*, they will bind. The antibodies are then detected using fluorescently labeled antidog antibodies.

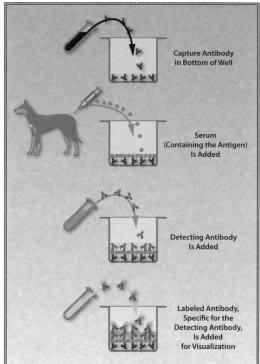

FIGURE 18.6. **Sandwich ELISA to detect antigens in the sera**

A monoclonal antibody to the antigen of interest (the capture antibody) adheres to the bottom of the well. The serum (containing the antigen) is added, and any specific antigen present binds to the capture antibody. A second antibody to the antigen (the detecting antibody) is added and reacts with bound antigen. A third, labeled antibody specific for the second antibody, allows for visualization of the bound complex.

erinary practice, including many for use in the clinic or field.

Indirect ELISAs are useful for detecting pathogen-specific antibodies in patients' sera, but there are times when one may wish, instead, to know the amount of antigen in patient sera. This amount can be determined using a variant of the ELISA technique called the sandwich ELISA. In a sandwich ELISA, an antibody against the test antigen (the capture antibody) is attached to the bottom of microwells in a microtiter plate. If the specific antigen is present, it will bind to the capture antibodies attached to the well after addition of serum (or other body fluid samples). A second antibody (the detecting antibody) that recognizes a different epitope on the same antigen is then added to detect bound antigen. Finally, a third antibody, labeled with an enzyme or fluorescent probe, is added to detect the second antibody (Figure 18.6). If all three antibodies used in this test are from different species, then no possibility exists that the tagged third antibody will give a false-positive result.

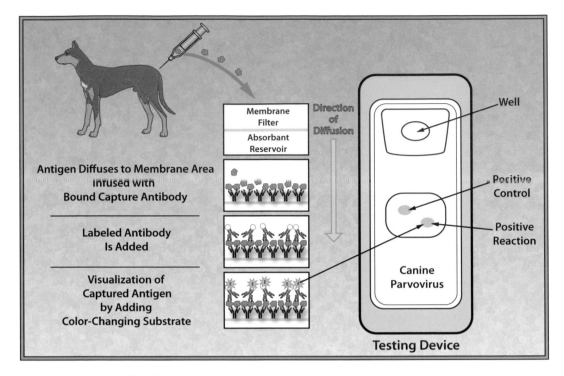

FIGURE 18.7. Immunofiltration technique

This technique is a variant of a sandwich ELISA using antibodies attached to a membrane to which the sample containing the antigen is added. A second labeled antibody forms the sandwich, which is detected by an enzymatic change in color of an added substrate. The right side of the figure depicts a well where the serum is added and two dots in the detection panel. One dot represents the test's positive control; the second dot is the positive reaction to the antigen (in this case, canine parvovirus).

Using the sandwich ELISA technique, several companies have also developed "pet-side" in-clinic assays, including the immunofiltration technique (used in SNAP ELISAs) and lateral flow tests (also called immunochromatography).

The immunofiltration technique is similar to a standard sandwich ELISA. An immobilized capture antibody attached to a membrane binds to the antigen in the sample (blood, urine, or serum), and a labeled detector antibody is added to measure the bound first antibody (Figure 18.7).

The lateral flow test uses the capillary action of a porous strip dipped into a sample. The sample (containing the antigen) flows along the strip until it comes to a line of unbound detector antibody (i.e., typically labeled with colloidal gold to produce a pink color or colloidal selenium to produce a blue color). The antibodies and antigens form complexes that continue to flow up the porous strip until the complexes come to a line of bound capture antibodies that "capture" the antigen–antibody complex, forming a sandwich among the detector antibody, antigen, and capture antibody. This reaction is visible as a line (pink or blue) on the strip. Negative samples will not bind the detector antibody, so no line will be produced (Figure 18.8).

IMMUNOBLOTTING

Immunoblotting (also called western blotting) is a common method used in research, but

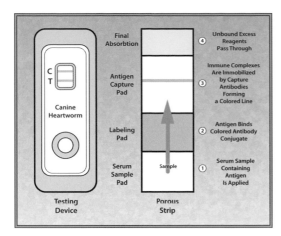

FIGURE 18.8. **Lateral flow test**

A porous strip is dipped into the antigen-containing sample and flows up the strip by capillary action. If antigen is present, it will bind to an unbound detector antigen, forming an antigen–antibody complex that will bind farther up the strip to a bound capture antigen to produce a colored line or dot.

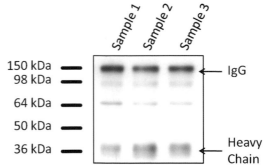

FIGURE 18.9. **Image of an immunoblot designed to detect IgG**

The line corresponding to the 150-kDa marker is IgG.

because of the length of time required to process immunoblots, it has limited use in routine diagnostics. Before immunodetection, protein mixtures (from serum or a tissue homogenate) are first separated on the basis of size using polyacrylamide gel electrophoresis, which stretches the sample over the length of the gel and in the process separates the proteins, with small proteins migrating farther than larger ones. It essentially produces a bar code–like pattern, with every band or stripe being composed of a different-sized protein. The separated proteins are then transferred from the gel onto a nitrocellulose membrane (which tightly binds to protein bands). Areas of the membrane that do not bind a protein from the sample are blocked with a generic irrelevant protein (such as albumin or casein) so they cannot further bind protein nonspecifically. To detect which band contains the protein of interest, the membrane is incubated in a solution containing an antibody (either monoclonal or polyclonal) raised against the particular protein of interest. The mem-

brane is washed and then placed into a solution containing a secondary antibody. The secondary antibody is an Ig able to bind the primary antibody (antiglobulin) and is coupled to a detection enzyme (usually horseradish peroxidase or alkaline phosphatase). These enzymes can convert a substrate into a colored product that stains the membrane or creates light (chemiluminesence) that can be detected on film or by a camera (Figure 18.9).

IMMUNOFLUORESCENT MICROSCOPY

Another antibody-based technique used in both diagnostics and research is immunofluorescent microscopy. This method of immunodetection uses fluorescently labeled antibodies to highlight protein antigens in cells or within histological sections (in situ). Immunofluorescence involves a primary antibody raised against the protein of interest, in combination with a secondary antibody (anti-Ig or anti–primary antibody) carrying a fluorescent tag. The fluorescent tag, when illuminated by a particular wavelength of light, emits light at a longer wavelength. Through the use of specific filters within the microscope, only the wavelength that is emitted by the given fluorescent tag on the secondary antibody passes through to the

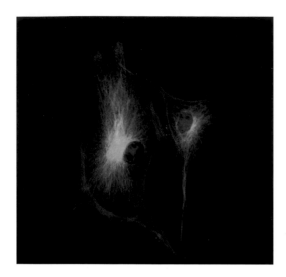

FIGURE 18.10. **A merged image generated by immunofluorescent microscopy showing the locations of two different cytoskeletal proteins (actin and tubulin) within two macrophages. Actin is shown in green, tubulin is shown in red and nuclei are stained blue.**

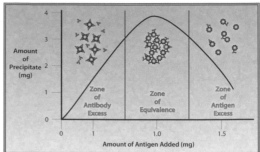

FIGURE 18.11. **Precipitation of antigen and antibody complexes in a precipitation assay exploits the concentrations of antibody and antigen (zone of equivalence) to measure their relative quantities (titers)**

eyepiece, giving an image corresponding to the location of the protein of interest.

One advantage of this technique is that, using multiple antibodies tagged with different fluorochromes, multiple proteins can be identified in a single tissue sample. By overlaying these images, it is possible to locate the various proteins relative to one another (Figure 18.10).

PRECIPITATION ASSAYS

As you have learned in previous chapters, under the right conditions antibodies and antigens can form immune complexes consisting of aggregates of antigen cross-linked with antibodies. Usually, these complexes are small and quickly disposed of via Fc receptors on RBCs, but, as with type III hypersensitivities, under the right conditions these antigen–antibody complexes can form large insoluble aggregates. In vivo, such aggregates can be life threatening, but in vitro, the complexes can form visible precipitates useful for diagnostic analyses.

To form a precipitate, the antigen of interest must be multivalent (i.e., contain multiple epitopes to which multiple antibodies can bind), and the relative proportions of antibodies and antigen must be optimal (the zone of equivalence). With too much of either antigen or antibody, the precipitate will not form (Figure 18.11).

A type of precipitation test used in diagnostics follows the diffusion of antigen and antibody within agar and is aptly called an immunodiffusion assay. Usually, the antigen and antibodies (typically serum samples or antisera) are deposited in separate wells in an agar gel. As the two proteins diffuse toward each other, their interactions form a visible area of antigen–antibody precipitate—the zone of equivalence. Where the precipitate forms relative to the antigen and antibody wells gives an indication of the concentration (or titer) of antibody, relative to the antigen (Figure 18.12). A specific example of an immunodiffusion assay is the Coggin's test. The Coggin's test is specifically used to detect antibodies against equine infectious anemia virus (a negative Coggin's test is required for horses to travel into or between most states in the United States).

Radial diffusion is a variant of the multiwell immunodiffusion assay, where either the antigen or the antiserum is incorporated into

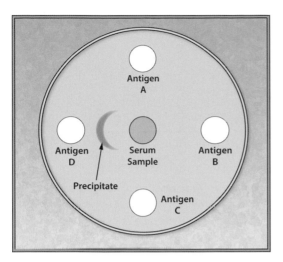

FIGURE 18.12. Example of an agar gel immunodiffusion assay (also known as Ouchterlony double immunodiffusion assay)

Here, an unknown serum sample is being tested to see whether it contains antibodies that recognize four different antigens (A, B, C, and D). In this example, a precipitate forms in the zone of equivalence between the serum well and the well that contains antigen D, indicating that the serum contains antibodies that can recognize and precipitate antigen D, but not antigens A, B, and C.

the agar itself and forms a precipitate with the test serum or antigen deposited in a well. The precipitate forms in a circle around the well as the sample diffuses out. The area of the circle is proportional to the concentration of the relevant antigen or antibody within the sample.

FLOW CYTOMETRY

Flow cytometry is a powerful technique used to characterize cells in fluid. In veterinary diagnostics and research, it is most frequently used to quantitate different immune cells in blood samples. Most basic complete blood cell counts in veterinary laboratories are now analyzed using flow cytometers and are typically done on unstained blood. Further information can be gathered by labeling immune cells with fluorescently labeled antibodies, which are increasingly being used in veterinary diagnostics to diagnose hematopoietic cancers (leukemia and lymphoma).

Flow cytometry analyzes a stream of cells suspended in fluid by passing them through a laser beam one by one. As the cells pass, they scatter the laser light in characteristic ways. There are two detectors. The first detector is positioned in line with the laser beam and detects light (forward scatter) blocked by a cell as it passes by. A second detector perpendicular to the laser detects light (side scatter) deflected by the cell.

In basic terms, forward scatter measurement gives information about the cell's volume (size), and side scatter measurement gives information about the cell's internal complexity (granularity and nuclear conformation). This information is then used to characterize immune cells in the blood. For instance, lymphocytes are small (low forward scatter) and have simple round nuclei with no cytoplasmic granularity (low side scatter). Neutrophils, however, are large (high forward scatter) and have complex nuclei and a high degree of cytoplasmic granularity (high side scatter; Figure 18.13).

Using forward and side scatter, flow cytometers characterize and count the various types of cells in a blood sample, providing very accurate information on the circulating population.

Both in research and in the diagnosis of hematopoietic neoplasms, more detailed information is needed on the immune cells than the cytometry of unstained cells provides. For example, one might want to know not only whether lymphocytes are present but also whether they are CD4+ or CD8+ lymphocytes. For these sorts of analyses, forward and side scatter data are combined with analyses of fluorescent antibodies attached to white blood cells. For example, CD4 is unique to Th lymphocytes, so fluorescently tagged anti-CD4 antibodies can be used to label those cells. As the cells pass by the laser beam, the fluorescent tags on the antibodies are excited by light,

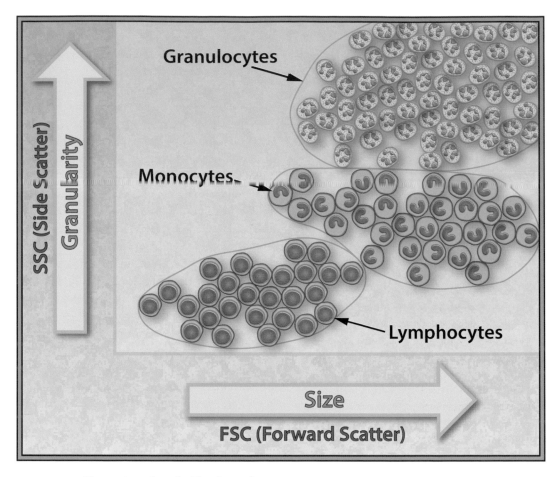

FIGURE 18.13. **Flow cytometry of a blood sample**

Large cells produce high forward-light scatter (size). Cells with a high degree of internal nuclear complexity and cytoplasmic granularity produce high side-light scatter.

causing the antibodies to fluoresce and emit a certain wavelength of light. This emitted light is concurrently detected along with forward and side scatter data (Figure 18.14).

IMMUNOHISTOCHEMISTRY

Immunohistochemistry is used principally on formalin-fixed tissues collected at necropsy or biopsy and submitted for histopathologic evaluation. It has become one of the most powerful tools pathologists have for identifying and characterizing tissues, structures, and infectious agents in tissue samples. Immunohistochemistry uses thin sections of formalin-fixed,

paraffin-embedded tissues; thin sections of frozen tissues; or cells attached to slides.

When antigen-specific antibodies labeled with an enzyme (typically a peroxidase) are added to the section or slide, they bind to any antigens present. The peroxidase is then visualized by a chemical reaction that produces a brown or red color change. The advantage of immunohistochemistry is that it does not disrupt the tissue architecture, so the location of the antibody reflects the in situ location of the antigen.

In veterinary diagnostics, immunohistochemistry is most often used to categorize tumors and to identify or detect the presence of infectious agents. Immunohistochemical analyses of

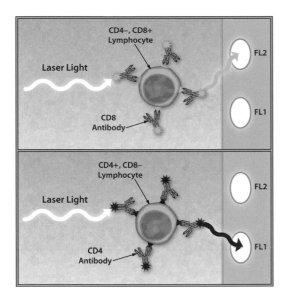

FIGURE 18.14. Flow cytometry using fluorescently labeled antibodies to detect subsets of cells

Anti-CD8 fluorescent antibodies bind to CD8$^+$ lymphocytes and not to CD4$^+$ lymphocytes. Anti-CD4 fluorescent antibodies bind to CD4$^+$ lymphocytes and not CD8$^+$ lymphocytes. FL2 detects the green fluorescence, and FL1 detects red fluorescence.

tumors use antigens unique to certain cell types. For instance, CD3 is unique to T cells and characteristic of T-cell lymphomas. Similarly, von Willebrand factor is characteristic of endothelial cells in hemangiosarcomas (Figure 18.15A).

Immunohistochemistry is especially useful for detecting infectious agents when no suitable sample is available for more traditional bacteriological, virological, or parasitological analyses. Immunohistochemical analysis uses peroxidase-labeled antibodies specific for an antigen unique to a particular organism. These types of analyses also pinpoint the tissue and cellular localization of pathogens (Figure 18.15B).

DIAGNOSIS OF BLOOD TYPE INCOMPATIBILITIES

One of the best ways of preventing or anticipating transfusion reactions due to blood type incompatibilities is to know the recipient's and donor's respective blood types and their compatibility. This can be achieved through blood typing or by cross-matching the patient's and donor's blood.

Blood Typing

Blood typing uses monoclonal or polyclonal antibodies that recognize the common erythrocyte antigens of a species. When these antibodies bind to the blood-type antigens on the surface of erythrocytes, they can start to cross-link these cells and cause them to visibly agglutinate. If the erythrocytes do not express that particular antigen, the antibody will have no effect on them. Thus, by simply observing whether erythrocytes agglutinate on a slide or in a test tube in the presence of a particular anti–erythrocyte antigen antibody, one can determine an animal's blood type. For example, to type feline blood, a drop of blood is added to a card or gel containing anti-A antibodies. When the erythrocytes are added, the anti-A antibodies bind to any erythrocyte A antigens present and cause the blood to clump or agglutinate, confirming the blood to be type A. If type B blood (that does not possess an A antigen) is added, the anti-A antibodies will not bind and thus no agglutination will take place. Similarly, blood added to a card with anti-B antibodies will cause agglutination of type B blood but not of type A (Figure 18.16).

With the increased use of blood products and blood banks in veterinary practice, blood typing for dogs and cats has become more available—offered in specialized diagnostic laboratories as well as in-clinic tests. Commercial, in-clinic blood group tests are available for canine DEA 1.1 and feline groups A, B, and AB. For horses, cattle, and other production species, blood typing is specialized and needs to be referred to a diagnostic laboratory. Currently, three methods are available for the in-clinic typing of blood: blood typing cards, typing gel, and membrane dipstick.

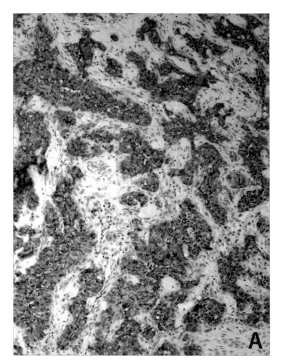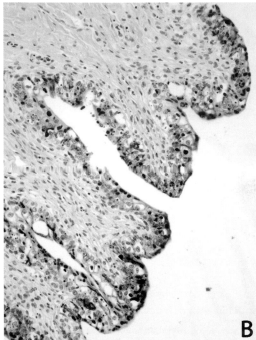

FIGURE 18.15A–B. **Immunohistochemical staining of a hemangiosarcoma using anti–von Willebrand factor antibodies (panel A) and transitional epithelium containing canine distemper virus (panel B) (courtesy of Dr. E. G. Clark)**

Antigen-specific antibodies labeled with horseradish peroxidase allow for visualization of antigens in situ as brown-colored areas on the cells.

Panel A shows anti–von Willebrand factor antibodies adhered to the cells of a hemangiosarcoma. Panel B shows anti–canine distemper virus antibodies attached to ureteral transitional epithelium. Inside the cytoplasm of many of these cells (and in some of the nuclei) are dark brown–staining aggregates of the canine distemper virus.

BLOOD TYPING CARDS

Blood typing cards are available for dog DEA 1.1 and cat AB blood group typing. These cards have monoclonal antibodies to DEA 1.1 or to feline A, B, and AB lyophilized in the card wells. Blood positive for the antigen being tested will bind to the lyophilized antibodies and visually agglutinate (Figure 18.17).

TYPING GEL

Typing gels use monoclonal antibodies suspended in gel matrices in test tubes. Blood placed at the top of the tube is allowed to filter through the gel. If the erythrocytes possess the antigen that the monoclonal antibody is directed against, the erythrocytes will agglutinate (similar to that on the cards). Agglutinated erythrocytes move less easily through the gel than individual erythrocytes and become suspended. Thus, negative samples pass through the entire tube unimpeded and end up forming a button on the bottom, whereas positive blood remains as a suspended line halfway up the tube (Figure 18.18). Typing gels are available for DEA 1.1 typing in dogs and A, B, and AB typing in cats.

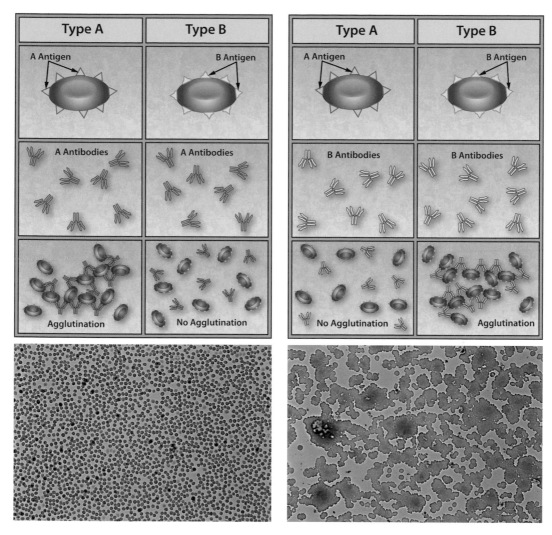

FIGURE 18.16. Blood typing in a cat

In a cat with type A blood, type A antibodies will bind to the A antigen on the surface of the erythrocytes and cause visible agglutination. Cats with type B blood will have no agglutination with a type A antibody. Similarly, type B cats will have agglutination using type B antibodies, and type A cats will have no agglutination. The images in the lower panels are of blood smears with no agglutination (left) and with agglutination (right).

MEMBRANE DIPSTICK

The membrane dipstick method uses monoclonal antibodies bound to lines on a dipstick. The dipstick is dipped into diluted blood, and erythrocytes move up the dipstick by capillary action. As the blood moves up the dipstick, antigen-positive RBCs will bind to the monoclonal antibodies at the corresponding line. Antigen-negative blood will move through, leaving no line (Figure 18.19).

Crossmatching

A more thorough and versatile method for testing for blood compatibility is a cross-match. Even when the blood types of two animals are

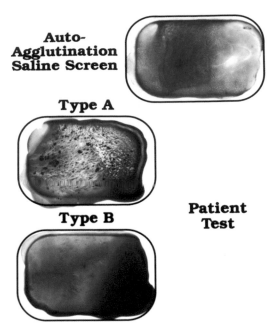

FIGURE 18.17. **Typing card for feline blood**

Macroscropic agglutination can be observed in the upper box labeled *Type A,* which is absent from the box labeled *Type B,* indicating that the A antigen is present on the erythrocytes and B antigen is absent. This cat has type A blood.

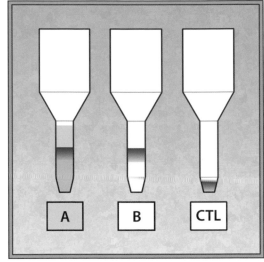

FIGURE 18.18. **Typing gel for feline blood typing**

The suspension of erythrocytes halfway down the tube indicates the presence of that antigen on the surface of the erythrocyte. The blood from the cat in this image has both A and B antigens and thus has an AB blood type.

known to be the same, a transfusion reaction (mediated by other types of antibodies) may still occur. For example, a DEA 1.1–positive dog may be transfused with DEA 1.1–positive blood but still have an immune reaction because of DEA 1.2 dissimilarity. A cross-match allows the veterinarian to prescreen for transfusion reactions before a transfusion and is a much more accurate determinant of compatibility. The disadvantage of cross-matching is that a compatible cross-match does not mean that both the donor and the recipient animals necessarily have the same blood type, just that no antibodies to that blood type are currently circulating. Thus, the recipient animal may still be susceptible to a transfusion reaction the next time that blood is used. Some dogs are also still susceptible to delayed and nonhemolytic transfusion reactions. Thus, a cross-match is necessary before any transfusion to prevent a transfusion

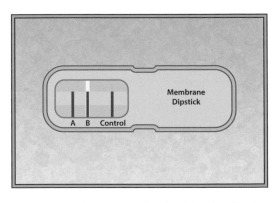

FIGURE 18.19. **Membrane dipstick blood typing for a cat**

The red lines on the stick correspond to spots where erythrocytes have bound to monoclonal antibodies. The first line, "A," contains anti-A antibodies; the second line, "B," contains anti-B antibodies; and the third line is the control. Thus, this cat has an AB blood type.

	Red Blood Cells from Individuals of Type		
Serum from Individuals of Type	A	B	AB
A Low-Titer Anti-B Antibodies	No Agglutination	Weak Agglutination	Weak Agglutination
B High-Titer Anti-A Antibodies	Agglutination	No Agglutination	Agglutination
AB	No Agglutination	No Agglutination	No Agglutination

FIGURE 18.20. Cross-matching of feline A, B, and AB blood types

The areas shaded in pink indicate cross-reactions evidenced by agglutination. In the white boxes, no cross-reaction occurs, indicating that the blood would be safe to transfuse.

reaction, and even then the cross-match is a relatively insensitive test and may fail to detect circulating antibodies in certain circumstances. In ruminants, in which a wide variety of erythrocyte antigens exist, a cross-match is generally more practical because it does not require specific antibodies raised against each of the many erythrocyte antigens.

A saline-agglutination cross-match is the most common type of cross-match performed in veterinary laboratories. Both major and minor cross-matches are performed. Briefly, EDTA-anticoagulated blood from both the donor and the recipient are individually centrifuged, and the erythrocytes removed. The centrifuged erythrocytes from both the donor and the recipient are then washed and resuspended in saline. Serum samples (which contain possible alloantibodies) from both the donor and the recipient are also obtained. The sera and erythrocytes are then mixed in a major and minor cross-match. In a major cross-match, the recipient's serum is mixed with the donor erythrocytes. This process will determine whether the recipient has any significant alloantibodies to the blood about to be transfused. In a minor cross-match, the donor's serum is mixed with the recipient's erythrocytes, which will assess for alloantibodies in the donor's serum that may lyse the recipient's erythrocytes. Both the major and the minor cross-matches are examined for hemolysis and agglutination, both macroscopically and microscopically (Figure 18.20). Some laboratories further evaluate the cross-match by adding in the Coombs reagent (see Diagnosis of Autoimmunity section), which allows a more sensitive assessment of bound antibodies than the cross-matches alone.

In the circumstance of equine neonatal iso-erythrolysis (a type of blood incompatibility between a mare and a newborn foal, in which antibodies against the foal's erythrocytes are in the colostrum; see the Clinical Correlation section at the beginning of this chapter), the cross-match method has been modified into the "jaundiced foal agglutination test." Here, instead of mixing the foal's erythrocytes with the mare's serum, the foal's erythrocytes and the mare's colostrum are mixed.

DIAGNOSIS OF IMMUNODEFICIENCIES

In general, immunodeficiencies are diagnostic possibilities when animals present with chronic or recurrent infections or infections with unusual agents that do not typically cause disease in an immunocompetent animal. Getting a precise diagnosis of immunodeficiency and where the defect lies can be difficult, but several tests can aid in the diagnostic process.

Serum Immunoglobulin Quantification

Several Ig deficiencies are relevant to veterinary medicine, including congenital hypo- or agammaglobulinemia (reduced or no Igs of all classes), selective IgG deficiencies in cattle and cavalier King Charles spaniels, selective IgA deficiencies in German shepherds, and acquired failure of passive transfer in foals. To diagnose these diseases, veterinarians need to be able to quantitate the total and relative quantities of Igs in the serum.

The radial immunodiffusion assay is the most common assay used to quantitate IgG, IgM, and IgA in sera. This assay is a precipitation test (see Principles of Antibody-Based Techniques section) in which anti-Igs against species-specific IgG, IgM, and IgA antigens are incorporated into an agar plate. The patient's serum is added into wells in the plate, where it then diffuses into the antiglobulin-impregnated gel. At the zones of antigen–antibody equivalence, immune complexes precipitate and form a visible ring. The width of the precipitation compared

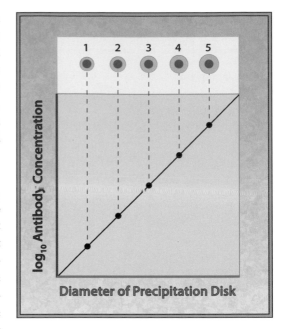

FIGURE 18.21. Radial immunodiffusion to measure serum levels of Igs

The greater the antibody concentration in the serum, the larger the ring formed around the well.

with a standard curve provides a measure of the serum concentration of a particular Ig (IgG, IgM, or IgA; Figure 18.21).

Phenotypic Analysis of Lymphocytes

Immunodeficiencies related to leukocyte abnormalities usually manifest as either a deficiency of a cell type or a deficiency of cell-surface receptors. In general, if a deficiency of a specific leukocyte type is present, it is apparent in a routine complete blood cell count and bone marrow examination. Morphologic abnormalities in some immunodeficiency diseases, such as Chediak-Higashi syndrome, are apparent on blood smears. Lymphocyte subset deficiencies are detected in flow cytometric analysis using antibodies reactive to specific lymphocyte-subset markers (CD4[+] T cells, CD8[+] T cells, and B cells).

Other Immunodeficiency Tests

BLAD and canine leukocyte adhesion deficiency (CLAD) result from inadequate levels of cell-surface proteins CD11b and CD18. Without these cell-surface proteins, neutrophils cannot adhere to endothelial cells and exit blood vessels. In diagnostic tests, this deficiency is apparent as the inability of neutrophils to adhere to plastic surfaces or to ingest particles opsonized with the complement component C3b. These deficiencies can also be diagnosed by flow cytometry using anti-CD11b and anti-CD18 markers.

DIAGNOSIS OF AUTOIMMUNITY

Antinuclear Antibody Test

The antinuclear antibody test (ANA) measures circulating antibodies against nuclear antigens. Although a number of different autoimmune diseases can produce antinuclear antibodies, the ANA test is most commonly used to establish the diagnosis of SLE—in veterinary medicine, a disease seen almost exclusively in dogs. SLE is one of the more enigmatic immune-mediated diseases in veterinary species, principally because its clinical presentation is so variable. Animals with SLE produce antibodies reactive with a number of self-antigens, including components of the animals' nuclei. These components include antibodies that bind to DNA, ribosomes, RNA, ribonuclear proteins, and components of the nuclear membrane. A strongly positive ANA reaction is useful in diagnosing this disease.

The ANA test is an indirect immunofluorescence assay (see Immunofluorescent Microscopy section). Serial dilutions of patients' sera are added to specialized plates with attached nucleated cells. If the dog has circulating antibodies reactive with nuclear antigens, the antibodies will bind to the nuclei of the cells on the bottom of the plates. The serum samples are then removed from each plate and replaced by an antidog IgG antibody tagged with a fluores-

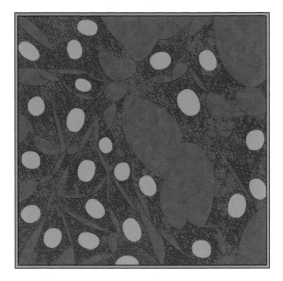

FIGURE 18.22. ANA positive serum sample

The nuclei of the test cells fluoresce green because of bound serum ANA antibodies. This fluorescence is a diffusely strong reaction and would be supportive of a diagnosis of SLE if other clinical features were present.

cent marker. The antidog IgG antibodies will bind to any antibodies bound to the cell nuclei in the plates and will fluoresce green when the appropriate wavelength of light is shone on them (Figure 18.22). Different patterns of staining may be seen, including diffuse, speckled, rim, or nucleolar staining. It appears that diffuse (homogeneous) staining may be linked to the diagnosis of SLE, whereas speckled staining is more often seen with SLE-related diseases. Regardless, the diagnosis of SLE on the basis of a positive ANA should be made with caution. ANA positivity is associated with a wide range of other autoimmune diseases and can be weakly positive in normal animals or animals with chronic disease.

A variety of secondary assays are available to detect the specific autoantibodies present in the serum of ANA-positive dogs (remember, the ANA test measures a variety of different autoantibodies that may target DNA, histones, RNA, ribonuclear proteins, or nuclear membranes). These tests include ELISAs, immunodiffusion

Coombs Test

The Coombs test is one of the oldest tests for immune-mediated diseases in existence. It was developed in 1945 by Cambridge immunologist Robin Coombs and his colleagues. The Coombs test, used in the diagnosis of IMHA, detects antibodies directed against erythrocytes. Depending on the reagents used, the Coombs test can also measure cell-surface–bound complement proteins. There are two Coombs tests that differ in their mechanism of action: the direct Coombs test (also known as a direct antiglobulin test, or DAT) and the indirect Coombs test (also known as an indirect antiglobulin test). The DAT detects antibodies and complement directly bound to erythrocytes, and the indirect antiglobulin test detects antibodies that are unbound and is more useful in antibody screening for blood transfusions and cross-matching. Both tests work on the principle that antibodies bound to erythrocytes can result in their agglutination. This agglutination can be visualized, which is the end result of this test. (One of the interesting effects of IMHA is that erythrocytes can also autoagglutinate. When autoagglutination occurs, the Coombs test is no longer useful.)

In IMHA, most of the Igs that bind to the erythrocyte surface are IgG and, less commonly, IgM. Many of these are incomplete antibodies. They sensitize and coat the erythrocyte and target it for premature destruction (by antibody-dependent complement activation, particularly C4 and C3) but do not cause agglutination. Polyreactive Coombs reagents in veterinary medicine commonly contain anti-IgG, anti-IgM, and anti-C3 antibodies.

In the direct Coombs test (direct antiglobulin test), erythrocytes are first washed in saline (to remove unbound antibodies and complement that may produce false-positive reactions). The antiglobulin reagent is added to the washed erythrocytes and then incubated. If the erythrocytes are coated with bound IgG, IgM, or C3, the added antibodies will bind to the erythrocytes and cause agglutination. The agglutination can be evaluated macroscopically and microscopically as a positive reaction (Figure 18.23).

The indirect Coombs test (indirect antiglobulin test) differs from the direct Coombs test because it measures serum levels of anti erythrocyte antibodies. In this test, erythrocytes are washed and incubated with the test serum (in the case of neonatal isoerythrolysis, washed erythrocytes would be from the foal and the test serum would be from the mare). If anti-erythrocyte antibodies are present in the serum, they will bind to the RBCs. The second step of the indirect antiglobulin test is much like the direct antiglobulin test. After incubation, the erythrocytes are washed again (to remove any unbound antibody) and are incubated with an antiglobulin antibody (e.g., in a horse, an antihorse IgG). If antibody binds during the first step, the anti-IgG antibody will bind in the second step and cause agglutination of the erythrocytes (Figure 18.23).

Antiplatelet Antibody Test

Immune-mediated thrombocytopenia is a common disease in dogs. Although a number of tests for this disease have been developed, the most sensitive (but least specific) are the direct immunofluorescent assays. These assays use platelet-rich plasma (prepared from an EDTA anticoagulated sample) to obtain purified platelets. The platelets are then washed and incubated with a fluorescein-labeled monoclonal antibody against canine or feline IgG. If autoantibodies are bound to the platelets, the anti-IgG fluorescently labeled antibody will bind to them and can be detected by flow cytometry. This test detects only Igs bound to platelets. It cannot differentiate which antigen the antibody is binding to and cannot differentiate auto-

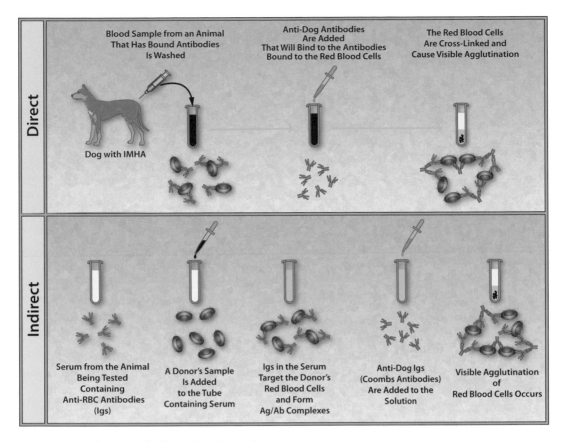

FIGURE 18.23. Direct and indirect Coombs tests

In the direct Coombs test, erythrocytes from an animal that has bound antibodies are washed. Antidog antibodies are added that will bind to the antibodies already bound to the erythrocytes, which will cross-link the erythrocytes and cause visible agglutination. In the indirect Coombs test, the antibodies to erythrocytes are not bound to the erythrocytes but are free in the serum (usually in the serum of a blood donor). The washed erythrocytes are added to the serum and antibodies are allowed to bind to the erythrocyte. Antidog antibodies are then added that will cross-link any bound antibodies and cause visible agglutination.

immune thrombocytopenia from other causes of immune-mediated thrombocytopenia.

Antithyroglobulin Autoantibody Test

Hypothyroidism is a common endocrine disorder of dogs. Approximately 50 percent of canine hypothyroidism cases result from lymphocytic thyroiditis, the pathogenesis of which is generally thought to be the autoimmune destruction of the thyroid gland. In some dogs with hypothyroidism, serum antibodies react-ing with thyroglobulin are observed. Antithyroglobulin antibody assays are available in some laboratories to aid in the diagnosis of hypothyroidism. This test is based on an indirect ELISA (see Principles of Antibody-Based Techniques section), in which the patient's diluted serum is added to purified canine thyroglobulin bound to the bottom of plastic wells in a microtiter plate. If autoantibodies to thyroglobulin are present in the serum, they will bind to the thyroglobulin. A second antidog IgG with an alkaline phosphatase tag is added to allow visualization of any bound antithyroglobulin IgG. Although a positive result here is indicative of an autoimmune disease, because of the potential importance of autoimmune T cells, a negative result does not rule out autoimmunity.

CLINICAL CORRELATION: FOLLOW-UP

Student Considerations

After reading this chapter and knowing that an animal can develop an acquired immune reaction against a blood type different from its own, you should be able to predict what will happen when incompatible blood is transfused. You should also be able to select two pretransfer diagnostic techniques you could use to avoid this reaction.

Possible Explanations

Transfusion reactions are similar to any immune response to a foreign antigen, in that antibodies bind to foreign antigens, in this case on the surfaces of erythrocytes. As mentioned earlier, these antibodies can be naturally occurring alloantibodies (i.e., present before the animal has any exposure to the foreign blood type, e.g., in cats) or created during a previous exposure to incompatible blood type (in an acquired immune reaction, e.g., in dogs and horses). Regardless of whether the antibodies are naturally occurring or generated, they are generally either IgG or IgM. Clinically, transfusion reactions can be either hemolytic transfusion reactions (in which transfused erythrocytes are destroyed) or nonhemolytic transfusion reactions.

Hemolysis of erythrocytes occurs as the result of antibodies binding to the surfaces of erythrocytes and can be either intravascular (occurring within the lumen of blood vessels) or extravascular (mostly in the spleen and liver). The severity of the hemolysis depends on the type of antibody and its ability to fix complement. For example, the binding of the hemolysin antibody to an erythrocyte surface activates the complement system, which results in

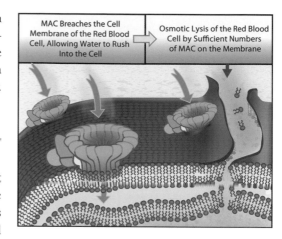

FIGURE 18.24. **MAC formed by complement proteins lysing a red blood cell (RBC)**

the production of a MAC. The MAC literally punches holes in the membrane of the erythrocyte, resulting in lysis, usually intravascularly (Figure 18.24).

Antibodies, either alone or in combination with complement proteins, can also opsonize erythrocytes. Bound antibodies or complement fragments (C3b) then enhance the phagocytosis of RBCs by leukocytes (principally macrophages). Either intravascular or extravascular hemolysis can result.

Hemolytic transfusion reactions can be acute or delayed. Acute hemolytic transfusion reactions typically occur within twenty-four hours of transfusion and result from preformed serum antibodies in the recipient animal, against the donor blood type (either naturally occurring, as in type B cats, or as a result of prior transfusion). Delayed transfusion reactions occur more than twenty-four hours after the transfusion and typically result from an acquired immune response to a previously exposed blood antigen in which the reactive alloantibody was weak or in very low concentrations. Alternatively, delayed reactions can occur several weeks after transfusion—sufficient time for the body to mount a new humoral response against the transfused erythrocytes. Typically, delayed

Inside the figure:
MAC Breaches the Cell Membrane of the Red Blood Cell, Allowing Water to Rush Into the Cell

Osmotic Lysis of the Red Blood Cell by Sufficient Numbers of MAC on the Membrane

transfusion reactions are clinically milder than acute reactions.

Less common are the nonhemolytic transfusion reactions. The two basic types of nonhemolytic transfusion reactions are fever and allergic (hypersensitivity type I) reactions. Fever reactions are typically thought to be due to the recipient's alloantibodies reacting to leukocyte antigens (rather than erythrocyte antigens) on the donor's lymphocytes, granulocytes, or platelets. Cytokines in the plasma of the donor's blood, believed to be released from platelets and leukocytes during storage, are also blamed. Allergic responses are thought to be associated with an immune reaction resulting from preformed recipient antibodies reactive with donor plasma proteins. As with most allergic (type I hypersensitivity) reactions, the onset of an allergic reaction is acute (within fifteen minutes of transfusion) and can include urticaria, pruritis, and erythema as well as vomiting, nausea, diarrhea, abdominal pain, and anaphylactic shock.

Although not all reactions can be predicted, particularly those that are nonhemolytic, most transfusion reactions can be anticipated and often avoided by performing blood typing or cross-matching.

acute-phase protein (APP). A serum protein whose abundance is altered in response to an acute inflammatory process.

adaptive immune system. A collection of organs and cells involved in generating adaptive immune responses, that is, those that involve T-helper and cytotoxic T cells.

adjuvant. Any of a number of chemical compounds or components of microorganisms that nonspecifically enhance innate and adaptive immune responses. Adjuvants are common components of vaccine formulations.

affinity maturation. The increase in antibody affinity to antigen observed during secondary and subsequent adaptive immune responses.

alternative pathway of complement activation. A pathway that leads to the activation of the complement cascade in response to the spontaneous deposition of complement (C3) on non host surfaces.

anaphylatoxin. Products of complement activation (mostly C3a and especially C5a) that cause local or systemic anaphylaxis—inflammation locally and anaphylactic shock systemically.

antibody-dependent cell-mediated cytotoxicity. NK cell–mediated killing of target cells decorated with antibodies.

antibody titer. The dilution at which a solution of monoclonal or polyclonal antibody generates one-half its maximum activity.

antigen-presenting cells (APCs). Cells capable of presenting antigenic peptides to T-helper cells.

antigens. Molecules that can stimulate an immune-specific adaptive response.

antiglobulin. *Anti*bodies that bind to another immuno*globulin* (antibody), for example, an antidog IgG.

antiserum. Blood serum that contains polyclonal antibodies.

basophils. Granulocytic white blood cells of low abundance thought to assist in the coordination of inflammation in a manner similar to that of mast cells.

B-cell receptor (BCR). Antigen-specific receptor molecule found on B cells. It is composed of two heavy chains and two light chains (an antibody molecule plus a membrane anchor) and Igα and Igβ, two molecules involved in signal transduction.

B cells. Bone marrow–derived lymphocytes that express antigen-specific receptors (BCRs) and, under appropriate circumstances, differentiate into antibody-secreting plasma cells.

blood typing. A group of techniques that determine the antigenic blood type of an animal before transfusion, reducing the risk of a transfusion reaction.

bovine leukocyte adhesion deficiency (BLAD). An autosomal recessive disease that affects Holstein cattle as a result of a mutation in the gene that encodes β_2-integrin (CD18), which results in an inability to effectively recruit leukocytes to areas of inflammation.

bronchus-associated lymphoid tissues. Secondary lymphoid organs found in the mucosal epithelia of the bronchi and the site of adaptive immune responses in the lungs.

B7. A molecule found on APCs. B7 comes in two forms, B7.1 and B7.2, also known as CD80 and CD86. When B7 on the APC binds to CD28 on T cells, it provides the second signal necessary for the activation of T cells.

β2-microglobulin. A small protein that associates with MHC class I α chains to form complete MHC class I molecules.

cathelicidins. Cationic antimicrobial peptides with an α-helical structure. Cathelicidins are secreted by certain immune and epithelial cells and contribute to the killing of engulfed microbes within the phagolysosomes of phagocytes.

CD28. Found on T cells; interacts with B7 to create the second signal necessary for activation of T cells.

central tolerance. Elimination of self-reactive lymphocytes in the thymus.

chemokines. Cytokines that induce chemotaxis in nearby cells.

chemotaxis. The directed movement of a cell in response to a chemical gradient (typically toward a chemoattractant such as a chemokine).

classical pathway of complement activation. A pathway that leads to the activation of the complement cascade in response to antigen–antibody complexes.

class II–associated invariant chain peptide (CLIP). Class II–associated invariant chain binds to nascent MHC class II molecules to prevent peptide binding in the endoplasmic reticulum. CLIP is the last portion of the invariant chain that remains bound until MHC class II molecules are in the endosomal compartment.

clonal expansion. The antigen-induced expansion of a single T or B cell into a large clone of identical cells.

colony-stimulating factors (CSFs). Produced by various cells, CSFs are cytokines that induce proliferation and differentiation of certain hematopoietic cells.

colostrum. Milk produced by mammals early in lactation that has high concentrations of maternal antibodies.

complement. A group of about sixteen plasma proteins arranged in a biochemical cascade that can be triggered in response to microbial surfaces or immune complexes. Activation of the complement cascade can result in the release of inflammatory mediators, opsonization of activating surfaces, and the direct lysis of microbes.

complementarity-determining regions (CDRs). Portions of antibody molecules that bind directly to antigens. The character of the CDRs determines the complementarity of the fit between antigen and antibody.

complement receptors. A group of proteins expressed on the surface of a variety of cells that can bind complement bound to surfaces or antigen complexes.

conjugate vaccines. Vaccines composed of two or more molecules conjugated together to enhance immunogenicity.

C-reactive protein. An APP that can bind to the surface of a pathogen or a damaged host cell, where it can activate complement or directly act as an opsonin.

cross-match. A technique that mixes the blood and serum of donor and recipient animals before a blood transfusion to predict a transfusion reaction. A major cross-match tests for alloantibodies in the recipient's serum by mixing the recipient's serum with the donor erythrocytes. A minor cross-match tests for alloantibodies in the donor's serum by mixing the donor's serum with the recipient's erythrocytes.

cross-presentation. The process whereby extracellular antigens taken up by dendritic cells (which would normally be presented on MHC II molecules) are processed and presented in MHC I molecules.

cytokines. Cell-derived soluble molecules that act on the cells that produce them and on other receptive nearby cells.

damage-associated molecular patterns (DAMPs). Molecular structures indicating tissue injury that are released from damaged and necrotic host cells, which can be detected by the innate immune system.

defensins. Cationic antimicrobial peptides with a β-pleated sheet structure. Defensins are secreted by certain immune and epithelial cells and contribute to killing of engulfed microbes within phagolysosomes of phagocytes.

delayed-type hypersensitivities. Hyperreactivities that involve T-helper or cytotoxic T cells but not antibody molecules and take days to develop.

dendritic cell. Any one of several cell types with a dendritic morphology that play important roles in antigen handling and antigen presentation during immune responses.

D-gene segments. DNA segments present in the TCR β gene and Ig H-chain gene families that add to the variety of TCRs and BCRs of T and B cells.

eicosanoids. A group of signaling molecules derived from the oxidation of fatty acids. Both leukotrienes and prostaglandins are eicosanoids that play important roles in mediating inflammation.

enzyme-linked immunosorbent assay (ELISA). A technique that uses antibodies labeled with enzymes, radioisotopes, or fluorescent markers to detect an antigen or, indirectly, an antibody.

Variants include the indirect ELISA and sandwich ELISA.

eosinophils. Granulocytic white blood cells important principally for defense against parasites such as helminths.

fever (pyrexia). The elevation of the core body temperature as a result of a higher-than-normal thermoregulatory set point within the anterior hypothalamus. Fever is commonly induced through the systemic release of proinflammatory cytokines (e.g., tumor necrosis factor–α and interleukin-1).

flow cytometry. A technique that characterizes cell types in a fluid by passing a thin stream of cells by a laser.

γ-interferon. A major proinflammatory cytokine.

granzymes. Serine proteases found in the cytoplasmic granules in cytotoxic T and NK cells that induce apoptosis once delivered to target cells.

gut-associated lymphoid tissues (GALT). Secondary lymphoid structures found in the mucosal epithelia of the gastrointestinal tract and the sites of gut-associated, secondary immune responses.

haptens. Small molecules that by themselves are not immunogenic but may, when coupled with other molecules, induce specific immune responses.

hematopoiesis. The production in the bone marrow of red blood cells, platelets, and white blood cells from hematopoietic stem cells.

high endothelial venules (HEVs). Specialized postcapillary venous swellings found in secondary lymphoid tissues. These structures are the sites where lymphocytes exit the blood and move into secondary lymphoid tissues and the lymphatic system.

humoral immune response. An adaptive response characterized by the production of antibodies.

hypersensitivities. Adaptive immune response directed toward innocuous substances such as self or pollen that induce damage to the host.

IgA. An isotype of antibodies characterized by α heavy chains. IgA appears in both monomeric (in the blood) and dimeric (mucosal secretion) forms.

IgE. An isotype of antibodies characterized by ε heavy chains and of particular importance in allergies and immunity to parasites.

IgG. An isotype of antibodies characterized by γ heavy chains. It is the most common antibody in many mammals.

IgM. An isotype of antibodies characterized by μ heavy chains. It is the predominant antibody in most primary adaptive immune responses.

IL-1. Any one of a family of cytokines that are strongly proinflammatory and some of which induce fever.

IL-2. A cytokine that stimulates T-cell division and is necessary for the development of most adaptive immune responses.

IL-3. A cytokine that stimulates the proliferation of bone marrow progenitor cells.

IL-4. A cytokine that stimulates B-cell division and induces production of certain immunoglobulin isotypes.

IL-6. A major proinflammatory cytokine.

IL-10. A cytokine with diverse effects in immunoregulation and inflammation. It suppresses the expression of T-helper 1 cytokines, MHC class II antigens, and costimulatory molecules on macrophages. It also extends B-cell survival, proliferation, and antibody production.

IL-12. A cytokine that stimulates the differentiation of naive T cells into T-helper 1 cells. It can also stimulate inflammation by enhancing production of IFN-γ and tumor necrosis factor–α from T and NK cells.

IL-17. A cytokine that is a powerful stimulator of inflammation.

immediate-type hypersensitivities. Hypersensitivities mediated by antibodies, including type I, type II, and type III hypersensitivities.

immune complex diseases. Type III hypersensitivities involving large antigen–antibody complexes that precipitate onto vessel walls and activate complement.

immune mediated. Any of a series of effects that result from the actions of innate or adaptive immune responses.

immune-stimulatory complexes. Combinations of antigens and other molecules (such as lipid micelles) that enhance the host immune response.

immunoblotting (western blotting). A technique that detects specific proteins in a fluid. Proteins are first separated using gel electrophoresis and are then transferred onto membranes, where they are incubated with labeled antibodies that can bind and identify specific proteins.

immunodiffusion assay. A technique that determines antibody or antigen concentrations in a fluid by diffusing them through an agar gel and detecting their zones of precipitation.

immunogens. Molecules or molecular complexes that induce immune responses.

immunoglobulin (Ig). Antibody molecules.

immunohistochemistry. A technique used to detect antigens of cells or infectious agents in a histologic section using labeled antibodies.

inflammasome. A multiprotein complex that can form in immune cells, such as macrophages, in response to inflammatory stimuli (typically PAMPs and DAMPs). The inflammasome catalyzes the maturation of proinflammatory cytokines IL-1β and IL-18.

inflammation. A term used to describe the process whereby immune cells, fluid, and protein accumulate in a tissue in response to infection or injury.

innate immune system. Complex collections of cells and molecules that preexist contact with pathogens and interact to produce protective immune responses such as inflammation.

integrins. Cell-surface proteins that mediate cellular adhesion to extracellular matrix or to other cells.

interferons (IFNs). A collection of cytokines that interfere with viral infection (IFN-α and IFN-β) and modulate immune responses (most notably IFN-γ).

Interleukins (ILs). Cytokines that are produced by one white blood cell (leukocyte) and act in autocrine and paracrine modes to alter leukocyte actions.

invariant chain (Ii). A polypeptide that occupies MHC class II molecules' binding sites to prevent peptide binding while the nascent MHC class II molecules are resident in the endoplasmic reticulum.

J gene segments. DNA segments present in TCR and BCR gene families that add to the variety of possible TCRs and BCRs with individual animals.

junctional diversity. Addition and subtraction of DNA bases that occur during the formation of junctions between variable-joining and variable-diversity–joining portions of TCRs and BCRs. It is responsible for dramatically increasing the variety of TCRs and BCRs found in individual animals.

lectin pathway of complement activation. A pathway that leads to the activation of the complement cascade in response to simple sugar residues commonly found on microbial surfaces.

leukocytes. White blood cells. Although this term technically encompasses only white cells that can be found in the blood (e.g., monocytes, neutrophils, eosinophils, basophils, NK cells, and lymphocytes), it is commonly used to describe all immune cells, including those not typically found in the blood (e.g., macrophages, mast cells, and dendritic cells).

leukotrienes. Lipid-based signaling molecules derived from arachidonic acid synthesized and released by sentinel cells and other cells. Leukotrienes play important roles in mediating inflammation.

lipopolysaccharide (LPS). A significant component of the outer membranes of Gram-negative bacteria, consisting of a complex of lipid and sugar residues. LPS is a major PAMP of the innate immune system and is often referred to as endotoxin.

lymph. The fluid that flows through the lymphatics.

lymph nodes. Small, oval, filtering secondary lymphoid organs that appear throughout the lymphatics.

lymphoid. Used to describe cells that are derived from the common lymphoid progenitor cells during hematopoiesis; includes B cells, T cells, and NK cells.

lymphoid follicles. Regions found in secondary lymphoid tissues where T and B cells interact.

macrophages. Large phagocytic immune cells found throughout tissues and at sites of inflammation; can function as sentinel cells, APCs, and antimicrobial effector cells.

major histocompatibility complex (MHC). The segment of animals' genomes that contains genes encoding MHC class I and MHC class II molecules.

mast cells. Granular immune cells found predominantly in connective tissues surrounding vasculature and nerves that act to initiate and amplify inflammation through the release of vasoactive compounds and other proinflammatory lipids and cytokines. Mast cells are also the principal cells associated with type I hypersensitivity reactions (allergy).

membrane attack complex (MAC). A structure that is assembled in membranes (typically of microbes) after the activation of the complement cascade. The MAC, which is composed predominantly of ten to sixteen molecules of C9, forms a barrel-shaped pore that compromises the integrity of the target membrane.

MHC class I molecules. Molecules composed of complex MHC class I α chain (derived from the MHC genes) and a smaller molecule, β_2-microglobulin. MHC class I molecules bind cytosol-derived peptides and present them to CD8⁺ T cells.

MHC class II molecules. Molecules composed of a complex of MHC class II α and β chains (both derived from MHC genes). MHC class II molecules bind peptide antigens present in cellular endosomes (generally derived from the extracellular spaces) and present these peptides to CD4⁺ T cells.

MHC class III genes. A classification sometimes used to describe MHC class I– and II–unrelated genes located among or between the MHC class I and II genes. Some MHC class III gene products are involved in immune responses but are in no way similar to the antigen-presenting activities of MHC class I and II molecules.

monoclonal antibodies. Antibodies derived from a single clone of hybridoma cells producing a single type of antibody with a single (or nearly so) antigenic specificity.

monocytes. Large circulating, mononuclear white blood cells that give rise to a variety of other cells, including tissue macrophages.

mucosal-associated lymphoid tissue (MALT). Secondary lymphoid tissues found in lung, gastrointestinal, and other mucosal epithelia.

myeloid. Used to describe cells that are derived from the common myeloid progenitor cells during hematopoiesis. These cells include monocytes, neutrophils, eosinophils, basophils, mast cells, macrophages, and myeloid dendritic cells.

naive T cells. A mature T cell expressing a TCR, CD3, and CD4 or CD8 that has not encountered an antigen reactive with the cell's TCR.

natural killer (NK) cells. Large granular lymphocytes that function as a part of the innate immune response against intracellular pathogens. These cells can recognize and kill virally infected host cells or tumor cells before an adaptive immune response is mounted.

negative selection. The process by which self-reactive lymphocytes are eliminated in the thymus.

neutralizing antibodies. Antibodies that bind to critical sites on toxins, viruses, and sometimes bacteria and prevent the toxin, virus, or bacterium from binding to its receptor on host cells.

neutrophil extracellular traps. Structures secreted from activated neutrophils at the site of inflammation that consist of DNA and antimicrobial proteins that can trap and kill extracellular microbes.

neutrophilia. The increased abundance of neutrophils in the peripheral blood. Neutrophilia is said to have a left shift when increased numbers of less mature neutrophils (band neutrophils) are released into circulation.

neutrophils. Granulocytic white blood cells important for innate defense against extracellular microbes such as bacteria. Neutrophils are rapidly recruited in acute inflammation when they can phagocytose and kill microbes and release antimicrobial products.

nonsteroidal anti-inflammatory drugs (NSAIDs). A class of pharmaceutical agents that aim to reduce inflammation, fever, and pain. Many NSAIDs are inhibitors of the cycloxygenase enzymes that are responsible for the synthesis of prostaglandins.

nuclear factor kappa-light-chain-enhancer of activated B cells (NFκB). A transcription factor that controls the expression of genes associated with proinflammatory responses and cell survival.

nucleotide-binding oligomerization domain (NOD)–like receptors. A family of intracellular PRRs that can detect pathogen-associated molecular patterns, such as peptidoglycan, within the cytosol of a cell. These receptors are particularly important for the detection of intracellular bacteria.

opsonization. Coating (generally of bacteria) with antibodies, C3b, or both to enhance phagocytosis and destruction of pathogens.

passive immunotherapy. Neutralization of toxins, viruses, or bacteria by injection of preformed antibodies, for example after a snakebite.

passive transfer. Movement of preformed antibodies from mother to fetus (transplacental or yolk sac passive transfer) or offspring (via colostrum and milk).

pathogen-associated molecular patterns (PAMPs). Evolutionarily conserved molecular structures that are common to groups of microbes and pathogens but are absent from the host species. The innate immune system can detect the PAMPs through PRRs.

pattern-recognition receptors (PRRs). Germline-encoded receptors expressed on or in many immune cells, particularly sentinel cells, that detect PAMPs, DAMPs, or both. These receptors include TLRs, NOD-like receptors, and RLRs.

peptidoglycan. A meshlike component of bacterial cell walls consisting of chains of alternating sugar residues cross-linked with short chains of amino acids. Peptidoglycan is recognized by the innate immune system as a PAMP.

perforins. Cytolytic proteins found in the granules of cytotoxic T lymphocytes and NK cells.

periarteriolar lymphoid sheath. Secondary lymphoid tissue of the spleen.

peripheral tolerance. Maintenance of tolerance to self antigens beyond the thymic mechanism of negative selection, including Treg cells.

phagocytes. Cells (generally white blood cells) capable of phagocytosis.

phagocytosis. Engulfment of pathogens or other particles into intracellular phagosomes.

phagolysosome. A hybrid organelle resulting from the fusion of a phagosome with lysosomes. The lumen of a phagolysosome is antimicrobial and degradative, which acts to kill and digest phagocytosed microbes and debris.

plasma. The liquid component of blood that has the red blood cells, white blood cells, and platelets removed. Clotting factors are still present.

polyclonal antibodies. Usually sera-containing antibodies of multiple Ig isotypes with multiple antigenic reactivities, produced by multiple clones of plasma cells in immunized animals, also known as antisera.

positive selection. The thymic process that results in elimination of T cells with unreactive TCRs and selection for T cells with functional TCRs.

primary lymphoid organs. Lymphoid organs in which lymphocytes arise or differentiate; in mammals, they include the thymus and the bone marrow.

proinflammatory cytokines. Cytokines that promote inflammation.

prostaglandins. Lipid-based signaling molecules derived from arachidonic acid synthesized and released by sentinel cells and other cells. Prostaglandins play important roles in mediating inflammation as well as in homeostatic processes.

proteasomes. Large molecular complexes that degrade proteins into their component peptides and amino acids.

pyrexia. See **fever**.

pyrogen. Any substance that induces fever. Pyrogens can be derived exogenously (e.g., LPS) or endogenously (e.g., tumor necrosis factor–α).

RAG1. A protein that acts in concert with *RAG2* to induce and direct recombination of TCR and BCR gene segments during T-cell and B-cell differentiation.

RAG2. A protein that acts in concert with *RAG1* to induce and direct recombination of TCR and BCR gene segments during T-cell and B-cell differentiation.

recombinant vaccines. Immunogens composed of antigen-encoding DNA incorporated into the genome of a viral vector. The purpose of the vector is to introduce the antigen-encoding DNA into the cytosol of host APCs.

RIG-like receptors (RLRs). A family of intracellular pattern-recognition receptors that can detect the presence of viral RNA in the cytosol of host cells.

secondary lymphoid organs. Sites of immune responses, including lymph nodes, spleen, and MALTs.

selectins. Cell-surface proteins that can bind specific glycoproteins displayed on other cells. Selectins can be expressed on vascular endothelial cells as well as several immune cells and are important in the recruitment of leukocytes to areas of inflammation.

serum. Plasma (from the blood) with the clotting factors removed.

somatic hypermutation. Rapid and random mutation of DNA bases in the regions of Ig genes that encode CDR1, CDR2, and CDR3 portions of the BCRs of B cells in lymphoid follicles.

T-cell receptors (TCRs). T-cell surface molecular complexes that bind antigens often in association with MHC class I or MHC class II molecules on APCs.

Th1 cells. CD4$^+$ T cells involved in inflammatory and antibody responses.

Th2 cells. CD4$^+$ T cells involved primarily in antibody responses.

Th17 cells. CD4$^+$ T cells involved primarily in inflammatory responses.

Thymocytes. T cells in the thymus.

thymus-independent antigens. Antigens capable of inducing T-helper cell–independent antibody production.

toll-like receptors (TLRs). A major family of intracellular PRRs that can detect a variety of PAMPs as well as DAMPs, which leads to the activation of proinflammatory responses.

transfusion reaction. A potentially life-threatening reaction after a blood transfusion in which the animal's immune system destroys transfused red blood cells from another (donor) animal.

transporters associated with antigen presentation. Molecular complexes that deliver cytosolic peptides into the endoplasmic reticulum for binding by MHC class I molecules.

T-regulatory cells (Tregs). Extrathymic CD4$^+$ T cells that help to regulate immune reactions to self.

V gene segments. DNA segments found in BCR and TCR gene families. These segments join with joining or diversity-joining gene segments to form the N-terminal, variable regions of the BCR heavy and light chains, and the TCR α/β or γ/δ chains.

Page numbers in italics indicate illustrations.

antithyroglobulin autoantibody test, 315–16

antivenins, 280, 281, *283*

antivenin therapy, type III hypersensitivities, 280, 281–82, *283*

antiviral capabilities, 27

antiviral vaccines, 255

APCs. *See* antigen-presenting cells

apoptosis: NK cells n, 7, 32; of tumors, 290–92

APPs. *See* acute phase proteins

acquired immune responses. *See* adaptive immune responses

arthritis: in goats, 139, 140; suppurative, *70*

Aspergillus sp., *42*

aspiration, bone marrow, 24–25

atopy, in dogs, 197

autocatalysis, 58

autoimmune diseases, autoimmunity, 121, 132, 156; antibody-mediated, 283–84; diagnostic tests for, *313–16*

autoimmune hemolytic anemia, 156

autoimmune regulator (AIRE), 156, 157

autosomal recessive diseases, 77

B-1 B cells, actions of, 191–94

β2-microglobulin, 320

B-2 B cells, 182, 260; BCR diversity in, 194–95

B7 molecules, 168–69, 320

bacteremia, in neonatal foals, *37–38*

bacteremia-induced systemic inflammatory response syndrome (SIRS), 37

bacteria, 14, 19, 21, 40, 44, 119; antibodies and, *13*, 194; exotoxins of, 224–25, *260*; Gram-negative, 37, 38, *224*; Gram-positive, 224; gut, 234–35, 237; phagocytosis of, *93, 94, 95*

bacterial infections, 77, 274; in dairy cattle, 67, 68, 86–87, 241, 251–52; in dogs, 17, 53, 161; exotoxins and, 224–25; in foals, *37–38*, 89–90, 181, 195–96

barriers, anatomical and physiological, 18–21

basophils, 3, 4, 27–28, 274, 319; production of, 22, 23, 112

basset hounds, *163*; XLSCID in, 161–62, 177–79

B-cell coreceptors, *202–203*

B-cell receptors (BCRs), 9, 111, 182, *201, 211*, 229, 230, 252, 299, 319; antigen binding, 199–200; diversity of, 183, *187*, 194–95, 239;

hypermutated, 207, 209–10; immunoglobulin isotypes in, 189–91; MZ B cells, 194, 203

B cells (B lymphocytes), 3, 9, 114, 117, 118, 120, 135, 236, 243, 259, 275, 319; affinity maturation of, 207–10, 230–31; antigen interactions, 199–203; as APCs, 133, *203–4, 229*; and BCRs, 182–83; in calves, 242, 249; clonal expansion of, 10–11; and complement system, 63–64; development of, 188–89, *214*; genetics of, 183–86; Ig isotype switching in, 206–7; and immunoglobulin isotypes, 189–91; marginal-zone, 194–95; maturation of, 33, 112–13; memory, 12, 212, 231, 238; production of, 23, 111; somatic hypermutation, *231, 232*; Th-activated, *204–7*, 210–13; and Th cells, 170, 171; variety of, 191–95; in XLSCID dogs, 162(table), 178–79. *See also* by *number designation*

BCRs. *See* B-cell receptors

bile, 20

birds, 43, 156; B cell development in, 182, 212; BCR gene diversity in, *184, 186, 187*; in ovo vaccination, 244, *245*; maternal transfer of immunity in, 243–44

black disease, 251

BLAD. *See* bovine leukocyte adhesion deficiency

blackleg, 251

bladders, urinary, 20

blood, 114, 182: crossmatching, 309–12; erythrocyte antigens in, 295–97; innate immune system cells in, 25–28; typing of, 307–9

blood cells, 3, 34; production of, 21–23, 111

blood counts, 24

blood flow, and acute inflammation, 73

blood groups, 296–97

blood smears, monitoring hematopoiesis, *24*

blood typing, 319; crossmatching, 309–12; methods of, 307–9, *310*

blood typing cards, 308, *310*

blood vessels, 236; immune complexes and, *281–82*; and inflammatory mediators, 72–73

B lymphocytes. *See* B cells

bobcats, FIV in, 271

bone marrow, 34, 82, *85*, 171, 212, 242; aspiration of, 24–25; B-cell

development, 182, 186, *188*, 189, *214*; hematopoiesis, 21–25, 110–11, *113*; immune cell production, 111–12, *152*

bordetella, vaccines against, 258, 266

Bordetella bronchiseptica, 266

Borrelia burgdorferi, ELISA for, 300, *301*

botulinum toxin, 224–25

bovine leukocyte adhesion deficiency (BLAD), 77, 313, 319–20

bovine respiratory syncytial virus infections, 84

bovines, 44, 84, 252; acute mastitis, 67, 68, 85–88; basophils, 27; BLAD in, 77. *See also* cattle

bovine viral diarrhea, 242

Brittany dog (Brittany spaniel), *54*; C3 deficiency in, 53, 64–65

bronchitis, in dogs, 197, 215

bronchopneumonia, 84

bronchus-associated lymphoid tissues, 119, 320

Bruton's tyrosine kinase (BTK), 181, 195–96

BTK. *See* Bruton's tyrosine kinase

Burnett, MacFarlane, 124, 288

bursa of Fabricius, 113, 114, 243; B-cell development, 182, 189

C3b, 53–63, 90–91, 198, 207, 210, 228, 277, 281, 311, 315

C3 convertase, 55

C3 deficiency, 53, 64–65

C5a, 54–62, 69, 71, 76, 277, 281, *282*

C5 convertase, 55

cachexia, 82

CAEV. *See* caprine arthritis encephalitis virus

calcivirus, live-attenuated vaccines and, 258

California Mastitis Test (CMT), 67, *69*

calves. *See* cattle

camelids, BCR genetics, 183, 186

cancer, 84; cell development, 288–89; and immune system, 287–88; immunotherapy for, 267, 292–93; research on, 124–25; tumor growth, 290–92

cancer drugs, and acquired immune deficiencies, 273

cancer therapy, 289, 292–93; immune stimulants as, 289–90

Candida albicans, 16

candidiasis, oroesophageal, 1, 16

canine leukocyte adhesion deficiency (CLAD), 313

canine pertussis vaccine, 266